Explorations in Medicine, Evolution, and Mind

By Dr. Anab Whitehouse

© Dr. Anab Whitehouse

Interrogative Imperative Institute

Brewer, Maine

04412

All rights are reserved. Aside from uses that are in compliance with the 'Fair Usage' clause of the Copyright Act, no portion of this publication may be reproduced in any form without the express written permission of the publisher. Furthermore, no part of this book may be stored in a retrieval system, nor transmitted in any form or by any means – whether electronic, mechanical, photo-reproduction or otherwise – without authorization from the publisher.

Published 2018

Published by One Draft Publications In conjunction with Bilquees Press

Man's mind cannot grasp the causes of events in their completeness, but the desire to find those causes is implanted in man's soul. And without considering the multiplicity and complexity of the conditions any one of which taken separately may seem to be the cause, he snatches at the first approximation to a cause that seems to him intelligible and says: "This is the cause!"

Leo Tolstoy -- Chapter 1, Book XIII of *War and Peace*

Table of Contents

Introduction – page 9

1) **Methodological Madness**

- A few questions – page 23

- Muddying the Waters – page 27

- The Burzynski Affair – page 33

- The SSRI Issue – page 89

- HIV/AIDS Ambiguities – page 119

2) **The Evolutionary Landscape**

- Setting the Stage – page 149

- Critique of An Abbreviated Textbook Perspective – page 169

- A Few Lessons Related to Archaea – page 195

- Deep Solutions for the Problem of Biological Origins – page 217

- Extinction – page 269

- The Evolution of Human Beings – page 287

- Some Evolutionary Roots of Psychology – page 305

- Evolution's Black Box – page 311

3) **The Mentality of Neuroscience**

- Glial Mysteries – page 329

- Mirror Neurons – page 359

- Memory – page 373

- The Computational Mind – page 413

- The Nature of the Unconscious – page 439

- A Few Notes on Consciousness – page 469

Some Closing Remarks – page 487

Bibliography – page 497

| Explorations |

6

For my mentor, Dr. Baig ... who taught me, among other things, that searching for the truth is essential to being human. He also taught me how important character is to such an undertaking.

I am unlikely to ever realize the truth in the way, or to the extent, that he did. Nonetheless, the fact that after more than four decades I am still deeply engaged in trying to bear witness to the foregoing process of searching – albeit in my own way and according to my very limited capacity -- is largely due to his example.

There are no words that adequately can convey the depth of gratitude I feel for the fact that he came into my life and helped make it better than it otherwise would have been. The words that follow are mere shadows of the truths that he tried to communicate to me, and I wish I had been a better student.

| Explorations |

Introduction

To date, I have written thirty-nine books. For a variety of reasons, the present work might be my last one.

Among other things, none of us knows when the word "Time" may be uttered in conjunction with one's life. As if participating in some SAT-like test, when the fateful word is said, one will be required to stop in mid-sentence, turn in one's test booklet along with an accompanying number-2 pencil to the monitors and, then, exit from the room.

Fortunate is the individual who is afforded the opportunities to give written expression to what flows through his or her being over the years ... and I have been one of those fortunate ones. However, I am well aware of the fact that the grains of sand that mark the time still left to me are quickly disappearing from the container of my life ... and this realization has had an essential role to play in shaping the structure of this book.

I have a few remaining creative projects awaiting my attention on my unofficial 'Bucket List'. Those entries might, or might not, be completed, but they are not likely to be even remotely as time-consuming as the present book has been.

More than six years ago I finished writing my last book (*Beyond Democracy*), and almost immediately began undertaking research for the current work. Some 50-60 books, 70, or so, articles, a variety of DVDs, and a great deal of reflection later, I am ready to try to fill up white space with black lettering – hopefully in a coherent, constructive, and insightful manner.

My last book (*Beyond Democracy*) explored areas of: history, legal philosophy, political science, constitutional law, and economics. The present book is poised to venture into topical areas involving: medicine, psychology, methodology, evolutionary theory, and neurobiology.

I envisioned the two works – *Beyond Democracy* and *Explorations* -- to be complementary, in certain ways, to one another. I suppose the readers, if any, of the two works will have to make their own judgments on the matter.

In the foregoing paragraph I said "readers, if any". I do not use the phrase advisedly because there is a very real possibility that no one might bother to read what I have written.

The foregoing possibility is not as ominous as it first appears to be. I am a writer, not an author.

Authors write for an audience. Writers, on the other hand, do what they do irrespective of whether or not there is, or will be, an audience to engage their efforts.

Don't get me wrong (and notice that in saying this I am acknowledging a hope that someone will be reading my words), I am happy when people buy my books. Over the years, I have sold thousands of books in a variety of countries, but some books have succeeded better in this respect than other literary creations of mine have done, and some of those 'successful' books even have ended up on library shelves in a number of countries, including several prestigious universities.

However, there are some exemplars of my literary progeny that lead relatively neglected lives. It is like in those movies where the hero or heroine has written a book and is approached by a member of the audience after a lecture, and the latter individual indicates how much he or she liked one or another book written by the hero/heroine and the latter says with an ironic smile: "So, you are the one."

A few years ago, I saw the film documentary: *Stone Reader* by Mark Moskowitz. The film delved into the somewhat strange case of an American writer, Don Mossman, who had written a novel entitled: *The Stones of Summer*.

For a number of reasons (e.g., the publisher went bankrupt shortly after the book came out, and there had been very little marketing for the book, and the writer suffered a nervous breakdown at some point following the release of his work), very few people ever purchased the book. The aforementioned movie contained interviews with a variety of people who had read it and thought very highly of the book.

My wife saw the movie with me and, as a result, was inspired to buy the book. However, although she is an avid reader (and every year at Christmas I buy her gaggle of books that constitute part of her reading list for the following year), she never was able to get very far with the Mossman novel.

In any event and for whatever reason, there might be many reasons why a book never goes anywhere. An independent bookseller in downtown Bangor, Maine has, on several occasions, been kind enough to display works of mine in his bookstore but has told me on each occasion that unless the book gets reviewed via one means or another, the chances of anyone purchasing my books are slim to none.

While some individuals seem to have the knack to induce others to become interested in what they are doing, I have never been one of those people – though, from time to time, I have tried to accomplish this but with almost invariably null results. Since I publish my own books and because there is no money in the budget to market them, the works tend to get tossed about by the cosmic winds ... like some lonely seed that lands on fertile or barren soil as fate decides the matter.

During my research for the current book, I repeatedly was amazed by the number of individuals in the history of science and mathematics who had discovered or created something of a very remarkable nature only to have their discovery/creation be ignored by fellow scientists and mathematicians for years, if not decades. I am not sure that what I have to say in this book can be considered to be all that remarkable, but it is strangely comforting to realize that even a very good work can go unnoticed for considerable periods of time.

Ultimately, however, even if no one were to read this book (or some of my other works), I am at peace with such a possibility. My writing is one of the ways that I try to bear witness to the truth – at least to whatever extent I have succeeded in accurately grasping some limited facet of reality's complexity, depth and vastness.

Howling at the moon, so to speak, through my written words is a sort of modulated primal scream. It is my way of giving expression to an essential dimension of the facticity of my existence.

When faced with a choice between, on the one hand, never managing to have written something or, on the other hand, having managed to write something that no one will ever read, I would always select the latter option. Of course, the best of all possible worlds would be to write something, have it read, and for that piece of writing to have a salutary effect of some kind for those who have encountered it, but I am prepared to live with just being able to write something that I have wanted to write, and the present book is something that I have wanted to write for some time.

Quite independently of whether, or not, someone else reads what I have to say, I have benefitted from every book that has bubbled to the surface from the deep reflective pools within me out of which those creations originate. Writing helps to organize and clarify my thinking, and, then, there is also the amazing experience of seeing ideas and insights emerge during the course of writing that I had not anticipated prior to their appearance in my surface consciousness – as if 'something' is teaching me as I go along.

Approximately eighteen years ago, I wrote a book that eventually (after several naming sessions) was given the title: *Evolution and the Origin of Life*. The work encompassed (through a fictionalized court case somewhat akin to *Inherit the Wind*) a critical overview of the arguments that were directed toward providing an account of pre-biotic or chemical theories concerning the origin of life.

I sent out copies of the book to a variety of people. Some of those individuals were inclined toward some version of Creationist theology, and some of those recipients were proponents of evolutionary theory.

Neither of the two sides appeared to be interested in what I had to say on the matter. Stated in a slightly different manner, if the individuals I sent the book to did have an interest, that interest was not sufficiently great to induce them to enter into some sort of dialogue with me.

I do recall a conversation with a professor of anthropology from the University of Toronto that took place several years prior to the release of the aforementioned book on evolution. The exchange occurred during a recess that had been called with respect to a meeting about textbook bias that was being held under the auspices of the Ministry of Education for the Province of Ontario.

The professor – I was a graduate student in educational theory at the time – was incensed at, and full of sarcastic contempt for, the idea that anyone (namely, yours truly) could be so ill informed and scientifically backward as to question the truth of evolutionary theory. I was not advancing a Creationist position during the conversation, but, rather, I had a lot of questions concerning an array of lacunae in the evolutionary position with respect to the issue of the origin of life on Earth.

The professor refused to listen to anything that I had to say. He was open-minded, objective, and empirically oriented in a way that all too many professors have been that I have encountered over the years (both as a student and as one of their colleagues) – which is to say: not at all.

Be that as it may, I subsequently decided to add my two cents worth in relation to the great debate on evolutionary theory, and the result was the book: *The Origin of Life*. The book was rooted in considerable research on the subject, and in the process I read, among other works: Watson's *Molecular Biology of the Gene*, Lehninger's *Principles of Biochemistry*, as well as textbooks on cell biology, cell physiology, developmental biology, membrane functioning, as well as a wide variety of technical research on evolutionary theory.

Upon completion of *The Origin of Life*, I believed that I would write a sequel to that work within a reasonably short period of time – and even intimated as much in an earlier version of the book's introduction. However, other projects and issues took priority, and, therefore, quite a few years passed by -- approximately nineteen years' worth -- before I could find an opportunity to even begin to pursue such a possibility.

By the time that window of opportunity had opened up, the original idea for a sequel to the book on evolution became reconfigured in my mind. Although an updated engagement of the evolutionary issue continued to form part of the intended project, I wanted to expand things in a way that also would include forays into methodology, psychology, neurobiology, and varies facets of medicine.

I have always been interested in searching for the truth – whatever the nature of such truth might be. Unfortunately, many people seem to feel there is an unbridgeable chasm between science and spirituality and that the two are involved in some sort of zero-sum game in which one or the other is the winner while the remaining side loses.

| Explorations |

To be sure, there are certain kinds of theological perspectives that do not fare well when critically examined in the light of various evidential considerations. Consequently, those individuals who have tied their intellectual fate to theologies that appear to be untenable when filtered through the light of scientific evidence often tend to feel threatened by, and antagonistic toward, the presence of science.

Nevertheless, I never felt that evolutionary theory, quantum physics, modern cosmology, or psychology constituted direct threats to the idea of God's existence. Instead, I entertained the possibility that the discoveries of scientists were inducements to re-think what I thought or believed I knew concerning the nature of my relationship to the Ground of Being.

Quite frankly, if one were so inclined (which I am not and this book is a testament to that fact), one could accept the vast majority of the basic tenets of modern science as true descriptions of the nature of reality and not encounter anything that demonstrated, or even remotely indicated, that God didn't exist. One might have to rework one's ideas about God's relationship to the universe or what the nature of the laws were through which God operated, but there was nothing in science or mathematics that couldn't be reconciled (and done so relatively easily) with a broader, richer, more nuanced understanding of the notion of an on-going Divine presence with respect to the manner in which the physical and biological universe is manifested in everyday life.

On the other hand, one also could critically examine the tenets of science and mathematics (which the current book does) and ask whether, or not, the best way to engage life should be limited to science and mathematics. Napoleon was once reported to have observed that there was nothing in a book on physics written by Laplace that mentioned the Author of the universe that was being described (the universe, that is, not the Author) by Laplace in the book at issue, and the scientist is reported to have said: "I have no need of that hypothesis", but, perhaps, Laplace was operating out of an extremely impoverished and distorted hermeneutical framework when he said what he did.

For example, however impressive Laplace's book on physics might have been, nothing in that book explained how life, reason, consciousness, intelligence, creativity, or language were possible, and, yet, all of these qualities helped make the writing of his book a reality. Therefore, at the very least, Laplace could be considered to have been a tad premature in concluding that he had no need for a hypothesis concerning Divinity with respect to the workings of the universe.

Furthermore, offering a description of something is not necessarily the same thing as providing an explanation for the phenomenon being described. Laplace could describe a variety of physical dynamics with a fair degree of accuracy, and, as a result, he could solve numerous problems in physics, as well as make reliable calculations concerning different phenomena.

Yet, Laplace had absolutely no explanation for what made any of the capabilities underlying his problem-solving and reliable calculations possible. Furthermore, Laplace could not explain why the universe was the way it was, but, instead, he was limited to describing the surface dynamics of only certain aspects of physical reality.

For instance, he could mathematically capture the effects of gravity. However, he had no idea (nor did Newton) what gravity actually was – only that it appeared to operate in accordance with a certain kind of regularity that could be described through mathematics.

Since the nineteenth century, scientists and mathematicians have added considerable detail that both altered and deepened, in a variety of ways, their understanding of such descriptions. Yet, there are still many, many unanswered questions concerning why the phenomena of the universe have the properties and qualities they do.

Given the foregoing, one is led to the following problem: How should one proceed? Are science and mathematics the best way forward, or should one entertain some other possibility, and, if so, what would the latter possibility entail?

In 1959, C.P. Snow, a chemist and novelist, delivered the Rede Lecture at Cambridge University. The first portion of his presentation addressed the idea of 'two cultures' and how those cultures seemed to be at loggerheads with one another in Western society and, as a result, were impeding the chances of making progress with respect to solving a variety of problems in the world.

The term: 'two cultures' alluded to the different kinds of social, intellectual, historical, and behavioral values that led to the rise, respectively, of the sciences and the humanities. Among other things, each culture seemed disgruntled with the 'fact' that individuals who were members of a given culture were largely illiterate concerning the nature of the culture to which they did not belong.

Scientists didn't appear to know much about the humanities, and proponents of the humanities didn't appear to understand much about the nature of science. When they talked with one another, their words seemed to tumble, unheeded, into the great darkness that surrounded and separated them.

I tend to believe the only culture that is worthy of being pursued is that which is dedicated to pursuing the truth. Neither scientists nor advocates of the humanities necessarily have priority when it comes to the issue of truth or the nature of reality ... although each set of individuals may have important (but far from exhaustive or definitive) contributions to make with respect to such an endeavor.

When I was an undergraduate at Harvard back in the mid-to-late 1960s, I wrote a thesis and was required to orally defend it. During these latter proceedings, a member of the examination committee noted that he didn't see much of current research reflected in my thesis, and he was right since I didn't feel that current research in my field (which was psychology) reflected much of reality ... although there were bits and pieces here and there that I considered to be of interest and value.

In other words, the criticism being advanced by my examiner appeared to be that I wasn't a true card-carrying member of the culture of psychology, and, apparently, this was in some way troubling to, or disconcerting for, that person. I encountered the same sort of mindset later on during graduate school (in two different programs at two different universities) and, as a result, spent sixteen years in exile before discovering a way -- and a set of people – that would permit me to tangentially touch down long enough in such a culture to be able to obtain a doctorate.

While I certainly can't claim that I have cornered the market on truth, the search for truth has always been close to my heart and mind.

| Explorations |

17

At different points in my life, the nature of the search was shaped and colored by my interests at the time.

For example, early on, I engaged things through religious filters. Then, over time, I tried on scientific, philosophical, psychological, political, and mystical glasses ... each pair of lenses filtering reality through its own unique qualities.

Despite various differences among the foregoing sorts of filters, all were framed by the same kinds of questions: Who am I? What is the purpose, if any, of life? What is the nature of reality? What is the good, or the just, or the moral? What makes reason, consciousness, intelligence, creativity, language, and life possible? What methods should I employ to seek the truth? How should I proceed in the face of incomplete and/or uncertain information?

When one is young, the future seems to be a matter of limitless possibilities. One feels confident that one has enough time within which to arrive at reliable answers for all one's questions, but funny things happen on the way to the forum.

Now, here I am, some five decades later, and I still am embroiled in the same questions, problems, and issues noted previously with no guarantee that I am any closer to the truth than I was all those many years ago. One major difference between then and the present, however, is that I strongly suspect that I don't have much longer to come up with an answer for the problem of reality ... the endless horizons of youth have been telescoped down to the ramshackle room of old age whose surrounding walls are moving relentlessly inward.

In some ways my situation reminds me of the television show *Jeopardy*. More specifically, after the contestants have gone through several rounds of providing answers in the form of questions, toward the end of the show the participants are confronted with the challenge of the 'Final Jeopardy' phase of the program.

During this facet of things, the contestants are given one last question by their host, Alex Trebek. The former individuals can bet as little or as much as they like from the funds they have available to them for having correctly answered questions raised in the earlier part of the program.

| Explorations |

The three participants contemplate their respective financial situations and reflect, in silence, on the answer that is to be given in response to the 'Final Jeopardy' question. If a person bets a lot and is wrong, then, depending on what other contestants do, he or she likely will not be the individual who will get to appear on the next edition of *Jeopardy* to defend her or his title. On the other hand, if an individual bets a little or a lot and gives a correct answer to the 'Final Jeopardy' question, then – and, again, depending on what other contestants do -- that person may come out on top and get to participate in a future show ... maybe even face off against a computer somewhere down the road.

The fact of the matter is: Whether we like it or not, we are all engaged in our own version of Final Jeopardy. The question for all of us is: What is the nature of reality? The bet we are placing is doled out in the denominations of our lives, and the period we spend contemplating our response – with or without the accompanying Final Jeopardy music -- represents the time we have left on this Earth to form an answer.

Of course, the existential challenge with which we all are faced is a lot more complex than the sorts of categorized factual questions that are asked by Alex Trebek. Consequently, it might be a little cumbersome for any of us – per program rules – to state our answer in the form of a question, and, therefore, perhaps the rules of the real life form of Final Jeopardy should be relaxed a little to permit contestants to write, in declarative form, as little or as much as they like in responding to the Final Jeopardy challenge.

This book represents, in a sense, my response to the aforementioned Final Jeopardy question – namely, what is the nature of reality? I have no idea whether the answer I am giving is right or wrong, but I am fully committed to the answer being expressed, and in that sense I am betting my life that the answer being stated herein is correct ... more or less.

Now, Alex Trebek is a pretty smart guy and has studied philosophy during his years of attending university in Canada. However, I'm not sure that he has been supplied by the 'powers that be' with the official answer to the foregoing Final Jeopardy question.

| Explorations |

However, at the risk of mixing metaphors, I have it on good authority that the following words of Ed McMahon have been heard reverberating in and around us as we contemplate the nature of our answers to the Final Jeopardy question:

"I hold in my hand the envelopes. As a child of four can plainly see, these envelopes have been hermetically sealed. They've been kept in a #2 mayonnaise jar on Funk and Wagnall's back porch since noon today. **No one** knows the contents of these envelopes, but you, in your borderline divine and mystical way, will ascertain the answers having never before seen the questions."

The Great Carnac supplied many questions to many answers. Our task is to supply one answer to one question.

Will the answer I offer match the one to which reality gives expression? Will the answer you give in response to the Final Jeopardy question reflect the nature of reality?

Some people might wish to claim that the whole Jeopardy analogy is irrelevant. In other words, irrespective of whether, or not, a person decides to answer the foregoing existential dilemma, there are no actual consequences with respect to how – or if – we respond to the Final Jeopardy question.

For example, such individuals might say none of us is in any actual jeopardy to lose opportunities in relation to participating on future shows. Or, no one is going to come along after the fact and be able to authoritatively inform a person that the answer she or he has offered is correct (or not). Or, irrespective of whether one is correct or incorrect, nothing follows from it ... we give our answers (or refrain from doing so) and that is the end of the matter.

Now, the foregoing sorts of considerations might, or might not, be correct. In a sense, they are the kinds of answers that some individuals might give in response to the Final Jeopardy challenge ... but that is all they are: Responses to the Final Jeopardy question.

They don't settle anything but are themselves in need of settlement. Furthermore, the people who give the foregoing kinds of answers are betting their lives that they are correct with respect to such matters.

Even if one were to suppose that this Earthly life is all there is to existence, the Final Jeopardy challenge remains relevant. How a person responds to the reality problem tends to shape his or her life, and, therefore, the manner in which such an individual spends her or his: Time, money, resources, and talents will be affected by how that person engages the Final Jeopardy challenge.

None of us knows when "Time" will be called in conjunction with our lives. Every moment of our existence is, in effect, spent in Final Jeopardy, and every moment of our lives – whether, or not, we are cognizant of this -- is confronted with the problem posed by the Final Jeopardy question: What is the nature of reality?

Moreover, irrespective of how one might feel about all of this, one is, nonetheless, required to give an answer to that question. This is so even if that answer – like those contestants on Jeopardy who do not answer the final question because they don't want to risk whatever funds they have -- is not to issue any formal response.

I have a preliminary – and, at this point, a fairly general -- hypothesis concerning how to go about answering the Final Jeopardy question. More specifically, as valuable as science and mathematics are, I do not believe they can provide an adequate response to the Final Jeopardy challenge with which we all are faced.

This is not to say that science and mathematics couldn't form part of any such answer. Rather, the foregoing claim is, in part, a way of alluding to the fact that science and mathematics are committed to the long game – that is, the process of searching for the truth over a period of decades, centuries, if not millennia.

Furthermore, the depictions of reality that science and mathematics provide tend to change on a fairly regular basis. This is not necessarily a bad thing ... especially if that changing understanding is able to describe different facets of reality with increasing accuracy.

Nonetheless, the average, current lifespan of a human being in the United States is 75 years, or so (a figure that varies in relation to such factors as: geographical location, gender, socioeconomic status, and so on). The truths that science and mathematics might discover 50 years from now will be of absolutely no assistance to the individual faced with the Final Jeopardy issue now – especially if those future "truths" change again another fifty years on further down the road of progress ... life demands its answer in the present, not in the future.

However, there is an additional set of reasons for why I do not believe that science and mathematics should form the essence of a person's approach to addressing the challenge posed by the existential counterpart to Final Jeopardy. Just like many theologians, some scientists and mathematicians often cannot distinguish between their theories and reality – not because the former necessarily reflects the latter but because there often tends to be all manner of interpretation that permeates those theories and weaves available "facts" into an understanding or filtering system that might not serve truth very well.

In fact, surprisingly, there seems to be a great deal of "magical thinking" in the mental processes that some scientists and mathematicians exhibit. In other words, there appears to be a tendency among some scientists and mathematicians to suppose that because they think that something is the case, therefore, this means that this is the way reality is, and, consequently, it is the way they want the rest of humanity to understand the nature of reality ... and they will go to considerable lengths to control political decisions, media presentations, academic programs, and the distribution of resources in order to serve their approach to things.

Quantum theory, special and general relativity, evolution, neurobiology, cosmology, and mathematics all – each in its own way -- suffer from the foregoing sort of malady. I believe that scientists and mathematicians can describe a great many phenomenal aspects of the universe with considerable accuracy, but I also believe that scientists and mathematicians actually understand, or are able to fully explain, much less than what they seem to suppose is the case.

Terms such as: randomness, infinity, space, time, dimensionality, evolution, field, energy, red shifts, mass, virtual particles, gravity, and so on are thrown around as if the individuals uttering them knew what they are talking about. However, I don't believe such people necessarily understand what they are saying ... even as they seek to convince other people that they do.

Much of what follows is a critique of the modern, scientific worldview, along with some commentary directed toward philosophy and education. During the process of exploring various facets of methodology, evolution, neurobiology, psychology, quantum physics, string theory, special relativity, general relativity, thermodynamics, cosmology, mathematics, philosophy, and education, I try to preserve what I consider to be of value in such areas while simultaneously attempting to point out what I believe are many of the problems and questions that permeate those same areas.

Along the way I seek to provide an overview of what I think a plausible and defensible response to the Final Jeopardy challenge might look like. That response includes science and mathematics, but it also goes beyond those pursuits in a variety of ways.

Beginning in the late 1950s, I have had a tendency – unplanned though it might have been – to focus on issues of science and mathematics from time to time. Usually, and for whatever reasons, those forays almost invariably have occurred during the last three or four years of a given decade, with an occasional overlap, here and there, that might have extended into the first part of the following decade.

Since I might not make it to the latter part of the present decade, I have jumped the gun somewhat and decided to put forth -- before the mid-point of the current ten-year period -- what might well be my final kick of the can concerning such matters. However, even if I were to live to the end of this decade -- and perhaps beyond -- I am not sure that I would have the energy, health, or command of faculties to undertake another go around in relation to science and mathematics ... so, carpe diem.

Should any actual readers decide to engage this book, I hope that engagement provides you with as many ideas to constructively reflect upon as the process has that encompassed my research and entailed the writing of this book. Whether you find yourself in full agreement, partial agreement, or substantial disagreement with the contents of this book, I hope that your answer to the Final Jeopardy challenge will serve your pursuit of the truth well in both the present and as well as in conjunction with your sojourn into the Big Sleep ... perchance to dream.

Chapter 1: Methodological Madness

A Few Questions

What is the difference between good and bad science? Is bad science even science?

Surely, there is a difference between, (1) someone who: Posits a hypothesis, rigorously tests that conjecture, but discovers that the contention is false while admitting as much after the fact, and (2) a person who: Makes a claim and either never bothers to determine whether the claim is true or false, or who undertakes a shoddy, error-ridden process of 'testing' that involves the manipulation of data, methods, and conclusions in order to be able to continue supporting the original claim. There is a difference between, on the one hand, being wrong about an issue but being willing to acknowledge the incorrect character of one's former idea in the light of new data or experimental results, and, on the other hand, a person who is unwilling to admit that a belief he or she holds is incorrect and who will intentionally alter or frame things in order to be able to continue to advocate for such a belief in some self-serving manner.

Various people have used different terms to refer to the process of intentionally undermining, biasing, distorting, obfuscating, or rendering dysfunctional the process of experimental methodology. For example some individuals speak of the foregoing sorts of activities as "bent science", while others talk about that kind of behavior in terms of the notion of "junk science".

Still other individuals use the phrase: "merchants of doubt" in an attempt to capture some of the flavor of the tactics that are used by those practitioners whose vested interests lie with something other than seeking the truth. In other words, there are individuals who use the tools of critical skepticism in a manner that is intended to cast doubt on any data, experiments, articles, and/or researchers that run counter to the perspective that the former individuals want to advance irrespective of how reliable such data, experimental results, articles, and researchers might be.

There is an important role to be played within the realms of science by the processes of posing reasonable doubts, exercising critical reflection, and operating through the filters of skepticism.

However, when such processes are used to muddy the waters and obscure matters rather than clarify them, then the purposes of science are no longer being served.

Someone might have the academic credentials of a scientist and, yet, not be a genuine scientist when it comes to issues of: intention, objectivity, sincerity, honesty, rigor, character, competency, thoroughness, judgment, and a sense of fiduciary responsibility to the truth. Something might be referred to as "scientific" and, yet, lack the many qualities that are necessary to be worthy of such a description.

Who is a true scientist and what constitutes real science are not always easy matters to determine. Even within the scientific community, these issues are often not straightforward but, instead, are subject to considerable disagreement, and, therefore, for those of us who are not members of the culture of science, the situation is even more problematic.

Moreover, relief does not necessarily always come in the form of identifying what the majority of scientists within a given community believe. Over the years, the vast majority of what scientists held to be true at any given time has been subject to change – sometimes in a minor manner, but also in much more dramatic ways.

In fact, one probably could claim, with considerable justification and without fear of exaggeration, that over the years scientists, as a group, tend to be wrong more often than they are right. What is found to be true is often the result of a long process of trial and error in which many missteps are taken before a path with firm footing is established, and, even then, what appears to be solid ground might subsequently be found to require a certain altering of the trajectory with respect to the path forward.

What lies at the heart of science are methodologies – both empirical and mathematical, but epistemological and moral as well – that, hopefully, permit one, in time, to differentiate between fool's gold and relatively pure, empirical and mathematical nuggets of value. Unfortunately, the results of methodological activity often become tainted by hermeneutical treatments of one sort or another that imbue those results with certain kinds of ontological status that might be consistent with such results but are not necessarily justified by them.

| Explorations |

Data is one thing. Interpretation of the data is quite another matter.

The word "science" is often extended to the process of interpreting data as well as extended to the process of interpreting the mathematical descriptions that are used to give representation to such data. However, for reasons that will be documented throughout this book, one might do well to try to maintain a clear distinction between, on the one hand, science as a set of methodologies and, on the other hand, 'science' as a hermeneutical exercise that seeks to impose meaning and 'reality' onto such data, along with accompanying mathematical descriptions, since in many ways, the aforementioned, hermeneutical process is not really science at all but a system of reification in which theoretical interpretations are afforded a degree of concrete, ontological status that is not necessarily warranted.

Just as "bad science" is not really science, so too, 'bent science' and 'junk science' do not constitute forms of science but, instead, are terms used to refer to processes or behaviors that tend to exclude the presence of, or are devoid of, actual scientific activity. Similarly, the hermeneutics of data generated through scientific means or the hermeneutics of data that is represented/modeled via mathematical notation is not really science, but a non-scientific process that is often tends to be done in tangential or asymptotic conjunction with the results that are generated through scientific methodologies.

Some theories are said to be scientific because they constitute a way of organizing scientifically generated data, along with mathematical treatments of that data, into a coherent understanding concerning some aspect of experience. However, philosophy also can provide ways of organizing scientifically generated data, along with mathematical treatments of that data, into a coherent (but not necessarily correct) understanding concerning various facets of phenomenal experience, so the ability to organize such things into various frameworks of coherency doesn't necessarily make something scientific.

Perhaps a theory is scientific because it is issued through scientists. Yet, scientists put forth many theories that turn out to be wrong, so the mere issuing of a theory via one or more scientists does not necessarily render that theory scientific.

Alternatively, maybe there is some critical number of scientists who must subscribe to a theory before one can refer to the theory as being scientific. If so, one would like to know what the relationship is between the numbers of scientists endorsing a theory, the truth of such a theory, and how the truth of the theory is a function of such numbers. Is the scientific nature of a theory really just a matter of some form of democratic voting procedure where the majority rules – irrespective of whether that majority is right or wrong?

Scientific theories are ways of engaging experience that suggest hypotheses that might be tested and, therefore, can be considered to have heuristic value in the manner in which they open one up to possibilities for deepening one's understandings. However, scientific theories also can be incorporated into various non-scientific ways of framing and biasing the understanding of a person in a manner that precludes entertaining possibilities considered incompatible with such theories and, therefore, in the process, closes one off to possibilities that might actually lead to the deepening of a person's understanding. As a result, so-called scientific theories can be a very "iffy' set of propositions.

In general terms, a theory that is referred to as scientific tends to signify little more than that a scientist (or a number of them) has (have) developed a theory of interpretation concerning the meaning and significance of a given set of data ... data that has been generated through methods of science. That theory might, or might not, be correct, and the theory might, or might not, have heuristic value.

Furthermore, even if a theory does contain features that correctly predict the behavior of a given facet of reality, and even if the theory does have heuristic value, neither of the foregoing 'facts' guarantees that the theory is an accurate reflection of the nature of reality. The theory is a way of looking at -- and trying to understand -- experience, and such a theory needs to be critically evaluated to determine precisely what it does and doesn't accomplish in those respects

This brings us back to where we started. How does one distinguish between truth and falsehood within science? What constitutes good science? What are the criteria that need to be displayed by a theory for it not only to be referred to as scientific but as giving expression to good science?

Muddying the Waters

Suppose a person hands you a "scientific result" that makes some claim concerning the nature of an aspect of reality. What sorts of issues should be considered in order to try to determine whether the result is worthy of merging with one's worldview (or attempting to) so that one might be able to better understand the nature of that which makes experience of certain kinds possible?

One avenue to pursue is to ask whether, or not, the result has been replicated. In other words, has someone independent of the individuals who generated the scientific result that has been handed to you also been able to produce the same or similar results in a separate experiment?

If a given result has not been independently replicated, then irrespective of however interesting and provocative such a result might be, it needs to be bracketed as merely a tentative possibility. Without replication, treating such a result as 'factual' or as a piece of knowledge is premature.

One could, of course, just go ahead and reconfigure one's worldview in order to accommodate the new information. However, when other individuals actively try to replicate the result and do not succeed, or another group of individuals runs a study that produces results that conflict or contradict the 'scientific result' that was first given to you, then, one might have wasted a lot of time trying to re-organize one's worldview to better reflect a result that might be destined to be added to a dust heap made up of ideas that never worked out.

Even if a given result has been replicated through apparently independent means, one could still ask about the identity of the individuals who have conducted the research and whether, or not, those 'researchers' were being paid by entities, corporations, institutions, or governmental departments that stood to gain, in some fashion (financially, commercially, politically, and so on) if the research came out one way rather than another. Replicated experimental work has been done that demonstrates how researchers are significantly more likely to produce results that support the interests of a company, institution, or agency when those researchers are funded by such entities than when individuals conduct research that is free from those kinds of financial, legal or political conflicts of interests.

The foregoing considerations often have had a substantial role to play when it comes to publishing in peer-reviewed journals. Although steps recently have been taken, and are continuing to be taken, in order to render research more transparent in all of its dimensions – including financial ones -- the individuals who are called upon to review research don't always have access to the myriad details that underwrite such research and, as a result, do not know whether, or not, conflicts of interests were present that might have led to subtle manipulations in the running of an experiment, or in relation to the gathering of data, or with respect to the analysis of that data and that could have led to results that were agreeable to whoever was paying for the research.

For example, let us assume that a research group runs five experiments concerning the performance of some given product. Let us also assume that four of those experiments led to results that indicated the product being marketed by the company paying for the research was ineffective or even dangerous, whereas the other experiment generated data that seemed to indicate that, at least, for some people, the product appeared to be effective and safe.

If the four negative results are buried (i.e., are never published or released for public consideration) and only the one 'positive' result is written up, submitted for publication, reviewed, and, eventually -- after a few rounds of corrections -- published, then, really, virtually everyone on the outside of the research (the journal, the reviewers, the public, and committees who base public policy decisions on such research) is being given a distorted understanding of the true research dynamic and context that led to the one, published result.

Alternatively, journals that publish research articles sometimes receive substantial amounts of money – for example through advertising or subsidies – from certain institutions, agencies, and/or companies that have a vested interest in having positive research published concerning their products. Unfortunately, some of those journals might not be all that motivated to rigorously observe their due diligence when it comes to exploring possible financial, political, and/or ideological entanglements between researchers and said entities.

The fact that a research study has been published does not necessarily, in and of itself, mean much of anything. Someone purportedly has: run an experiment, generated data, analyzed that data, drawn conclusions, written an article that organizes the whole experimental process, and, then, submitted the article to various journals. Someone at the place to which the article was submitted has sent the article off for review, and one or more of these latter individuals has perused the article, written up a response, and sent the material back to a publisher for further consideration.

Problems that are rooted in financial, ideological, institutional, and political conflicts of interest can enter into each and every step of the process leading to the publication of an article – that is, with: the researchers, the editors of a journal, and even the peer review process. The individual who reads an article after it surfaces in this or that journal is often not privy to any of the foregoing activities and, therefore, is not necessarily in a position to judge the actual worth of the research.

People with scientific credentials have done research and produced results that are labeled "scientific". People with scientific credentials have reviewed that work in an allegedly rigorous – but, actually, unknown -- manner. People with scientific credentials have published that material. People with scientific credential often read the finished product.

Yet, the significance of the whole process is still fairly ambiguous. No one is quite certain whether a given journal article is a matter of information, disinformation, facts, drivel, knowledge, propaganda, or something else.

The murkiness of the situation is often further exacerbated when newspapers enter the fray and publicize such results. Fewer and fewer papers have the requisite resources -- or even inclination -- to hire individuals with the appropriate academic background and/or industry experience that are capable of conducting serious investigatory journalism on their own, and, therefore, all too frequently, the 'news' pieces about 'scientific' research that appear in the papers might be little more than rewrites of the marketing releases of the companies/institutions/agencies that have paid for the research to be done in the first place and who stand to benefit in various ways from such publicity.

When this occurs, what is transpiring is actually advertising in the guise of news reporting. The real story lies hidden in the activities of an array of "scientists", institutions, agencies, companies, and the like whose actual behavior is usually never reported on and, therefore, remains hidden from the public.

Another matter that needs to be considered when reflecting upon the value of research revolves around the idea of "expertise". For example, court cases sometimes feature the testimony of experts, and, indeed, those experts are employed by opposing sides in an attempt to try to convince a jury, judge, or both that one form of expertise is closer to the 'truth' than some other expression of expertise is.

However, oftentimes, the battle of "experts" amounts to little more than a tug of war among credentialed individuals who have some degree of facility with a given subject matter and are capable of providing testimony that can be woven into the story being constructed by the lawyer or lawyers for a given side. Scientific and technical experts are not necessarily dispensers of the truth, but, instead, are merely individuals who have an informed opinion concerning some specific topic, and that opinion might -- or might not -- give expression to the truth of a matter.

Lawyers who call upon such witnesses will seek to draw out all of the relevant information from the "expert" that might support the lawyer's version of a case. Opposing council will seek to probe all of the lacunae, alternative possibilities, and uncertainties that lie along the horizons of that same testimony.

Although, on the surface, the point-counterpoint nature of the legal questioning might appear to be about trying to get at the truth of a matter, this is not necessarily what is transpiring. Frequently, lawyers are in the business of trying to find ways to push or pull jurors and judges in one direction or another. In other words, the task of lawyers is often more along the lines of an exercise in perception management rather than being a process that is intended to uncover the truth.

The value of such testimony might not even be a function of the degree of truth to which 'expertise' gives expression. Sometimes individuals who seek to glean their understanding from so-called 'experts' are more impressed with style and form than they are with content. For instance, an expert witness who is: Confident, charismatic, has a pleasing vocal timbre, and is attractive/handsome might be perceived by some individuals to be more believable than an expert witness who does not exhibit those qualities to the same degree.

Race, gender, ethnicity, religion, and educational pedigree might also influence a person's perception of the value of testimony. Yet, none of these factors necessarily has anything to do with determining the degree of truth that might, or might not, be present in a given case.

The foregoing comments are not intended to suggest there is no such thing as: Independent, objective, rigorous, judicious, reliable, and considered research or expertise present in the world. Rather, the foregoing possibilities are part of a cautionary tale that should be kept in mind whenever one engages research results and attempts to gauge the value and significance of that material.

Moreover, even under the best of circumstances – that is, when no external financial, institutional, political, ideological, or economic influences are undermining either a research process or the publication of the results generated through such a process – one should not forget that scientists (even good ones) possess their own set of biases and assumptions with respect to how they believe the universe operates. Such biases and assumptions tend to shape how those individuals go about choosing what to do research on, or how they go about conducting research, or how they go about interpreting the data that arises through research, or how they go about presenting their conclusions concerning that research to the public.

The presence of biases and/or assumptions, in and of themselves, does not necessarily invalidate research. Every investigative undertaking has starting points that orient, direct, and motivate that activity, and while those starting points deserve to be critically scrutinized, even Archimedes felt the need or desire to discover a place to stand so that he might try to move the world.

Assumptions and biases often constitute the ground on which a researcher stands in her or his attempt to leverage reality and lift its veil to one degree or another. However, once a scientist or expert takes a stand in the foregoing manner, then the reliability, plausibility, quality, and reasonableness of that in which such a position is rooted is open to being critically engaged.

As one contemplates what answer to write down in response to the Final Jeopardy challenge that was outlined in the Introduction, one is inundated with an array of information whose value needs to be questioned. Newspapers, magazines, journals, books, television commentators, radio programs, movies, educators, politicians, scientists, commercial enterprises, technical experts, researchers, celebrities, economists, religious officials, family, think tanks, friends, and social media are all engaged – directly or indirectly -- in the process of shaping one's perceptions and understandings ... caveat emptor (buyer beware).

The Burzynski Affair

Explicating the 'Burzynski Affair' will take a bit of time. It is a story that runs across nearly 50 years of intriguing twists and turns ... and, unfortunately, at this point, it doesn't have a happy ending.

While this saga has its own intrinsic, existential dimension of interest, the 'Burzynski Affair' also has a great deal of value to offer to the issue with which this book is concerned – namely, the reality problem in the context of the Final Jeopardy challenge. I will present a few summary comments concerning such matters toward the end of this portion of the first chapter, but, in the meantime, the reader might do well to engage the following material by reflecting on what it might have to offer one concerning how to go about responding to the issue of Final Jeopardy.

Sergeant Rick Schiff is a veteran of the San Francisco police office who has been decorated for bravery. On February 29, 1996, he testified before a Congressional Subcommittee Hearing that had been called in order to investigate the activities of the FDA in relation to its persistent attempts to put an American medical doctor, Stanislaw Burzynski, in prison (more on this later).

Sgt Schiff spoke about his twin daughters. One of them was seven, still alive, and with him at the Congressional proceedings, while the other daughter, Kristen, had died a few months earlier.

Kristen had developed a malignant brain tumor when she was four years old. Eventually, the malignancy spread into her spine.

Doctors gave Sgt. Schiff and his wife two options in relation to addressing Kristen's condition. Either the young girl could undergo an intensive regimen of both radiation treatment and chemotherapy, or the girl should be taken home to die.

Whatever Kristen's parents decided to do, the doctors had indicated that the prognosis was bleak. The medical experts believed the girl would die in the near future irrespective of how the parents decided to proceed.

Having been persuaded by the doctors that the only chance – small though it might be – for Kristen's recovery was a course of radiation and chemotherapy, they proceeded with that treatment. The effects on Kristen's body from the effects of the allegedly therapeutic process were so toxic that her parents had to use rubber gloves when changing her diapers.

Following six months of the foregoing combination of chemotherapy and radiation treatment, the girl was still alive – although she had suffered second degree burns to her scalp and skull due to the effects of the radiation treatment and, as a result, had lost most of her hair. Unfortunately, the cancer remained, and the girl's doctors believed she only had a few months to live.

Unwilling to accept the disheartening prognosis that had been pronounced by Kristen's doctors, her parents began to look for alternative possibilities. During their search, they came across the work of Dr. Stanislaw Burzynski who had been born and educated in Poland but was now working in America.

Dr. Burzynski had graduated first in his class of medicine in 1967. Approximately a year and a half later he also obtained a doctorate in biochemistry.

When Dr. Burzynski was studying for his doctorate in biochemistry, he began to explore a group of peptides (a molecule consisting of two or more amino acids … amino acids also are the building blocks for proteins). These peptides were referred to as Antineoplastons and had not been previously received very much attention or study.

Subsequently, Dr. Burzynski realized that the blood and urine of people who suffered from cancer seemed to display an absence of the very kinds of peptides that he earlier had discovered and been studying. Healthy people (or, at least, those who were cancer free), on the other hand, seemed to possess considerable quantities of those same peptides.

Initially, Dr. Burzynski hypothesized that if he could extract the aforementioned peptides from healthy patients, and, then, transfer that extract to individuals suffering from cancer, then, perhaps, he might be able to help the latter group of people in some way. However, there was resistance to his idea almost from the very beginning, and, among other things, some individuals believed that Dr. Burzynski was nothing more than a medical fraud.

During Sgt Schiff's eleven years as a police officer, he had acquired some expertise with respect to being able to detect whether, or not, fraud might be present in a given case he was investigating. He undertook his own inquiry into the life of Dr. Burzynski and came to the conclusion that not only was the doctor not a fraud, but, as well, irrespective of whether, or not, the cancer treatment advocated by Dr. Burzynski might prove, ultimately, to be successful, the procedures had been judged by the FDA to be non-toxic.

Kristen's parents arranged to have their daughter participate in Dr. Burzynski's medical protocol ... a procedure that revolved around the use of Antineoplastons (more on this later). Following 18 months of treatment, Kristen's parents took their daughter off the Antineoplastons protocol since all available evidence indicated that the girl's body was cancer free.

Within a month of removal from the Antineoplastons protocol treatment, the cancer returned. Against the advice of the original doctors (who had recommended traditional treatments of radiation and chemotherapy), Sgt. Schiff and his wife put their daughter back on the Antineoplastons protocol and within nine weeks the tumor had, once again, disappeared.

In July of 1995, Kristen died. However, she had not succumbed to the effects of the Burzynski approach to treating cancer.

Instead, she had died as a result of neurological necrosis. In other words, Kristen's brain had deteriorated due to the cumulative effects of the radiation treatment she previously had undergone before switching over to the Burzynski protocol.

An autopsy of Kristen's body demonstrated that she had been cancer free at the time of death. Of the 52 people who have been diagnosed as having suffered from the same kind of cancer as Kristen, not one of them had died cancer free except Kristen Schiff.

Antineoplastons appear to interact with, and affect, an array of genes that have been demonstrated to play substantial roles in the growth and development of various forms of cancer. More specifically, there are two broad categories of genes that, under certain conditions, allow cancer to grow ... (1) oncogenes and (2) tumor suppressor genes.

People who develop cancer tend to exhibit a higher number of oncogenes that have been switched on while, simultaneously, displaying a larger number of tumor-suppressing genes that have been switched off. Antineoplastons appear to have the capacity to not only help switch oncogenes back off, but, as well, to help turn tumor-suppressing genes back on.

While a number of drugs already approved by the FDA have the capacity to target specific cancer-related genes, Antineoplastons seem to be able to have an impact on more cancer-related genes than do most, if not all, of the drugs that currently are available on the market. In fact, most gene targeting drugs act on only a single gene, whereas Antineoplastons have been found to affect at least a hundred genes at a time, and, as a result are far more powerful than other gene-targeted drugs.

In the early 1990s, Dr. Burzynski received confirmation from the National Cancer Institute that seven patients who were being treated by him had proven to be either completely free or substantially free from the cancers that had beset them. Those clinical trials were FDA approved.

The foregoing patients who were being treated might be referred to as 'hard cases'. In other words, during clinical trials, Dr. Burzynski often focused on various kinds of brain cancer precisely because they were among the most difficult forms of cancer to treat and, as a result, had proven to be largely resistant to conventional approaches to cancer treatment (i.e., radiation and chemotherapy). Furthermore, Dr. Burzynski hoped that if he could make progress with respect to such hard cases, then, perhaps, the medical world might take notice and begin to co-operate with him rather than resist and undermine his efforts.

Let's take a look at some specific cases. For example, on May 15, 2000 Jodi Fenton was diagnosed with an inoperable, grade III condition of anaplastic astrocytoma, and the young woman had been given a life expectancy of approximately 6 to eighteen months.

At the time of her diagnosis, a standard form of treatment would be to undergo a round of chemotherapy using temozolomide, followed by treatment with radiation. The median survival for patients treated through this form of chemotherapy was about 13.6 months, but there was a possibility that she might be able to survive for as long as five years, but even if an individual lasted that long, there still was a strong likelihood that the person would have to undergo additional rounds of the same sort of treatment.

Ms. Fenton had heard about Dr. Burzynski's work through a friend. However, Ms. Fenton has been warned by a neurosurgeon that she should steer clear of Dr. Burzynski and, in addition, she was told by that same neurosurgeon that Antineoplastons therapy did not work.

Normally, the FDA would not permit people to participate in Dr. Burzynski's clinical trials unless they first had gone through a course of treatments involving chemotherapy and radiation. However, Ms. Fenton's tumor was so aggressive and her prospects so grim, she was granted Special Exception status so that she might participate in Dr. Burzynski's clinical trials despite not having undergone either chemotherapy or radiation treatments.

Ms. Fenton decided to opt for the Antineoplastons approach to cancer treatment. She began undergoing treatment in June of 2000.

Within one month of beginning the Burzynski treatment, the most aggressive portion of her tumor had discontinued growing. By December of 2000, the sole remaining trace of her cancer was some scar tissue, and by October 2001 she discontinued the Antineoplastons protocol altogether.

During the following eight-year period, she had annual MRIs. On each occasion, the evidence indicated that some scar tissue was all that remained of her tumor.

Jodi Fenton is not an isolated, anomalous case. Comparisons have been made concerning the outcomes of conventional versus

Antineoplastons treatments in relation to a number of individuals who have been diagnosed with anaplastic astrocytoma.

In 2005, the following results were recorded. Of fifty-four individuals who had been treated through chemotherapy and radiation, five (9%) were considered to be cancer free.

In 2008, a clinical trial report indicated that among the 20 people who had participated in an Antineoplastons-only protocol, five (25%) were designated as being cancer free. Moreover, one should keep in mind that unlike chemotherapy and radiation treatments, Antineoplastons do not appear to cause any toxic side effects.

There were further indications of the potential effectiveness of cancer treatments using Antineoplastons. This involved brain tumors in children that, usually, prove to be fatal.

For instance, brainstem glioma tends to emerge far more frequently in children than in adults. Every year in the United States roughly 500 children are diagnosed with this form of cancer.

More than 90% of the children who suffer with this disorder die within two years of diagnosis, and the median survival time for brainstem glioma is less than one year. It constitutes the leading cause of death in children who suffer from various forms of brain cancer.

The normal course of treatment involves a radiation protocol of some sort. Even then, the prognosis is not promising since, at best, radiation only slows down, to some extent, the growth of the tumor rather than being able to eradicate the malignancy.

In fact, if one were to search the medical literature in relation to the foregoing form of cancer, the results would prove to be quite depressing. Using traditional forms of treatment, there is no record of even one patient who has either been proven to be cancer free following conventional, standard of care treatments or who has managed to live as long as five years following diagnosis and undergoing a traditional form of cancer.

In March 1996, an eleven-year old girl, Jessica Ressel, was diagnosed, via MRI, with brainstem glioma. The tumor had become interwoven with healthy tissue and, therefore, was inoperable.

Even if the young girl underwent radiation treatment, the outlook was not promising. Her prognosis for survival was between 8 and eighteen months.

In addition, the side effects of the radiation 'therapy' were considerable. The beams of radiation would be shot through her ears, and, as a result, not only would the ears become burnt and deformed, but she would become deaf as well.

The treatment also would compromise, if not destroy, the girl's pituitary gland that, among other things, helps regulate growth. Moreover, it was very likely that due to the toxic effects of the radiation treatment, Jessica might end up in a vegetative or semi-vegetative condition, requiring constant care for whatever period of time she might continue to live.

Since the prognosis for treating her glioma through radiation was not good and because the quality of life issues were so grim, the Ressel family decided to look in a different direction. As a result of their search, they selected the Burzynski Clinic and sought to enter into a clinical trial with Antineoplastons.

By November 1996, approximately 8 months after being diagnosed with an inoperable and incurable disease, Jessica Ressel's condition had improved considerably. In fact, within one month of being placed on an Antineoplastons regimen, her tumor had disappeared.

However, the nature of her form of cancer was particularly aggressive. Consequently, it returned within a few months and continued to establish itself.

At that point, the protocol was changed. The level of Antineoplastons she was receiving was doubled, and a month later, the tumor had, once again, disappeared.

Unfortunately, the tumor reappeared in January of 1997 and persisted for another three months. Finally, by May 1997 the tumor disappeared for good and has remained absent through 2001.

Jessica is now in her twenties, married, and has several children. She remains cancer free.

FDA-supervised clinical trial data have been collected for individuals who were afflicted with Childhood Brainstem Glioma. In

| Explorations |

2006 a comparative tabulation of results showed that only 1 of the one hundred and seven individuals (0.9%) treated via chemotherapy and radiation were considered to be cancer free following treatment, whereas 11 of 40 participants (27.5%) who were involved in the Antineoplastons trials were said to be cancer free upon completion of the clinical protocol.

The one person from the radiation/chemotherapy trial who was deemed to be cancer free, died following the termination of treatment. On the other hand, eleven individuals in the Antineoplastons trials survived beyond five years, and, in fact, within this latter group, those individuals who were not required to undergo a round of chemotherapy or radiation treatment prior to being placed in the Antineoplastons clinical trial have been able to go on and live a full life without cancer and without having to live with the toxic side effects associated with radiation and chemotherapy treatments.

Let's take a look at a different form of cancer – namely, adrenocortical carcinoma. A six month-old infant, Kelsey Hill, not only had been diagnosed with a baseball-sized form of the foregoing cancer growing in her abdomen, but, as well, doctors discovered that the disease had metastasized into the baby's kidney, liver and lungs, and as a result, Kelsey's parents were told that their daughter only had a few months to live.

Surgery was performed. Although the full tumor was removed, in the process, young Kelsey lost her left adrenal gland and left kidney.

Following surgery, doctors recommended that Kelsey be given a cocktail of four drugs, all of which had a potential for generating horrifically toxic side effects. Included among those toxic possibilities was the emergence of leukemia as well as the possibility of incurring significant damage to other organs in her body.

Kelsey's parents decided against the chemotherapy treatment. At some point they found out about the Burzynski Clinic and asked an endocrinologist associated with their daughter's case about Antineoplastons, and the parents were told that Dr. Burzynski was a medical fraud.

Despite the warnings, the Hills decided to give Antineoplastons a try and enrolled their daughter in a clinical trial at the Burzynski

Clinic. If their daughter only had nine months, or so, to live, they felt that the non-toxic dimension of the Burzynski treatment process represented a much better option than subjecting their daughter to a cocktail of chemicals that were likely to provide a very low quality of life for both their daughter and themselves with respect to whatever time their daughter might have left to live.

By the time the Hills had been given permission to participate in clinical trials through the Burzynski clinic, a cancerous lesion had shown up on Kelsey's liver. The Antineoplastons protocol was begun in early 2006, and by August 2007, the cancer in Kelsey's liver had disappeared.

Prior to treatment with Antineoplastons, there also had been 6 tumors in Kelsey's lungs. Over the next several years of continued Antineoplastons therapy, the tumors in her lungs went away, and, eventually, only one small spot was left that was considered to be inactive and, most likely, merely constituted scar tissue.

| Explorations |

Since the beginning of his work with Antineoplastons, Dr. Burzynski has treated a vast array of different forms of cancer. His approach to treating that set of diseases has led to the saving of thousands of lives and has proven to be far more effective than the treatment protocols developed by billion-dollar pharmaceutical companies who, quite frequently, are subsidized by tax-funded grants given through the National Cancer Institute.

The National Cancer Institute has an annual budget of over five billion dollars. Antineoplastons protocols often have proven to be far more effective than any combination of chemotherapy and radiation treatments and with none of the toxic side effects of the latter kinds of treatment, but, nevertheless, pharmaceutical companies continue to be rewarded with tax dollar subsidies for their largely ineffective and toxic treatments.

Furthermore, the federal government has consistently pursued a policy which has stipulated that no tax-payer money might be distributed to either the Burzynski Clinic or the Burzynski Research Institute in relation to whatever Phase II, FDA-supervised and approved clinical trials are conducted by Dr. Burzynski in conjunction with cancer research. Those trials are very expensive (around twenty-five million dollars) and unlike many of his competitors, Dr. Burzynski must pay for them out of his own funds.

In the beginning (back in the late 1970s and early 1980s), Dr. Burzynski's research was funded by the National Cancer Institute and the Baylor University College of Medicine. After he decided to open his own research institute and clinic in order to pursue independent research, the funding dried up, and Dr. Burzynski was forced to subsidize his research via bank loans, patient fees, and payments from insurance companies.

Institutions (like the National Cancer Institute or the Baylor College of Medicine) sometimes seem to forget the alleged purpose of their existence and, as a result, they appear to become more concerned with the issue of money and/or the perceived potential of something (such as someone setting up an independent laboratory) to adversely affect them in a financial, economic or political way than they are concerned with actually solving problems or curing diseases. Unfortunately, this sometimes leads to actively trying to keep certain kinds of independent individuals (such as Dr. Burzynski) on the periphery of power in whatever way those institutions can and through whatever means they might deem to be appropriate.

Therefore, sometimes, a person who decides to strike out on his or her own risks becoming ostracized both professionally and financially. Grant applications are rejected. Articles are denied publication. Negative evaluations of character and competence are spread about quite independently of corroborating evidence.

Cancer is a serious business in the United States. Being a serious business, means that a tremendous amount of money is up for grabs (in the way of tax dollars, foundation grants, charitable donations, and substantial profit margins) by those companies and individuals who are ensconced within the bowels of power involving cancer research and treatment.

For a variety of reasons, the work of Dr. Burzynski often has been perceived by some individuals in the cancer industry to be a direct threat to the foregoing potential for financial gain, and, indeed, Antineoplastons protocols might even be able to cause the metastasized forms of malignant financial and political growth that exist in the cancer industry -- and have existed for quite some time -- to disappear. Consequently, although Dr. Burzynski has been making every effort, since 1977, to accommodate the FDA, the FDA and other related institutions have not reciprocated.

A vast network of: researchers (both biochemical and medical), academics, oncology programs, journals, pharmaceutical companies, hospitals, manufacturers of medical equipment, doctors, charities, government agencies, lawyers, stock holders, banks, and insurance companies make up the cancer industry. Collectively, they siphon off billions of dollars annually, and, yet, the benefits to the public that have been generated by the foregoing multi-generational set of researchers, manufacturers, educators, and practitioners have been, for the most part, fairly negligible. Moreover, as already indicated on several occasions, whatever forms of treatment that have been developed through the cancerous, hydra-headed industrial Leviathan that prowls the American countryside tends to be accompanied by fairly toxic side effects as well.

| Explorations |

In order for the cancer industry Leviathan to continue feeding, the dollars must continue to pour in. Therefore, anything – such as the research of a Dr. Burzynski – that potentially threatens to disrupt the financial supply lines that fill the feeding troughs of the cancer industry is likely to be subject to the full rage and circumspection of those who feel they are being deprived of what they consider to be rightly theirs – i.e., money, power, position, and prestige.

The FDA (Food and Drug Administration), a federally funded agency, is one of the primary guardians of the cancer industry. There are 18 committees that advise the FDA with respect to, among other things, drugs that are to be evaluated for possible approval.

The membership of those committees consists of individuals who work outside the federal government. However, many of those members also serve as consultants who are paid by pharmaceutical companies.

In the event of a potential conflict of interest between, on the one hand, an advisor's task to fairly evaluate a given drug and, on the other hand, that advisory member's role as a consultant for some pharmaceutical company, an advisor is supposed to recuse himself or herself. Yet, often times, the FDA will exempt members of the advisory committee and permit them to evaluate a drug that is being developed by the very same company that is paying that advisor to be a consultant.

In 1992, Congress passed the Prescription Drug User Fee Act that required pharmaceutical companies to pay a certain amount to the FDA for each drug that is to be considered for approval by that agency. As a result, hundreds of millions of dollars poured into the FDA from the very companies that the FDA is supposed to regulate ... indeed, by 2010, these user fees amounted to more than half a billion dollars.

The idea for the change in user fee did not come from either Congress or the FDA. The drug companies, themselves, were the ones who were advocating for a change in the way 'business' was done.

The new user fee arrangement induced the FDA to place many drugs on a fast track for timely approval – which, in effect, was what the FDA was getting paid for by pharmaceutical companies. After all, the more drugs that are approved by the FDA (and done so quickly), then the more money will be paid to the FDA by pharmaceutical companies and, in turn, the more quickly will drugs begin to realize a commercial return for the drug manufacturers.

According to a study conducted by the George Washington University Medical Center in Washington D.C. and that was commissioned by Pfizer, there was a significant reduction in the median review period for priority drugs when one compares the approval times both before and after the passage of the Prescription Drug User Fee Act. Priority drugs are ones that are to be used in conjunction with diseases that are either serious or life threatening and for which existing treatments have been relatively ineffective (and this included treatments for cancer).

The aforementioned George Washington University Medical Center study indicated that the median review period decreased from approximately 21 months in 1993 to about six months in 2004. Furthermore, following the passage of the aforementioned Prescription Drug User Fee Act many other drugs were approved for use in as little time as 3-4 months.

Unfortunately, due to the financially-based incentives for the FDA to do things quickly, there is a considerable amount of this fast tracking that is done without sufficiently rigorous oversight or that is done with compromised oversight. This especially might be the case when members of various FDA advisory committees are permitted by the agency to by-pass potential conflicts of interests and approve (possibly) drugs for companies that also pay those same individuals consultant fees.

| Explorations |

46

Unfortunately, there are other means through which the FDA can impact research. Indeed, that agency has a variety of ways in which it can insinuate itself into the affairs of on-going research ... often at the behest of various representatives of the pharmaceutical industry who also are serving on advisory committees for the FDA.

In the late 1970s, before Dr. Burzynski began treating people with Antineoplastons, he discussed his intentions with a number of attorneys. More specifically, he wanted to know whether there were any legal prohibitions against his use of experimental drugs – namely, Antineoplastons – in his private practice or whether there were any legal impediments to a private, biomedical company becoming involved in cancer research.

After exploring the matter, the lawyers advised Dr. Burzynski that what he wanted to do with respect to setting up a clinic and research institute would not be in violation of any existing law or laws. The attorneys indicated that on both the state and federal levels there were no legal obstacles to treating patients with Antineoplastons or conducting cancer research in conjunction with Antineoplastons, but Dr. Burzynski would not be permitted to engage in interstate commerce with respect to distributing his drug outside of Texas.

Once Dr. Burzynski established his clinic and research institute, word began to spread concerning his early success in treating various kinds of cancer. As a result, people from all over the United States began to travel to Texas to be treated with Antineoplastons.

Dr. Burzynski later found out that representatives from the Texas State Board of Medical Examiners had visited with some of his patients in order to encourage the latter individuals to file complaints against Dr. Burzynski and his method of treating cancer. These agents didn't just visit with clients undergoing Antineoplastons therapy who lived in Texas, but they also went in search of clients who lived outside of Texas and who might co-operate with the Texas State Board of Medical Examiners.

In 1986, Dr. Burzynski received a letter indicating that the Texas State Board had initiated an investigation into his activities. Although no formal complaint had been issued by patients, nevertheless, Dr. Burzynski was told that he should appear -- with legal counsel if he wished -- at an 'informal' disciplinary hearing in order for him to have an opportunity to rebut whatever allegations might be voiced at that time ... allegations that could affect the status of his medical license.

Eventually, the Texas Board of Medical Examiners told Dr. Burzynski that if he would provide it with information concerning instances of successful, Antineoplastons treatment, the Board would have those results examined by a number of oncologists. If, in turn, those doctors concluded that the treatments were safe and effective, then, the Board would discontinue its investigation of Dr. Burzynski.

During November 1986, Dr. Burzynski entered into an agreement to provide the Texas Board of Medical Examiners with more than 40 cases of successful treatment involving Antineoplastons. These cases were quite varied with respect to the kinds of cancer that were being treated.

For two years following the foregoing agreement, there was no contact between the Texas Board of Medial Examiners and Dr. Burzynski. Finally, the Board contacted him and acted as if the cases submitted to them in November 1986 by Dr. Burzynski were not examples of treatment success but, instead, constituted failures and the State Board further alleged that he was not in compliance with a certain law – a law that actually didn't exist – and, therefore, there were grounds to suspend or revoke his medical license.

Despite the absence of any evidentially-based case against Dr. Burzynski, the State Medical Board filed its first amended complaint in 1990. Two years later – although still without any evidence or justifiable grounds -- the Board filed a second amended complaint.

In 1993, over sixty clients of Dr. Burzynski filed legal documents indicating that they wished to intervene on the side of Dr. Burzynski in the case involving the Texas State Board of Medical Examiners. The Board of Medical Examiners tried to strike that petition from the record.

In May of 1993, the foregoing case between Dr. Burzynski and the Texas State Board of Medical Examiners went to trial. Apparently, the purpose of the legal proceeding was to stop Dr. Burzynski's research and treatment of patients despite a complete absence of any evidence indicating that Dr. Burzynski was either operating in contravention of

| Explorations |

the law or that his treatment protocols were not successful and/or safe.

In fact, during the trial, the prosecution did not bring forth even one expert witness who could counter Dr. Burzynski's work or research. On the other hand, Dr. Burzynski's legal counsel did call to the witness stand Dr. Nicholas Patronas, from Georgetown University, who also was Chief of Radiology at the National Cancer Institute.

Dr. Patronas had reviewed seven cases involving treatment by Antineoplastons. He testified that all seven individuals suffered from some form of brain cancer, but, now, five of them were living cancer free and that he had never seen any other kind of treatment work so well with such difficult-to-treat forms of cancer.

One of the patients was Paul Michaels whose mother testified on behalf of Dr. Burzynski. Paul was only four or five years old when he developed brain cancer and his doctors had indicated there was nothing they could do for him ... that Paul was going to die from his cancerous tumor -- and, yet, in 2011, at the age of 25, the boy was still alive and cancer free due to his treatment involving Antineoplastons.

The judge in the case ruled for Dr. Burzynski and against the Texas State Board of Medical Examiners. In his ruling, the judge noted that the state had not presented any evidence during the trial indicating that Antineoplastons were either ineffective or unsafe. Furthermore, the judge indicated that Dr. Burzynski had not been shown to be in contravention of any state laws with respect to either the manufacture of his own drug or the use of that drug in conjunction with treatment of his patients.

The foregoing judgment did not dissuade the Texas State Board of Medical Examiners to cease and desist in its efforts against Dr. Burzynski. In spite of having no legal or medical basis to support its position, it continued to try to stop Dr. Burzynski's research into, and medical use of, Antineoplastons.

In 1995, the Texas State Board of Medical Examiners took Dr. Burzynski to district court. They were seeking to revoke Dr. Burzynski's medical license on the grounds that appropriate medical authorities had never sanctioned the use of Antineoplastons in the treatment of cancer patients.

| Explorations |

The Board indicated that the efficacy of Antineoplastons was irrelevant to its concerns. It was claiming, instead, that Dr. Burzynski was acting in a rogue fashion and, therefore, independently of the approval of appropriate medical authorities.

The case eventually ended up at the Texas State Supreme Court in 1996. A state Supreme Court judge placed Dr. Burzynski on probation for ten years, but one wonders how plausible and defensible the grounds were that allegedly justified such a ruling since there still was no evidence that Dr. Burzynski had violated any laws or did any harm with respect to his patients.

Why – despite a lack of evidence – would the Texas State Board of Medical Examiners continue to flog a dead horse over so many years? It turns out, apparently, that the FDA had been pressuring the Texas Board to revoke Dr. Burzynski's medical license.

In addition, certain members of the FDA were intent on trying to find a way to imprison Dr. Burzynski and bring his work with Antineoplastons to a complete halt. After all, if his research were ever given a fair and impartial hearing, then, both the pharmaceutical industry and the FDA might be at risk of losing a great deal of money in relation to the manufacture and approval of drug treatments that were, for the most part, neither particularly effective nor necessarily safe and non-toxic.

For example, in January of 1982, Dr. Richard J. Crout, Director of the FDA Bureau of Drugs, went on the record in *The Spotlight* and stated: "I never have and never will approve a new drug to an individual, but only to a large pharmaceutical firm with unlimited finances." The foregoing statement might, or might not, have been directed toward Dr. Burzynski, but whether, or not, this was the case, it gave expression to the mind set that would come to be focused on Dr. Burzynski by the FDA.

Aside from the issue of who, if anyone, was the object of the 1982 statement by Dr. Crout, one also wonders about the propriety of that statement. His words give priority to money and large corporations without even a mention of efficacy, safety, or service to the public.

Maybe, somewhere along, or beneath, the horizons of Dr. Crout's statement, there might be a rationale that makes sense if it were to be

| Explorations |

spelled out. However, as it stands, the foregoing statement is little more than an endorsement of the sort of thing that Dr. Marcia Angell, former editor of the New England Journal of Medicine, has complained and warned about for a very long time – namely, that drug companies possess an unacceptable level of control over the policies, practices, and decisions of the FDA.

In 1983 the FDA attempted, through civil litigation, to close down Dr, Burzynski's research and treatment facilities. Prior to a decision being rendered in the case by District Judge Gabrielle McDonald, the FDA wrote to her and stated that if the court did not grant injunctive relief as requested by the United States government in relation to Dr. Burzynski's activities involving Antineoplastons, then other "less efficient" means (that were alluded to in the letter to the judge) would have to be pursued

Quite irrespective of what the other, less efficient steps might be, the federal government and its lawyers seemed to be oblivious to the unethical, if not illegal, character of their letter to the judge. In effect, they were seeking to influence the judge's decision in the case.

Despite the inappropriate actions of the federal government prior to the issuance of a legal decision, District Judge Gabrielle McDonald ruled that Dr. Burzynski was entirely within his rights to produce Antineoplastons, as well as to use them in conjunction with his patients. However, she indicated that Dr. Burzynski could not ship his drugs across state lines.

Following up on the not-so-veiled threats concerning Dr. Burzynski that were stated in the aforementioned letter to Judge McDonald, In 1985, the FDA brought took steps to convene a grand jury. The impaneled grand jury would hear testimony that was intended to lead to an indictment of Dr. Burzynski.

Prior to the convening of the aforementioned grand jury, the FDA arranged for a raid to be carried out with respect to Dr. Burzynski's clinic. Among other items, all of his medical records were confiscated ... an action that interfered with, and undermined, the ability of Dr. Burzynski to properly treat a variety of clients -- many of whom were quite ill.

| Explorations |

Whatever the grand jury might have been exposed to during its sessions, the information given to them obviously didn't appear to be all that impressive. The grand jury refused to issue an indictment against Dr. Burzynski.

Furthermore, during this period of time, it was discovered that when a variety of people contacted the FDA in relation to the work of Dr. Burzynski, those individuals were told that criminal investigations were being conducted in relation to Dr. Burzynski. When a judge learned about the foregoing practice, a cease and desist order was issued instructing the FDA to discontinue that sort of behavior.

Later on, the FDA changed its tactics and no longer passively waited for people to call the agency. Instead, they were 'proactive' and used information acquired during its raids of Dr. Burzynski's clinic to contact clinics and institutes all over the world informing the latter that grand juries were being impaneled in conjunction with the work of Dr. Burzynski.

In 1986, the FDA conducted another raid on Dr. Burzynski's clinic. Tens of thousands of more documents and medical records were confiscated.

Another grand jury was convened. Once again the grand jury refused to issue an indictment.

In 1990 a third grand jury was assembled. On that occasion, Dr. Burzynski was brought in to give testimony, and, once again, after all was said and done, no indictment was issued.

A fourth grand jury was convened in 1994. The outcome was the same as the previous three grand juries – namely, no indictment.

In March of 1995, a fifth grand jury was convened. Following a television program later that month which carried interviews with some of the patients of Dr. Burzynski – all of whom gave positive testimony concerning the Antineoplastons treatment protocol -- the FDA again raided the Burzynski clinic and carted away more documents.

Further subpoenas were issued in conjunction with the latest grand jury proceedings. Further confiscated documents were introduced, and further testimony was given before the latest grand jury.

| Explorations |

During the period of time when many of the foregoing grand juries were being convened, Dr. David Kessler was the Commissioner of the FDA. At one point a question was asked of Dr. Kessler by one of the members of a 1995 Congressional Oversight and Investigations Subcommittee Hearing that was looking into the conduct of the FDA vis-à-vis Dr. Burzynski.

While acknowledging that the FDA had every right to convene a grand jury to investigate possible wrongdoing, the Congressman asking the question wondered how many times various grand juries would have to end with a 'no finding of fault' judgment before someone like Dr. Kessler would instruct the members of the FDA to cease and desist in their activities concerning Dr. Burzynski. Dr. Kessler responded by asking his own question of the Congressman -- namely: How did the Congressman know that there had been no finding of fault in any of the grand juries?

The Congressman responded by saying that no indictments had been issued in any of the grand jury proceedings. Dr. Kessler then replied in the following manner: Just because no indictment had been issued, one was not entitled to further conclude that there had been no finding of fault … and he appeared to further suggest that this was the case as a matter of law.

One might describe Dr. Kessler's comment as a distinction without a difference. The Congressman who engaged in the back and forth with Dr. Kessler might have agreed with the assessment with which this paragraph begins since he was baffled by Dr. Kessler's response … as was also the case with at least one other member of the Subcommittee who indicated that since a person had once proposed that one could indict a ham sandwich via a grand jury, the fact that no indictments had been issued in any of the grand jury proceedings concerning Dr. Burzynski would seem to indicate that, perhaps, there was just nothing there to pursue.

Dozens of former patients of Dr. Burzynski came from across the United States, at their own expense, to give testimony before the aforementioned Congressional Subcommittee. They were all unanimous in their support and praise of the work of Dr. Burzynski, as well as expressing outrage concerning the past conduct of the FDA.

| Explorations |

On November 20, 1995, the FDA achieved what it had been pursuing for such a long period of time. A grand jury finally issued an indictment against Dr. Burzynski.

The indictment charged him with having committed -- over a period of many years -- 75 specified acts that constituted either instances of violating federal law or instances of having committed fraud. If he were convicted of those charges, Dr. Burzynski could be sentenced for up to 290 years in prison and levied with millions of dollars in fines.

In early 1996, a further round of Congressional Subcommittee Hearings was convened for the purpose of investigating the FDA's aggressive pursuit concerning Dr. Burzynski treatment of cancer patients. Once again, many of his former and current patients traveled to Washington, D.C. in order to be able to testify during those Hearings.

There were a number of recurrent themes in the testimony of those individuals. Firstly, Dr. Burzynski had made no promises to any of them, and only informed them that his clinic had had some success in treating a variety of forms of cancer. Secondly, Dr. Burzynski's form of cancer treatment had helped his patients in significant ways that conventional protocols involving chemotherapy and radiation had not been able to do. Thirdly, the patients indicated that treatment with Antineoplastons had none of the toxic and damaging side effects that traditional cancer treatments tended to have. Finally, without continued access to Antineoplastons treatment, the patients felt they would be relegated to their original condition prior to entering into treatment with Dr. Burzynski – namely, a prognosis of death within a relatively short period of time that had been issued by various doctors who said there was nothing that could be done for them ... except to subject those patients to toxic forms of treatment.

On March 29, 1996, Dr. David Kessler, Commissioner of the Food and Drug Administration (FDA) made a statement, carried by C-Span, about a set of four guidelines that were being issued through the Executive Office and the FDA. These proposals were advocating the implementation of new procedures that would decrease the amount of time needed to test and approve new, promising drugs in relation to the treatment of cancer.

The indicated proposals were as follows:

"First, for patients with refractory or hard to treat cancers ... instead of requiring evidence of clinical benefit -- such as survival -- the FDA would rely on objective evidence of partial response – e.g., tumor shrinkage -- as an initial basis for approval. This will allow us to rely on smaller, shorter studies for the initial approval of cancer drugs."

"Second, we will expedite the availability of promising medications that have been approved in certain other countries

"Third, we will include representatives of cancer patients in the FDA's Cancer Advisory Committees, and, thereby, make sure that their views are heard when it comes to recommending approval or non-approval of cancer drugs."

"And, fourth, we will eliminate unnecessary paperwork that used to delay or discourage cancer research by non-commercial, clinical investigators."

What is ironically intriguing about the above four proposals is the way they resonate with Dr. Burzynski's research and medical treatment programs, and, yet, the FDA continued to be fully engaged in the pursuit of criminally prosecuting Dr. Burzynski. For instance, in line with proposal one above, patients treated with Antineoplastons not only had provided objective evidence of positive response to such treatments, but, as well, had provided clinical benefit – that is, the patients had survived and flourished. Moreover, in line with the second of the foregoing four proposals issued by the FDA, Dr. Burzynski's Antineoplastons therapy had been approved by, and was being used in, many foreign countries, but, nevertheless, those same kinds of treatments were under relentless attack by the FDA in America. Furthermore, in line with the third of the four FDA guidelines noted above, for years, hundreds of Dr. Burzynski's patients had been contacting the FDA and/or testifying before Congressional Subcommittees concerning the value, effectiveness, and non-toxicity of Antineoplastons, but the FDA had consistently disregarded such testimony. Finally, in line with the fourth of the aforementioned FDA proposals, the FDA had gone out of its way and spent millions of taxpayer dollars in an attempt to obstruct, delay, and discourage -- as well as proliferate the paperwork and official red tape associated with -- Dr. Burzynski's research into Antineoplastons.

Putting aside the Dr. Burzynski aspect of things, a cynical individual might suppose that however high-minded the new FDA guidelines sounded, something else was actually taking place. In effect, the FDA was opening up some new streams of income for itself (remember, following passage of the 1992 Prescription Drug User Fee Act, a new fee structure was established that required drug companies to pay a certain amount of each drug for which they sought approval), while simultaneously making it easier for pharmaceutical companies to release more products into the market place even more quickly than previously had been the case.

More disturbingly, perhaps, the new FDA guidelines meant drug companies didn't even have to prove their products actually helped people survive or that those products eradicated cancer. Now, those companies only had to show there was some sort of objective evidence (determined how, and by whom, and according to what criteria?) that indicated some kind of improvement might have occurred.

The new FDA guidelines were, in effect, lowering the bar as far as quality of cancer treatment was concerned, but, at the same time, the returns for satisfying such a lowering of standards were being increased. This was equally true for both the FDA as well as for pharmaceutical companies.

In the question and answer period that followed the FDA's announcement of its new four-part initiative, Dr. Kessler was asked how the guidelines would affect Antineoplastons research. Dr. Kessler proceeded to re-state the first proposal noted earlier and indicated that he didn't want to get into particular cases but went on to elaborate on how a given drug would have to have been part of a clinical trial in order to be considered to have satisfied the criteria for the first guideline he stated during his opening statement.

Dr. Kessler further stipulated that any drug that was to be considered in conjunction with the first guideline of the new FDA proposals concerning possible cancer treatments would have had to be the result of a certain set of scientific procedures. There needed to be a scientific way of assessing the effectiveness of whatever information was connected to use of a given drug ... one couldn't just take an agent here and there and try to draw conclusions from that ... it had to be part of a clinical trial.

| Explorations |

A follow up question concerning Antineoplastons was asked. Dr. Kessler responded by saying: "The agency has approved trials for patients with Antineoplastons."

Apparently, as a result of pressure from many people who had benefitted directly from treatment with Antineoplastons, as well as due to the impact of several Congressional Hearings concerning that issue, patients who were being treated with Antineoplastons were going to be permitted by the FDA to be part of Phase-II clinical trials. Eventually, this led to Antineoplastons being used in relation to 72 Phase-II clinical trials.

Notwithstanding having made some progress in relation to the FDA's willingness to permit Antineoplastons to be explored via FDA-approved Phase-II clinical trials, the FDA was continuing to press for the criminal prosecution of Dr. Burzynski. The FDA didn't dispute the fact that Antineoplastons had been demonstrated to be effective and non-toxic, but, rather, the agency seemed to be concerned with the fact that Dr. Burzynski was a rogue element when it came to big Pharma culture, and as such, he constituted a potential – perhaps very real – threat to the way that culture sought to control the cancer industry, in particular, and medical practice in general.

The FDA saw Dr. Burzynski as a means for generating a 'teachable moment'. More specifically, by prosecuting Dr. Burzynski, the FDA hoped to teach practitioners and researchers – both in the present and the future -- a lesson about what would happen to them if any of those individuals were not willing to comply with the way the cancer industry was operated and regulated in the United States.

For the FDA, the issue was not primarily a matter of the effectiveness or safety of medical treatments. If this had been the case, the FDA would have behaved quite differently toward Dr. Burzynski across the several decades that it sought to harass him and place obstacles in the way of his research.

Rather, the essential issue for the FDA was one of control and money. The FDA's public acknowledgment that Antineoplastons were: Saving lives, effective, and safe belied everything else that organization was trying to claim concerning its reasons for acting in the way it had been doing with respect to Dr. Burzynski.

| Explorations |

The FDA isn't necessarily in the business of regulating things for purposes of safety, effectiveness, and saving lives. The FDA is in the business of regulating things on behalf of certain powerful business interests, and Dr. Burzynski was a fly in that economic and political ointment.

How else can one explain the perspective of Assistant U.S. Attorney Mike Clark when he indicated prior to the Burzynski trial that the effectiveness of Antineoplastons was not germane to the criminal proceedings being brought against Dr. Burzynski? In fact, in a December 5, 1996 article by T.D. Elias in *The Washington Times* Mr. Clark is reported as having said in an October 11, 1996 court filing that the issue was: "irrelevant, emotional, prejudicial, and misleading ..."

Obviously, the fact that Antineoplastons are effective and safe is <u>*irrelevant*</u> to the desire of the FDA to stop Dr. Burzynski for reasons that have nothing to do with safety and effectiveness but that have everything to do with control and with who really stands to benefit if Dr. Burzynski is removed from the picture. To be sure, the use of Antineoplastons generates <u>emotional</u> outbursts both on the part of the people whose lives are saved through Antineoplastons treatments, as well as in relation to those who are losing money as a result of the success of such treatments. In addition, the fact that Antineoplastons are effective and non-toxic is certainly <u>prejudicial</u> toward those who want money and power to be the central issues, not effectiveness and safety. Furthermore, the issue of the effectiveness of Antineoplastons is quite <u>misleading</u> because it confuses people by inducing those individuals to wonder why money and control are considered to be more important than effectiveness and safety.

The FDA vendetta against Dr. Burzynski cost $60 million dollars. To defend himself against the criminal charges, Dr. Burzynski spent more than $2 million dollars.

Proponents of neoclassical liberal economics might claim that the trial increased GNP by millions of dollars. Proponents of any sane version of economics might contend that the efforts of the FDA to criminally prosecute Dr. Burzynski were a waste of time, money, and resources that could have been directed toward the saving of lives through repurposing such sums for the treatment of people with various forms of cancer.

On March 4, 1997 Judge Lake, who was presiding over the criminal case involving Dr. Burzynski, declared a mistrial. The federal jury that had been impaneled to deliberate on the case had reached an impasse and become deadlocked.

Moreover, Judge Lake further stipulated that during the trial proceedings the federal government had failed to meet the burden of proof in relation to a variety of counts involving mail fraud – which came to nearly half of all the charges for which Dr. Burzynski had been indicted originally. Consequently, Judge Lake issued a directed verdict of acquittal concerning those counts.

The FDA was not prepared to disengage from the matter. They pushed for a further trial to be held.

Initially, the federal prosecutors who were working on behalf of the FDA sought to seek convictions in relation to all of the charges that had not been dismissed by Judge Lake in the previous trial. However, shortly before the new proceedings were set to start in May of 1997, the federal prosecutors shifted gears and decided to drop all but one criminal charge against Dr. Burzynski.

On May 19, 1997, the case in the second trial was handed over to the jury for deliberation. Those individuals took approximately three hours to reach a verdict and indicated that Dr. Burzynski should be acquitted of the final charge still outstanding against him.

The National Cancer Institute entered the Burzynski affair in October 1991, first in the form of Dr. Nicholas J. Patronas who, eventually, testified on behalf of Dr. Burzynski during proceedings involving the Texas State Medical Board of Examiners (discussed earlier). Prior to the occasion of giving testimony, Dr. Patronas had taken a delegation from the National Cancer Institute to conduct an on site visit of the Burzynski facilities in Texas.

The delegation was quite impressed with what it learned during the trip with respect to Antineoplastons. In a subsequent letter, the National Cancer Institute indicated an interest in carrying out confirmatory trials with respect to Antineoplastons that would be conducted under the sponsorship of the National Cancer Institute.

| Explorations |

59

The trials were to involve many top-caliber medical doctors, including Michael Friedman. At the time, he was an associate director for the Cancer Therapy Evaluation Program at the National Cancer Institute.

On October 31, 1991, Dr. Friedman issued an internal memorandum to the Director of the Division of Cancer Treatment suggesting that based on what Dr. Friedman knew already, the potential efficacy of Antineoplastons deserved further study. On December 2, 1991, a Decision Network Meeting at the National Cancer Institute gave the go ahead for government approved clinical trials to be held in conjunction with several Antineoplastons.

The future looked very promising. Then, everything came to a grinding halt.

A few months later, plans for clinical trials in conjunction with Dr. Burzynski's work seemed to be placed on a back burner while Élan Pharmaceutical appeared to show up out of left field, so to speak, and was given approval to conduct clinical trials involving one of the metabolites (phenylacetate) associated with Antineoplastons. Earlier Élan had agreed to enter into a partnership, licensing arrangement, and royalty agreement with the Burzynski Research Institute and Clinic with respect to the latter's research into, and use of, certain Antineoplastons

However, quite abruptly on September 24, 1990, Élan decided to terminate the foregoing arrangement. In its notice of termination, the company indicated that it felt there might be some difficulties surrounding the issue of patent rights in relation to Antineoplastons.

At some point – either slightly before, or shortly after the foregoing date of termination – Élan recruited Dr. Dvorit Samid to work on Antineoplastons. Dr. Samid was a medical professor from Maryland who had been hired earlier by Dr. Burzynski as a consultant for the purpose of studying Antineoplastons. Apparently, Dr. Samid first came into contact with Élan through Dr. Burzynski.

Subsequent to her Burzynski-related work on Antineoplastons, Dr. Samid spoke about that research at the 9th International Symposium on Future Trends in Chemotherapy that was being convened in Switzerland. News of the research on Antineoplastons, along with the aforementioned presentation in Switzerland, appeared in the July/August 1990 edition of *Oncology News*.

(1) The July/August 1990 *Oncology News* item about the talk on Antineoplastons that was given by Dr. Samid in Switzerland, along with (2) Élan's September 1990 termination of its agreement with Dr. Burzynski, as well as (3) the subsequent recruitment of Dr. Samid by Élan following her work with Dr. Burzynski, together with (4) the later (and aforementioned) announcement concerning the fact that Élan was going to be running some clinical trials involving Antineoplastons might all have been coincidental. Nonetheless, the whole situation does tend to make one wonder about what might have been going on behind the scenes.

In addition to recruiting Dr. Samid, Élan Pharmaceutical entered into an agreement with the National Cancer Institute to conduct clinical trials on Antineoplastons. Dr. Samid had not only served as a consultant for, and worked with, Dr. Burzynski, but she also worked at the National Cancer Institute, including as a Section Chief.

The clinical trials that were to be conducted by Élan Pharmaceutics in conjunction with the National Cancer Institute were to be done using a metabolite (phenylacetate) associated with Antineoplastons. Dr. Burzynski's lawyers had informed him early on that the foregoing metabolite could not be patented (the molecule was already an established part of the pool of common knowledge available to the world of science), but, in point of fact, that metabolite was not central to the discoveries that Dr. Burzynski eventually made with respect to the critical activity and structure of Antineoplastons that extended far beyond the phenylacetate molecule.

Dr. Burzynski already knew by 1980 that phenylacetate, by itself, possessed limited efficacy with respect to the treatment of cancer. Dr. Burzynski had been studying other, more promising Antineoplastons for quite some time.

Li-Chuan Chen, a scientist at the National Cancer Institute began to work with Dr. Samid in 1994. Dr. Samid did not inform him that the compound being used in their research had any connection with Dr. Burzynski, and, instead, she just showed Dr. Chen the published research involving phenylacetate and some of its anti-cancer capabilities.

The aspect of the research that most intrigued Dr. Chen involved the analog molecules that were related to phenylacetate. If one is studying a certain molecule that has some anti-cancer properties, and, then, other analog molecules begin to emerge, one begins to feel that one might be on to something of value ... especially if those analog molecules were to display considerable biological activity in relation to cancerous tumors.

Researchers at Johns Hopkins University also had been working along lines somewhat similar to the work of Dr. Samid. The former researchers tried to take out patents on some of the analog compounds they had been studying but were prevented from doing so by Dr. Samid.

Dr. Chen noted that Dr. Samid decried the behavior of the Johns Hopkins researchers for, seemingly, going behind her back and attempting to register patents for some of the compounds involved. Yet, the pattern of behavior displayed by the Johns Hopkins researchers appeared to be quite similar to what had transpired following Dr. Samid's work with Dr. Burzynski.

On October 21, 1991, Dr. Samid, in conjunction with the Department of Health and Human Services of the United States, filed a patent involving phenylacetate-related Antineoplastons and indicated that the compounds were methods for treating cancer. That patent was eventually granted on March 14, 2000.

Another patent involving phenylacetate-related Antineoplastons was filed on October 12, 1993 and, subsequently, was approved on June 3, 1997. This patent not only listed Dr. Samid as the inventor and the Department of Health and Human Services as an Assignee, but the name of Élan Pharmaceuticals also appeared in the application.

The patent application indicated that the 'invention' was to be used for more than cancer treatment. The methods for therapy and prevention being outlined in the patent were intended to treat a variety of pathologies, including: cancer, AIDS, and anemia.

A third patent was filed by Dr. Samid and the Department of Health and Human Services on March 3, 1994 and approved on February 25, 1997. This was their most extensive filing (over a hundred pages long) on phenylacetate-related compounds up until

| Explorations |

that time and was described in terms of "compositions and methods for treating & preventing pathologies, including caner."

A fourth patent was filed on October 12, 1994 and approved on December 22, 1998. The patent was intended to cover: 'phenylacetate and derivatives alone or in combination with other compounds against neoplastic conditions and other disorders.'

On June 6, 1995, Dr. Samid, in conjunction with the Department of Health and Human Services, filed three more patents. The very next day – June 7, 1995 – further patents involving phenylacetate compounds were filed. Those patents were approved, respectively, on January 20, 1998, and March 2, 1998.

However, the entire set of filings that had begun in 1991, together with their subsequent approvals, was something of a Pyrrhic victory. The patents only covered compounds that already had been proven by Dr. Burzynski to be of limited value in the treatment of cancer, but the wording of the patent filing might have been an attempt to provide a precedent for later claiming -- in, say, some sort of legal proceedings -- that because Dr. Burzynski's Antineoplastons were sometimes entangled with phenylacetate analogs, then, there might be some sort of patent infringement issue involving the phenylacetate compounds.

According to the first patent application noted above (October 21, 1991), the "invention" that was described within the application could be "manufactured, used, and licensed by, or for the Government for governmental purposes without the payment to us of any royalties thereon". The patent and its wording might explain some of why Élan Pharmaceuticals and the National Cancer Institute behaved in the way they did with respect to Dr. Burzynski in relation both to previous, as well as the following, descriptions of events dealing with Phase-II clinical trials involving Antineoplastons.

On April 29, 1993 Patricia R. Schettino, a clinical research pharmacist, distributed a memorandum concerning the minutes of a meeting that had been held on the issue of Antineoplastons. The minutes indicated that concern had been expressed about the political fallout surrounding Antineoplastons. The name of Congressman Berkley Bedell was specifically mentioned during the meeting as someone who felt people at the National Cancer Institute might be taking Antineoplastons away from Dr. Burzynski.

| Explorations |

The minutes of the aforementioned meeting also clearly stated knowledge about the fact that Dr. Burzynski held patents on Antineoplastons. The minutes went on to state the since phenylacetate-related compounds might be a key, active component in Antineoplastons, there were some concerns surrounding the issue.

Although the aforementioned Dr. Chen of the National Cancer Institute continued to work with Dr. Samid into 1995, he had begun to have some concerns about what was taking place. For example, in the first published article concerning phenylacetate, Dr. Samid indicated in the methodology section of the paper that materials for the research had been obtained from BRI in Houston, Texas.

However, Dr. Burzynski's name was not mentioned in either the references or acknowledgments that were contained in the paper. According to Dr. Chen, this was inconsistent with proper procedure in scientific research.

Quite irrespective of the possible improprieties circulating about the Élan/Dr. Samid/National Cancer Institute triangle when it came to the research concerning phenylacetate, the line of research they were collectively pursing already had been proven to be, for the most part, a dead end as far as finding effective treatments for cancer are concerned. Nevertheless, those institutions and individuals were in the process of wasting years, along with millions of dollars, doing research that would lead nowhere, while Dr. Burzynski's much more promising and effective research continued to be neglected and prosecuted.

The reason why the aforementioned triumvirate was focusing on phenylacetate was because all of the Antineoplastons that actually possessed any degree of real promise in relation to cancer treatment were already under patent to Dr. Burzynski. Dr. Samid and the other two members of her troika would rather try to search in vain for the possibility of discovering gold in a mine that already had been demonstrated to be depleted of value rather than to acknowledge that the potential for successful cancer treatments might be found in a place that they did not control or to which they did not own the mining rights.

Eventually, however, after a lot of wasted time, efforts, resources, and money, the National Cancer Institute decided to revisit the idea of honoring their original commitment to Dr. Burzynski. This was the same commitment that had been pushed aside a number of years earlier while various people (such as the National Cancer Institute) had become caught up in the misplaced gold-fever frenzy that surrounded their research into phenylacetate.

However, there was a catch to the proposal. The National Cancer Institute wanted to alter the cancer treatment protocols that Dr. Burzynski had dedicated several decades of research and clinical practice in order to work out effective procedures.

Dr. Burzynski rejected the National Cancer Institute's offer. He indicated that unless protocols in which he had confidence were used in the proposed trials, then, he was not prepared to supply the National Cancer Institute with Antineoplastons.

Dr. Michael Friedman, who as Director of the Division of Cancer Treatment at the National Cancer Institute had indicated in 1991 that Antineoplastons deserved further study, was now expressing surprise and confusion in relation to Dr. Burzynski's insistence on the use of specific, established protocols for the proposed clinical trials involving Antineoplastons. In an October 1993 letter to Dr. Burzynski, Dr. Friedman stipulated that while the Institute would seek to have the designated researcher involved in the clinical trial act in compliance with Dr. Burzynski's concerns, nevertheless, if Dr. Burzynski did not provide the necessary Antineoplastons for the proposed study, then, the National Cancer Institute would use alternative means to secure the Antineoplastons (or active components) it needed to run the proposed clinical trials and, then, proceed on with things on its own.

Dr. Burzynski replied to the foregoing letter by indicating that he was appreciative of the National Cancer Institute's willingness to comply with the protocols that already had been established as effective agents in the treatment of cancer. Nonetheless, Dr. Burzynski expressed surprise that Dr. Friedman was apparently prepared to engage in patent infringement if Dr. Burzynski did not supply the Institute with the necessary Antineoplastons within a short period of time.

Eventually, the differences were ironed out. The two sides came to an agreement on the protocol that would be used in the clinical study.

| Explorations |

However, more than a year passed and according to Dr. Mario Sznol – Head, Biologics Evaluation Section, Investigational Drug Branch, Cancer Evaluation Program, Division of Cancer Treatment, National Cancer Institute -- the clinical trial was apparently experiencing difficulty in acquiring a sufficient number of patients to participate in the study. Oddly enough, in the interim period more than 15,000 individuals across the United States had been diagnosed with precisely the same form of cancer that was the focus of the clinical trial being run.

The Institute seemed to use the 'insufficient number of participants' issue as justification for permitting Memorial Sloan-Kettering Cancer Center to change the protocols that had been agreed upon in relation to the proposed clinical trials. Unfortunately, The Institute did not feel obligated to inform Dr. Burzynski about those changes.

When Dr. Burzynski learned about what was going on, he sent a letter to Dr. Michael Friedman on March 29, 1995 that outlined his objections as well as insisting that the original agreed-upon protocols be used. Among other concerns, Dr. Burzynski indicated that if the protocols were changed, then, different Antineoplastons with different dosages needed to be used.

Dr. Sznol wrote back that the decision concerning the change in protocol had already been approved. The change had been made because the original protocol was considered to have been "overly stringent" and created unnecessary eligibility criteria.

On April 20, 1995, Dr. Burzynski replied by saying that based on his more than two decades of working with Antineoplastons, changing the protocols in relation to the proposed clinical trials was likely to lead to ineffective outcomes. In other words, if the protocols were changed, then the form of treatment also had to be altered, and, yet, the researchers were apparently planning on doing the former without changing the nature of the associated treatment. In fact, Dr. Burzynski indicated that the dosage of Antineoplastons needed to be three times as great as the researchers were supposedly planning to provide in conjunction with the changed protocols.

On the one hand, Dr. Friedman claimed that he wanted to test the hypothesis concerning Antineoplastons. Yet, on the other hand, in

| Explorations |

effect, he – or the Institute for which he worked – wanted to arbitrarily alter the character of the hypothesis being tested.

The original hypothesis to be tested was akin to the following: Given protocol 'A', treatment 'B' will show effective results with respect to the sorts of cancer that are treated in conjunction by means of the stated protocol. Apparently, Dr. Friedman believed that one could restate the hypothesis as: Given protocol Z, treatment 'B' will still show effective results ... despite the fact that Dr. Burzynski had indicated there is a causal connection between, on the one hand, the type of treatment dosage and Antineoplastons that are used in any given case and, on the other hand, the degree of success one is likely to witness when treating cancers that fall within different kinds of protocols.

On May 8, 1995, Joan Mauer issued an internal memorandum at the National Cancer Institute with respect to the Phase-II clinical trials involving Antineoplastons. The memorandum informed the recipients of the communiqué that the Clinical Trials Monitoring Service and been instructed not to share any Antineoplastons trial data with either Dr. Burzynski or anyone who might inquire about such data. Moreover, in the event that anyone did inquire about the data, the individual was to be directed to Dr. Michael Friedman of the National Cancer Institute.

On June 6, 1995, Dr. Friedman wrote to Dr. Burzynski and indicated that the National Cancer Institute was under no obligation to seek any kind of permission or consent with respect to the nature of the protocols that were to be used in the Phase-II clinical trials involving Antineoplastons. Dr. Friedman further stated that Dr. Burzynski's attitude toward how those trials should be conducted were both "presumptuous and inappropriate."

According to Dr. Friedman, final authority concerning the conduct of the clinical trials belonged to the National Cancer Institute. The Institute had a responsibility to act in the best interests of the American people.

On June 22, 1995, Dr. Burzynski responded by pointing out that the National Cancer Institute was not fulfilling its responsibilities because its actions were placing people's lives at risk on the basis of arbitrary and frivolous grounds. Furthermore, the National Cancer

| Explorations |

Institute had reneged on some of its promises ... including that of providing Dr. Burzynski with relevant data from the clinical trials.

Over the next six months, or so, Dr. Burzynski set about trying to force the National Institute of Cancer to release the medical records of the patients involved in the clinical trials. When that information finally did become available, it was clear that the National Institute of Cancer had completely disregarded the agreed-upon protocol.

The failure to abide by the original protocol had a variety of effects. For instance, a number of patients were required to discontinue treatments because of fluid retention.

Dr. Burzynski was curious about the fluid retention aspect of things because his experience had indicated that the use of Antineoplastons tends to lead to dehydration, not excessive fluid retention. He subsequently discovered that the intravenous fluids being given to the patients didn't contain Antineoplastons.

In October 1995, the Cancer Information Service of the National Cancer Institute and National Institute of Health issued a statement about the Antineoplastons clinical trials. The statement stipulated that: "because these studies were closed prior to completion, no conclusions can be made about the effectiveness or toxicity of Antineoplastons."

However, in February 1999 -- four years after the foregoing National Cancer Institute sponsored trials drew to a close and two years following the complete exoneration of Dr. Burzynski with respect to all criminal charges that had been finagled by the FDA – an article appeared in the *Mayo Clinic Proceedings* bearing the names of a number of researchers who proceeded to claim that the original National Cancer Institute Phase-II clinical trials involving Antineoplastons had shown that none of the patients in the trial "demonstrated tumor regression."

Not only did the foregoing article fail to reflect the actual status of the original study – namely, that the trials had been discontinued prior to completion -- but, as well, the article appearing in the *Mayo Clinic Proceedings* failed to point out that the protocol used in the National Cancer Institute sponsored clinical trials involving Antineoplastons had been changed over the objections of the individual (Dr. Burzynski)

| Explorations |

who was most knowledgeable and experienced concerning the relationship between protocol and an effective choice of treatment.

The people who wrote the February 1999 article were, in a sense, re-writing history. In the process, those individuals were – perhaps unintentionally -- both distorting history and, as well, potentially misleading anyone who might read their article.

Furthermore, the *Mayo Clinic Proceedings* is a peer-reviewed publication. Nevertheless, to whomever the staff of the *Mayo Clinic Proceedings* decided to entrust the responsibility for reviewing the article in question prior to its being accepted for publication, that person or persons – for whatever reasons – did an extremely poor job.

Upon critically examining the Antineoplastons-related article that had appeared in the February 1999 edition of the *Mayo Clinic Proceeding*, Dr. Burzynski and some of his associates discovered that the people who were running the original National Cancer Institute sponsored Phase-II clinical trials had been drastically diluting the amount of Antineoplastons that were being administered to the participants of the study. Not only had the so-called researchers changed the protocol, but, they also had changed the dosage of Antineoplastons being administered ... diluting them, when, according to Dr. Burzynski, that amount should have been increased significantly.

The change in dosage also helped to explain another anomaly that showed up in the Phase-II clinical trials. As noted earlier, a number of patients had been forced to discontinue treatment because of severe fluid retention, and such fluid retention tended to make sense in the light of the extremely diluted dosages of Antineoplastons the participants had been receiving during treatment since Antineoplastons were associated with dehydration, not fluid retention.

By arbitrarily altering the protocol for the clinical trials and by arbitrarily altering the dosage of Antineoplastons being administered, a very definite result came about. The participants in the Phase-II clinical trials all died.

Dr. Burzynski's research and clinical practice had shown again and again that if one administered an appropriate dosage of Antineoplastons for a given protocol involving a certain cancerous

| Explorations |

condition, then one often saw effective results. By altering the protocol and the dosage, the researchers involved in the National Cancer Institute sponsored Phase-II clinical trials of Antineoplastons guaranteed that the participants in that study would not receive effective treatments, and, as a result, people died from forms of cancer that might otherwise have been helped if the appropriate protocol and dosage had been observed.

According to the aforementioned Li-Chuan Chen who had been employed at the National Cancer Institute from 1991 until 1997, whenever the National Cancer Institute became involved in the clinical testing of alternative, therapeutic approaches to cancer treatment – such as Antineoplastons – the decision was always made to change the protocol and, as a result, bring about the failure of, or negative results in relation to, such alternative cancer therapies. Dr. Chen feels that the purpose of such practices was to undermine the credibility of those kinds of treatments.

Dr. Chen goes on to note that he feels many scientists might not be sufficiently rigorous in their examination of the foregoing practices to detect what was actually was taking place at the National Cancer Institute with respect to its examination of alternative treatments for cancer. Dr. Chen's assessment of the situation seems quite apropos given that the authors of the aforementioned February 1999 article in the *Mayo Clinic Proceedings* did not do due diligence with respect to what actually had happened in the original Phase-II clinical trials on Antineoplastons that had been sponsored by the National Cancer Institute. In addition, apparently, the reviewers who were assigned the task -- by the staff of the *Mayo Clinic Proceedings* -- to critically review the quality of the foregoing article did not do his, her, or their due diligence in that respect either.

Everything, on the surface, can appear quite scientific – so-called scientists appearing to do science, and alleged scientists writing about something called science, and presumptive scientists evaluating activities said to be related to science. Yet, underneath it all, an epistemological cancer of enormous proportions is being permitted to flourish right before the eyes of an array of supposed scientists, scientific journals, and scientific institutions.

| Explorations |

In the summer of 1995, one of the individuals who had played a prominent role in helping to derail the Phase-II clinical trials involving Antineoplastons – namely, Dr. Michael Friedman – left the National Cancer Institute and became the Deputy Commissioner of Operations for the FDA. His new boss was Dr. David A. Kessler ... the individual who had been attempting to imprison Dr. Burzynski for quite a few years.

A few months following Dr. Friedman's appointment, the FDA was finally able -- after more than a decade of efforts -- to help bring about a indictment involving criminal charges of Dr. Burzynski ... the same charges for which Dr. Burzynski was later completely exonerated. Once again, Dr. Friedman was associated with an organization that was supposed to serve the American people but was doing its "best" to undermine the opportunity of Americans to have ready access to a form of cancer treatment – in other words, Antineoplastons – that had exhibited considerable success and promise when engaged rationally rather than through self-serving ulterior motives.

One month after the criminal trial of Dr. Burzynski began in 1997, the first of the aforementioned patent applications – which had been filed by Dr. Samid, in conjunction with the Department of Health and Human Services, back in 1991 -- was approved. Shortly following the acquittal of Dr. Burzynski, two more of the phenylacetate-related patent applications filed by Dr. Samid and the Department of Health and Human Resources were approved, while the remaining nine phenylacetate-related patent applications were approved over the next three years.

There are a few questions that might be raised concerning the ethical character of the manner in which Dr. Samid obtained her initial 'ideas', knowledge, and understanding concerning phenylacetate-related compounds. Nonetheless, whatever her method of 'invention' might have been, neither she, nor Élan Pharmaceuticals, nor the National Cancer Institute, nor the Department of Health and Human Services, nor the FDA seemed to understand – or, perhaps, they didn't care -- how they were all engaged in a journey down a cul-de-sac as far as effective cancer treatments were concerned.

Moreover, there was considerable hypocrisy (if not criminal collusion) surrounding the whole affair. On the one hand, various

| Explorations |

government agencies were busily engaged in trying to discredit and prosecute Dr. Burzynski for his research on, and highly promising results with, a variety of Antineoplastons, while, on the other hand, those same government agencies (along with several pharmaceutical companies) were doing whatever they could to assist Dr. Samid to file patent applications involving several compounds (in other words, phenylacetate and phenylacetylglutamine, along with their analogs) that had been 'acquired' under questionable circumstances and, even more importantly, already had been proven to have limited effectiveness with respect to the treatment of cancer.

Once Dr. Burzynski had been cleared in relation to all charges of criminal wrongdoing, the attempts to discredit him did not come to an end. Whether out of maliciousness, ignorance, envy, fear, and/or having bought into some propaganda campaign or another, individual doctors, as well as various medical organizations – such as the American Cancer Society and the American Medical Association -- continued to attack Dr. Burzynski's credibility in relation to his research and clinical practice involving Antineoplastons.

However, by 2009, enough proof had accumulated with respect to the effectiveness and safety of Antineoplastons in conjunction with a variety of Phase-2 trials (which had been done independently of the National Cancer Institute) that Antineoplastons were permitted to enter into Phase-III clinical testing. In reaching this stage of the testing process, Dr. Burzynski became, thus far, the only scientist in U.S. history to gain access to the federally operated drug approval system in relation to a proprietary form of cancer treatment despite the complete absence of support from pharmaceutical companies (other than his own), the established cancer industry, or the federal government.

Should Antineoplastons survive this round of testing and continue to demonstrate their effectiveness and safety in relation to an array of cancer treatments, then, they – presumably -- would get the FDA seal of approval. Unfortunately, Phase-III testing is expensive ... the estimated cost is in the vicinity of approximately $300 million dollars.

In addition, there is also a troublesome rider attached to the Phase-III trials that extends beyond the foregoing price tag. More specifically, the FDA insists that it would be unethical not to treat children suffering from an inoperable brainstem glioma with radiation quite independently of whatever Antineoplastons might be administered ... despite the fact that radiation treatment is largely, if not completely, devoid of success with respect to the treatment of such tumors ... and despite the fact that radiation treatment has proven to be highly toxic and destructive in the collateral damage it tends to impart to the individuals being treated with it ... and despite the fact that Antineoplastons have been shown to be the only treatment to register some degree of success in treating such malignancies (between 30 and 50%) ... and despite the fact that Antineoplastons have been demonstrated to be completely non-toxic and safe.

One wonders what the criteria were that were being used by the FDA to determine the quality of ethicalness with respect to the use of radiation treatment in children who have been diagnosed with brainstem glioma. If radiation treatment has been shown to be ineffective with respect to that kind of cancer and if radiation treatment has been shown to be toxic and unsafe in such cases, then just what is the basis for claiming that to refrain from the use of radiation in relation to brainstem glioma would be unethical?

The foregoing issue of ethicality becomes even more baffling when one understands that as of 2013, just two drugs – namely, Temodar (temozolomide) in 1999 and Avastin (bevacizumab) in 2009 -- have been given FDA-approval to be used in the treatment of malignant brain tumor. Although neither of the aforementioned drugs was able to demonstrate sufficient qualities of safety or effectiveness to be given final approval in conjunction with the treatment of brainstem glioma (Avastin did, however, receive preliminary approval to be used in the treatment of brainstem glioma as a result of fast track legislation that had been passed in the 1990s).

What is puzzling is that, unlike Antineoplastons, the foregoing drugs have not been shown to be all that effective with respect to the treatment of brain tumors. Even more puzzling is the fact that those drugs were given initial, preliminary approval without having to undergo any of the randomized Phase-III trials that were required of Antineoplastons

Temodar and Avastin were required to undergo such randomized Phase-III trials only after they already had been made available to the public. As was indicated in the previous paragraph, when those drugs were finally put to the test in relation to the more rigorous requirements of randomized Phase-III clinical trials, they failed to demonstrate sufficient effectiveness and freedom from toxic side effects to be given final market approval with respect to the treatment of brainstem glioma.

Yet, between 1995 and 2008, Antineoplastons had gone through a series of FDA-approved Phase-II clinical trials with respect to cases involving brainstem glioma. Of the 169 patients who participated in those trials, 33 of them were either cancer free or had lived for a five-year period after being diagnosed with that form of cancer.

The foregoing degree of success was something that none of the, then, available 'standard of care' treatments – including Temodar or Avastin -- had been able to remotely approach. Nonetheless, Temodar and Avastin were given fast track approval to be used in the treatment of brain tumors and to avoid – at least initially – having to be subjected to Phase-III trials, whereas Antineoplastons – which unlike the other two drugs had shown considerable success and promise in Phase-II trials (and, as well, had proven to be non-toxic) – were denied fast-track status and had to immediately proceed to Phase-III trials.

If, according to the FDA, it would be unethical not to require patients suffering from brainstem glioma to receive radiation treatments in addition to Antineoplastons, then why wouldn't it also be unethical not to require Temodar or Avastin to also have to be used in conjunction with radiation therapy – especially in light of the fact that neither of the latter two drugs have demonstrated anywhere near the level of safety or efficacy that Antineoplastons have shown in Phase-I and Phase-II clinical trials. The foregoing issue is, of course, quite independent of the question of why anyone who suffered from brainstem glioma would be required to be subjected to a form of treatment – namely, radiation – that had proven to be neither effective nor safe when used in conjunction with patients suffering from brainstem glioma.

In either event, there was, and continues to be, a significant bias at the FDA concerning Antineoplastons. Drugs -- such as Temodar and Avastin, which had shown little evidence of effectiveness or non-toxicity -- were pushed right through the approval process and, at least temporarily, were made available for public consumption, whereas Antineoplastons, that had shown themselves to be both effective, to some extent, and non-toxic, were held back from availability to the general public.

Despite the fact that across three decades of research and treatment the use of Antineoplastons has demonstrated considerable success and promise and despite the fact that even when unsuccessful, these compounds have been shown to do no harm to the patients to whom they are administered, nevertheless, by 2013, only a small fraction (10%) of the individuals seeking treatment involving Antineoplastons are permitted to receive treatment as a result of the federal governments regulatory oversight of the situation ... a form of control that in the case of Antineoplastons has been shown to be rooted in little more than ignorance, fear, self-serving agendas, jealousy, arbitrary use of power, and greed.

The federal government insists on subjecting those individuals who are seeking Antineoplastons cancer treatments to undergo a process of intensive scrutiny concerning their medical history and condition. Furthermore, unless those prospective candidates can provide evidence that they already have undergone one, or more, rounds of traditional forms of chemotherapy and radiation treatment, those individuals, generally speaking (there have been some exceptions), are excluded from participating in any form of treatments based on Antineoplastons.

The foregoing sorts of restrictions might appear to be important safeguards with the best interests of the patient in mind. After all, if chemotherapy and radiation were well-established as being the treatments of choice or the standard of care because they were generally successful and non-toxic, and if Antineoplastons lacked a track record with respect to being able to treat various forms of cancer successfully and/or do so in a safe and non-toxic manner, then, it might make sense for the federal government to insist that prospective candidates for treatments with Antineoplastons should exhaust the options that already have been approved by the federal government, the cancer industry, and the medical establishment before moving on to experimental forms of therapy.

However, none of the foregoing hypothetical assumptions are true, and this is especially the case in the matter of the brain tumors on which the Phase-II clinical trials involving Antineoplastons focused. To begin with, chemotherapy and radiation treatments generally lead to very poor outcomes when used with patients suffering from different forms of brain cancer – not only because those treatments don't seem to be very effective, but, as well, because they often inflict a great deal of collateral damage to the individual undergoing them.

Furthermore, Antineoplastons are not exactly a Johnny-come-lately in the treatment of cancer. For more than 30 years, Antineoplastons have been demonstrated, among other things, to be able to treat -- with varying degrees of success -- forms of cancer that are beyond the capabilities of traditional medical treatments (such as chemotherapy and radiation) ... and to be able to accomplish this without exposing patients to toxic side-effects, and, yet, for those same 30 years, the federal government, the cancer industry, and the medical establishment in America have sought to place one obstacle after another in the way of the U.S. public gaining access to treatment with Antineoplastons.

A drug that is approved for Phase-III clinical testing must be used in trials run by facilities, hospitals, and the like that are completely independent of the individuals who are manufacturing that drug. When the FDA gave Dr. Burzynski the go ahead for his Antineoplastons to be able to participate in Phase-III trials, he contacted every major hospital in America, Canada, and England to see if any of them would be willing to run trials focusing on brainstem glioma, and, without exception, they all turned him down.

The Texas State Board of Medical Examiners, the National Cancer Institute, the FDA, the AMA, the American Cancer Society, along with an array of so-called scientists, researchers, media personnel (including some of those involved with professional journals), and pharmaceutical companies have all done an effective job in helping to discredit Dr. Burzynski and Antineoplastons. Their collective resistance to Antineoplastons was not necessarily rooted in science or reasonable concerns but all too frequently was due to the human conditions of: ignorance, fear, self-centeredness, greed, jealousy, and the willingness to let other people control the way those individuals think about such issues ... the very antithesis of the process of science.

Collectively, they had created a hostile environment concerning Dr. Burzynski and Antineoplastons. Even when the hospitals and medical centers contacted by Dr. Burzynski were not unduly influenced by that atmosphere of hostility and antagonism that had been manufactured in conjunction with Antineoplastons, those hospitals and medical clinics often expressed skepticism concerning the likelihood that parents would be prepared to let their children be subjected to the Phase-III conditions mandated by the FDA – namely, that all patients would have to undergo radiation treatments ... treatments that often resulted in considerable disabilities being imparted to the brains and bodies of the patients undergoing that kind of treatment.

Many people who express skepticism concerning the effectiveness of Antineoplastons claim that this class of drugs has never undergone systematic, rigorous, randomized clinical trials and, in the process, demonstrated their effectiveness and safety. Such people claim that all of the reports of success involving Antineoplastons are purely anecdotal and not scientific.

Aside from the fact that organizations such as the National Cancer Institute and the FDA have done their level best to try to ensure that Antineoplastons are never properly tested in the aforementioned scientific sense or have tried to ensure that when Antineoplastons are tested scientifically that they were set up to fail (such as requiring all of their patients be subjected to ineffective, but highly dangerous, forms of radiation treatments), it is entirely inaccurate to claim that the alleged anecdotal nature of clinical experience does not contribute significantly to the develop of scientific understanding.

If over time, one matches certain medical protocols with various levels of drug dosage that prove to be effective and safe in case after case, then, although, on the one hand, such knowledge might not be a function of randomized tests, nevertheless, that knowledge is not merely arbitrary, useless information either but, instead, is tied to hypothetical conditionals which demonstrate that when certain circumstances or treatment protocols are established and when specific things are done in relation to those circumstances, then some very interesting and beneficial events tend to follow.

If one proceeds in the foregoing manner just once, one would be justified in referring to the results as anecdotal. However, if one pursues the foregoing sort of methodology again and again with different people and, yet, one observes similar positive results across those patients, then, the results are no longer anecdotal, but highly promising and suggestive ... in fact, the information generated by such clinical work is the sort of outcome one looks for when considering what kind of randomized clinical trial to pursue.

Dr. Hideaki Tsuda, a professor at Kurume University in Japan, was interested in, and intrigued by, the clinical results that Dr. Burzynski had obtained. Nonetheless, at the same time, Dr. Tsuda believes that "science must be born in doubt", and, therefore, he had questions

| Explorations |

concerning Antineoplastons ... questions that could be expressed and tested through the methodology of science.

Dr. Tsuda first wanted to determine how safe or non-toxic Antineoplastons are. In other words, as in other Phase-I studies, he wanted to establish what levels of dosage were capable of being safely tolerated by patients.

Using both an oral and an injection formula of several Antineoplastons (A-1- and AS2-1), he worked with 43 patients. He established safe dosage levels with respect to those patients and, in addition, he found that approximately 50% of the patients were responding, to some degree, to the foregoing combination of Antineoplastons.

After publishing the results of their Phase-I toxicological study on cancer patients treated with Antineoplastons, Dr. Tsuda and his colleagues transitioned to Phase-II clinical studies – that is, research that was directed toward determining whether, or not, Antineoplastons actually worked. Since the patients in the Phase-I studies who seemed to respond best to Antineoplastons were individuals with cancer of the liver, the research group decided to focus its efforts in the Phase-II trials on that form of cancer.

The Phase-II study conducted in 1999 showed promising results. Use of Antineoplastons seemed to help bring about both a disease-free interval as well as an enhanced likelihood of long-term survival.

Given that Antineoplastons had been demonstrated to be somewhat efficacious in Phase-II testing, the decision was made to enter into Phase-III research. This research was conducted in the form of randomized studies involving individuals with colon cancer that had metastasized into both the lungs and liver.

The study involved 65 patients who were randomly divided into an experimental and control group. The 32 individuals in the experimental group were treated with chemotherapy and Antineoplastons, while the 33 patients in the control group were treated with chemotherapy only.

Approximately 50% of the people in the control group (those treated with just chemotherapy) lived for about 36 months. Around 50% of the individuals in the experimental group – that is, they were

| Explorations |

treated with Antineoplastons as well as chemotherapy – lived nearly twice as long (around 70 months).

Obviously, the presence of Antineoplastons seemed to make a constructive difference. Just as obviously, not everyone treated with Antineoplastons benefitted equally well since some people lived for a shorter period of time than others did even though they both were being treated with Antineoplastons.

One would have to do further statistical analysis to acquire a deeper understanding of the extent – if any -- to which there were significant differences between the control group and experimental group when it came to the 50% of the respective groups that lived for less than 36 months in the case of the control group or lived for less than 70 months in the case of the experimental group. Conceivably, there might have been a consistent trend of life extension that was present among the members of the experimental group relative to the length of life exhibited by individuals in the control group even among the 50% of the patients in the two groups who did not fare as well as on their respective forms of treatment as others did.

There also are all manner of questions that could be raised with respect to the foregoing Phase-III study. For example, what might have occurred if the control group had been treated with some standard of care form of chemotherapy, whereas the experimental group was treated with just Antineoplastons (sans chemotherapy)? Alternatively, what might have taken place if the study had been done with patients who had not already undergone metastasis? Or, what might have transpired if the patients had been given higher dosages of Antineoplastons?

Despite the fact that Dr. Tsuda's research group has proven, via scientific methods, that Antineoplastons appear to have the potential to be effective and safe ways of treating at least certain kinds of cancer, nevertheless, things might have been taken as far as they can with respect to how the world operates in such matters. For example, in December of 2012, Dr. Tsuda indicated that due to the power that the FDA wields in markets around the world, Japanese pharmaceutical companies were not likely to unilaterally make Antineoplastons commercially available to the Japanese public since if this step were taken, those same companies might, very likely, face retaliatory

| Explorations |

measures, of one kind or another, from the FDA with respect the acceptance of Japanese pharmaceutical products into not only the US market, but in other markets around the world as well.

While acknowledging the very real nature of the power struggle in which the Japanese pharmaceutical companies might be entangled vis-à-vis the FDA, the fact of the matter is there are still things that could be done. For instance, what is to stop Dr. Tsuda, or other researchers, from following up on the earlier Phase-III studies and broadening the research to include other kinds of protocols and dosage levels involving different categories and populations of cancer patients?

At the present time, the commercial possibilities might be quite limited. However, the scientific possibilities are virtually unlimited, and they need to be pursued until – hopefully – the epistemological culture (or lack thereof) in the FDA and other medical institutions changes with respect to – among other things -- Antineoplastons.

| Explorations |

On January 7, 2013, representatives from the FDA arrived, unannounced, at the facilities of the Burzynski Clinic. Soon, thereafter, the FDA ordered that all patient information that was, in some way, connected to the use of Antineoplastons had to be removed from the Burzynski clinic website.

The people from the FDA 'made themselves welcome' at the Burzynski Clinic for nearly a month and a half. During that period of time, they questioned many of the staff members who worked at the Clinic, as well as went through Clinic documents that went back some 25 years.

In addition to ordering that the Clinic's website must eliminate certain kinds of information involving Antineoplastons, the FDA made a further stipulation. More specifically, until further notice, no new cancer patients could be treated with Antineoplastons anywhere in America despite the fact that neither the FDA nor anyone else has been able to demonstrate that Antineoplastons are neither safe nor effective.

The FDA, along with an amalgamation of institutes, agencies (both governmental and private), universities, hospitals, journals, associations, charities, medical doctors, professors, lawyers, legislators, judges, and pharmaceutical companies are not necessarily engaged in service to either the American people, or to the people of the world. Instead, they are all too ready to be in the service of greed and power.

The foregoing amalgamation apparently doesn't care what the truth is. Despite their protestations to the contrary, they do not seem to be interested in making medical breakthroughs that will save lives.

It just wants to keep the financial spigots open. If people have to die or suffer in order for this to continue on, then, apparently, so be it.

| Explorations |

At the present time, no one really knows what causes oncogenes to turn on or what causes tumor-suppressing genes to turn off. There are a variety of carcinogenic agents that might play a role in either of those two possibilities ... or, maybe, agents are carcinogenic because they adversely affect the proper functioning of a system of Antineoplastons that is responsible for controlling the on/off switches for oncogenes and tumor-suppressing genes.

No one – not even Dr. Burzynski – seems to know why Antineoplastons are naturally abundant in healthy individuals, or why Antineoplastons are relatively absent in individuals who suffer from cancer. One might hypothesize that because Antineoplastons seem to have the capacity to either turn various oncogenes back off or to turn different tumor-suppressing genes back on, then, perhaps, in those individuals suffering from cancer, there is some unknown process that undermines the capacity of those people's bodies to properly manufacture and/or regulate the activity of Antineoplastons.

If so, then, cancer might not be a function of irregularities in oncogenes and/or tumor suppressing genes per se. Instead, cancer might be a symptom of an underlying problem with the generation and regulation of Antineoplastons.

At this time, no one in the world of science knows how oncogenes and tumor-suppressing genes came into existence. At this time, no one in the world of science knows how the regulatory and functional properties of Antineoplastons came into existence. At this time, no one knows what goes wrong to bring all of these interlocking parts into dysfunctional alignment.

One can add to the foregoing list of unknowns the fact that, at this time, no one knows why Antineoplastons seem to help some people but not others. Moreover, no one knows whether being treated with Antineoplastons helps, in some direct manner, to restore normal manufacturing and regulatory activities of those peptides and, therefore, permits a person to remain cancer free once treatment stops, or, whether being treated with Antineoplastons helps people suffering from cancer in an indirect manner and, thereby, assists such individuals to be able to bridge or survive the period when the normal process of manufacturing and regulating is dysfunctional and that once the problem of cancerous growth disappears, then, the normal activity of Antineoplastons comes back on line.

There are many unknowns surrounding Antineoplastons. However, there are two things that are known about the set of peptides to which the term "Antineoplastons" has been given.

First, Antineoplastons are non-toxic. Therefore, quite independently of whether, or not, Antineoplastons help cure cancer, they comply with the most fundamental law of medicine – namely, to do no harm.

Second, Antineoplastons have been shown – both clinically and in randomized trials – to help treat cancer. In fact, they have been shown to achieve a level of care with respect to some forms of cancer (e.g., brainstem glioma) that the currently accepted 'standard of care' modes of cancer treatment cannot successfully treat.

So, what does the Burzynski affair tell us about the nature of the reality problem with which this book is ultimately concerned? What does it have to tell us about the issue of 'Final Jeopardy'? I believe the answer to both of the foregoing questions is: 'quite a lot'.

To begin with, it seems there are two kinds of groups of individuals that are, in some way, connected to the process of science. There are those people who seek the truth concerning a given matter, and there are those individuals who are not interested in the truth but who, instead, do whatever they do for the purpose of serving their own interests rather than the interests of truth.

As the research team put together by Dr. Hideaki Tsuda at Kurume University in Japan demonstrated in the late 1990s, it is relatively easy to scientifically test whether, or not, Antineoplastons work. This task of proof is made even easier by the fact that Antineoplastons have proven to be non-toxic and safe to use.

The Texas State Board of Medical Examiners, the FDA, the National Cancer Institute, along with a bevy of allegedly scientific/medical: organizations, associations, clinics, institutes, researchers, foundations, university departments, consultants, scientists, medical doctors, government agencies, journals, and pharmaceutical companies were not interested in finding out whatever truths might be hidden in the world of Antineoplastons. Instead, they all were pursuing their own self-serving agendas, and as a result, they either actively, or passively, placed obstacles in the way of establishing the truth concerning Antineoplastons.

Those individuals and groups might have all kinds of degrees in science and/or medicine, and they might have acquired numerous credentials or have received any number of professional honors, and they might run about in neat, white lab coats or work with all manner of spiffy technological equipment or have had articles published in this or that prestigious journal, or have been awarded grants from various notable charities and foundations, but none of them is a scientist in the only way that matters: being dedicated to uncovering the truth about the nature of reality.

Instead, they chose to occupy themselves with attempts to: ostracize, persecute, discredit, penalize, obstruct, undermine, demean, control, lie about, and prosecute a person whose primary goal was to help people with cancer get healthy again. If those individuals and groups believed that Dr. Burzynski was wrong about the efficacy and safety of Antineoplastons, then they easily could have dispensed with all the stupidity to which their actions gave collective expression, and just gone about testing the issue scientifically ... and the very fact that they all shied away from engaging events in a scientific manner with respect to the matter of Antineoplastons demonstrates the extent to which none of them deserves to be called a scientist or a medical doctor – their likely protestations notwithstanding.

They are disciples of Svengali and Machiavelli. They are part of a system of mind control whose function is to obfuscate, bury, distort, and undermine any effort to uncover the truth of things, and they do this for the sake of financial gain and political power.

They are counterfeiters. They are engaged in a massive process of epistemological fraud that seeks to pass off various worthless, ineffective, toxic denominations of information as if the latter were backed by a real knowledge that is rooted in truth.

They are the most egregious of thieves. They seek to steal the truth.

What those credentialed individuals do is not bent science or junk science. No matter what the nature of the technical language might be that is used to describe what is going on with them, such activity is not science of any kind.

It is a form of systematic abuse. It involves a process that is no different than the sort of dynamic that takes place in: domestic, physical, sexual, or spiritual abuse in which some people are forced to suffer so that the desires of the perpetrator of the abuse might be satisfied.

Unfortunately, there are all too many people in the world who refer to themselves as scientists but who would present their 'Final Jeopardy' response in a form that like the picture of Dorian Gray gives expression to only the monstrous and grotesque representation of the kind of truths to which no one in his or her right mind and heart would want to claim ownership. They have sold their souls for a few trinkets, some cheap thrills, and the illusion of being someone that matters in the universe.

Of course, people are free to choose the foregoing sort of 'Final Jeopardy' response. And, in doing so, they will give expression to a certain dimension of the nature of reality since human beings certainly do have the capacity to act in the most: Abysmal, mean, callous, hateful, biased, hurtful, blind, ignorant, abusive, selfish, and sickening of ways. History has shown the foregoing sorts of behavior to encompass a most unsettling set of truths that has manifested itself rather relentlessly since human beings first appeared on the face of the Earth.

If a person is honest with herself or himself, an individual can sometimes catch glimpses within one's being involving a potential to be drawn to, if not inclined toward, such an unseemly existential landscape. It is like there is some hidden maelstrom within which possesses currents of varying degrees of intensity and subtlety that swirl all about one and seek to pull one down into the black heart of its deadly, turbulent embrace.

The individuals that sought to oppose the research on Antineoplastons and, in the process, deny the possibility of either life-saving treatment or put an end to the suffering to a variety of cancer patients could be any one of us. All one has to do is make the wrong combination of choices that little by little -- or, perhaps, all at once --

induce one to become indifferent to the truth and/or what happens to one's fellow human beings.

I recognize the potential for ugliness that exists in human beings. Part of that ugliness comes from the willingness to seek to hide or deny or distort or oppose the idea that such a potential exists in each of us.

I also recognize the capacity for beauty that exists in human beings. Part of that beauty comes from a willingness to seek to uncover the nature of truth irrespective of where such an endeavor might lead with respect to how one understands the nature of reality.

It is the truth that needs to be sought or adhered to. It is falsehood that needs to be avoided or discarded.

Science is the process of striving to distinguish between the two foregoing possibilities. Science is not necessarily about generating a worldview or providing a theory of how reality might function but, rather, is an on-going attempt to push back the horizons of ignorance by differentiating between what is true and what is not.

Accounts that purport to constitute the best scientific understanding of a given phenomenon are only scientific to the extent that they can be shown to be true. If one cannot do this, then the account is not scientific but an expression of hermeneutics – that is, it is a theory of understanding concerning the proposed epistemological status of a given body of information, and, as such, it is not necessarily actually true but is merely believed to be true.

Consequently, at the heart of my Final Jeopardy response is the issue of truth. Irrespective of whether, or not, I have attained the truth in any given set of circumstances, my response must demonstrate a commitment to uncovering the truth and jettisoning whatever is false

This means that I must try to do everything I can to distance myself from the tactics, methods, behaviors, practices, and processes of thinking that might lead me into the type of epistemological quagmire that resulted from the sort of engagement exhibited by all too many people who sought to undermine and oppose the search for truth in relation to the issue of Antineoplastons. The individuals who opposed Dr. Burzynski for more than three decades – despite possessing a complete absence of any actual scientific facts that would warrant or justify such opposition – constitute the sort of negative exemplars that tell one a great deal about what not to do if one is interested in finding the truth about something.

One of the most disturbing facets of the Burzynski affair is the manner in which it indicated just how epistemologically corrupt – and corruptible -- so much of the so-called scientific and medical community is. One must be very, very careful as one travels through that landscape.

To be sure, there are individuals – such as Dr. Burzynski (and his colleagues) or Dr. Tsuda (and his colleagues) – who have demonstrated (and, hopefully, will continue to demonstrate) that the quest for doing real science (that is, the desire to differentiate between truth and falsehood) is still very much alive in the world. Unfortunately, there are other individuals who – though they come in the guise of scientists and technical experts – cannot be trusted.

Learning who can be trusted is as important as discovering what can be trusted. Character (for example, as manifested through qualities of objectivity, honesty, fairness, resistance to corrupting influences, and so on), or the lack thereof, plays an important role in the search for truth.

If truth is uncovered concerning the lack of character of someone who claims to be a scientists or researcher, then, one should understand that the likelihood of any form of truth – other than that of being a negative example with respect to the issue of character – ever being manifested through such an individual is very limited. When an individual displays a lack of character in the way he or she conducts himself or herself with respect to the quest for truth, then, such people tend to prove to be an obstacle to discovering any kind of truth other than that concerned with the individuals own lack of character.

| Explorations |

The SSRI Issue

My mother had quite a few physical problems, ranging from: severe rheumatoid arthritis, to: some form of Addison's disease, food allergies, and a few other physical ailments thrown in for good measure. The doctors prescribed quite a few medications in their attempt to treat different symptoms of her various maladies.

At some point, she began to worry about what was going on and, as a result, she purchased a fairly comprehensive reference guide to pharmaceuticals. Whenever a doctor prescribed a drug, she would do some research in her book and proceed to express whatever concerns she might have to the doctor who had written out the prescription (such as raising questions about whatever contraindications were listed in conjunction with a given drug or, perhaps, talking about the possibility that there might be problematic synergistic effects when a given drug was used in combination with certain other drugs).

My mother found out at least two things when she did this. First, her doctors – or, at least, some of them -- seemed to resent the fact that someone was looking over their shoulders, so to speak, and raising questions about treatment. Second, the doctors often didn't know all that much about the drugs they were prescribing.

From time to time, some of my mother's doctors would criticize her behavior and belittle her concerns. Those same doctors would often treat my mother with a certain amount of contempt ... as if she were a petulant child complaining about irrelevancies rather than someone who was the object of whatever treatments were being administered and, consequently, she would be the one who would have to suffer the consequences if there were problems entailed by the cocktail of medications being imposed on her.

Doctors, of course, are busy people. Among other things, this means they don't have the time to do a great deal of research concerning the developmental history of a particular drug ... let alone hundreds of such pharmaceutical agents.

What they know about those drugs is frequently limited to what a drug company representative might have related to them, or what other doctors might have told them over, say, lunch, or what they have heard about such drugs at a medical conference, or that information

| Explorations |

might be based on having read an article appearing somewhere in a medical journal, newsletter, or circular.

Oftentimes – and, sometimes, this is true even in the case of specialists – general practitioners do not look at the original research that led to the approval of a given drug, nor are they likely to have done their own independent and rigorous research on the matter. Most of their understanding concerning those drugs is based on little more than hearsay testimony from various formal and informal sources ... including their own clients/patients.

Drug representatives often leave samples of a drug with the doctors they visit. Those samples constitute part of Phase-IV testing when drugs, with the approval of the FDA, are released for purposes of public consumption and statistics begin to be compiled on: how well different patients/clients safely tolerate those drugs, or what problems, if any, show up with respect to those drugs, and whether those drugs seem to work effectively outside the confines of the laboratory.

Although a number of steps are taken by government regulators (such as the FDA) in order to protect the public and, hopefully, to try to ensure that drugs are both safe and effective by the time they reach the public, Phase-IV testing is, nonetheless, still part of an experimental process. In effect, the general public constitutes a group of guinea pigs that are not always properly informed about the on-going experimental character of the process through which they are being prescribed drugs.

When guinea pigs – like my mother – speak out, all too frequently they are treated as if they had no more rights than a mouse does who is judged to be acting in an ethically-challenged manner should it decide to object to the questionable drugs to which it is being introduced in some pristine, high-tech laboratory. The system works best – at least for the doctors, insurance companies, and the pharmaceutical companies -- when the experimental subjects keep their mouths shut and just go along with the "normal" order of things.

There are other considerations beyond the foregoing one. Suppose a medical doctor takes his responsibilities seriously and actively seeks out to learn about the drugs by attending a number of talks being given at a medical conference of some kind.

What does that doctor know about the background of the speakers? For example, does he or she know whether, or not, the speakers are getting paid by a pharmaceutical company in order to promote such a drug – a practice that tends to occur fairly often.

Or, suppose that a medical doctor makes the effort to read the relevant literature concerning a given drug. Does that doctor know how many of those articles have been ghost written for the author(s) of such articles by individuals who have been hired by a pharmaceutical company to give the drug a positive spin or that the author gets various financial or other considerations for allowing her or his name to appear on those articles?

Alternatively, what about the process of receiving FDA approval? How many of the individuals who are on the review committees that advise the FDA are merely advocating for drugs or products that are manufactured by companies for whom those people are consultants, and what, if anything, does a given medical doctor – even a conscientious one who desires to exercise a certain amount of due diligence with respect to the drugs she or he prescribes – know about the actual dynamics that underlie the approval of a given drug?

Let us assume that our heroic medical doctor – the one who is trying to do right by his/her clients with respect to the drugs that are being prescribed -- comes across a report that pits some, unknown clinician against the powers that be with respect to possible problems surrounding use of a given drug. The unknown clinician is being criticized by an array of established and well-known medical organizations, university professors, and foundations for having uttered various critical remarks concerning, say, the safety or efficacy of a given drug ... remarks that are considered to be unprofessional and without foundation.

What should our medical doctor think about that difference of opinion? This question becomes more complicated when considered in the light of the fact that there have been quite a few historical examples in which the people of power have sought to discredit some individual, not because the latter person was wrong in what she or he was saying, but, quite the contrary, because that individual was speaking the truth and those with vested interests were trying to

| Explorations |

weather the storm by seeking to discredit, if not destroy, that person in the eyes of the general public.

Consider the case of Dr. Martin Teicher, a psychiatrist, who worked at McLean Hospital in Belmont, Massachusetts. Up until 1988, he had used a variety of approaches in conjunction with the treatment of depression – including tricyclics, MAO (monoamine oxidase) inhibitors, and electroshock therapy – with varying degrees of success but, as well, with varying kinds of unwanted side-effects.

In 1988, he began to hear about a new drug – Prozac – which was an SSRI ... that is, a selective serotonin reuptake inhibitor. Serotonin is a neurotransmitter, and SSRIs have the capacity to prevent or inhibit serotonin from being reabsorbed back into surrounding neurons and, thereby keep them actively available in the synaptic spaces that separated the terminal portion of neurons (referred to as an axon bulb) from one another.

According to one of the initial hypotheses involving SSRIs, people who suffered from depression exhibited diminished levels of serotonin, and, consequently, the possibility was entertained that increasing those levels might relieve some of the symptoms associated with depression. Since SSRIs had been discovered to increase the levels of serotonin – at least in certain synaptic areas – drugs like Prozac were being hailed as the next generation with respect to, allegedly, state of the art treatments for depression.

Before continuing on with the Martin Teicher saga, there are several preliminary considerations to keep in mind. For example, no one has explained why levels of serotonin tend to be diminished in individuals who are suffering from depression. In addition, no one has explained what role the absence of serotonin plays in generating the symptoms of depression. Moreover, no one has explained why – even if one were to suppose that increasing levels of serotonin is the right thing to do – that enhancing the quantities of serotonin in synaptic areas is the way to go. Finally, no one has explained how the process of elevating levels of serotonin in synaptic areas actually engages the problem of depression.

Notwithstanding the foregoing pieces of information, and prior to Prozac even being approved by the FDA in January of 1988, quite a few clinicians had begun to experiment with Prozac in relation to their patients/clients. A sufficient number of those clinicians had indicated how use of the drug was producing remarkable results, and consequently, a considerable buzz began to swirl about the drug.

After earning a medical degree from Yale University and a PhD in developmental psychology from Johns Hopkins, Martin Teicher had worked his way up through the ranks at McLean Hospital, long considered one of the preeminent psychiatric facilities in America. He started out as a psychiatric resident, then became a staff psychiatrist, and, eventually, was appointed to be the director of the fledgling bio-psychopharmacological research program that had been established at the hospital. In addition, he was a member of the faculty at the Harvard Medical School.

After he began hearing about the seemingly 'miraculous' successes that Prozac appeared to be enjoying, he decided to give the drug a try and began to administer it to a few of his patients. Although Dr. Teicher might have done some manner of homework concerning the biochemistry of Prozac, it is more likely that his willingness to experiment with the drug was based on the word-of-mouth reports he was hearing about in relation to the practice of various psychiatrists because the fact of the matter was that no one really knew how Prozac worked ... to whatever extent it did.

In any event, after working with the drug for a period of time, Dr. Teicher was not all that enamored with its efficacy. Although he continued to prescribe it, he didn't feel the drug was particularly effective.

In addition, he started to wonder if there might be a dark underside to the drug. He began to harbor these concerns when he observed that a number of his patients who had never exhibited any inclination toward, or ideation about, suicide began to become preoccupied with thoughts about ending their lives.

The foregoing changes could just be a function of a deteriorating, condition of deepening depression. On the other hand, those changes might have something to do with the drug that they were taking.

Dr. Teicher began to collaborate with several other staff members at McLean Hospital, each of whom had noted similar anomalies in a number of other patients. Their concerns were heightened when one of these other patients -- who had never expressed any thoughts about suicide prior to taking Prozac but who began to harbor such thoughts after beginning to take Prozac – was taken off Prozac and the suicidal ideation stopped.

The three staff members – Dr. Teicher, Dr. Jonathan Cole (head of psychopharmacology), and Carol Glod (who was a nurse) – wrote up an article that provided an overview and analysis of six cases involving changes in ideation and/or behavior with respect to suicide and the use of Prozac. They submitted their article ('Emergence of Intense Suicidal Preoccupation during Fluoxetine Treatment') to *The American Journal of Psychiatry* and, eventually, after recommended revisions were completed, the article was accepted for publication ... appearing in the February 1990 edition.

After the publication of the foregoing article, Dr. Teicher was contacted by hundreds of people from various parts of the world who had lost – or nearly lost -- a family member or friend to suicide after the loved one had been placed on Prozac (Fluoxetine) by a psychiatrist or medical doctor. The FDA also had received nearly 15,000 complaints in conjunction with Prozac ... significantly more than had been the case with other drugs that had been released.

In September 1991, the FDA decided to hold hearings on the issue via its Psychopharmacological Drugs Advisory Committee. Dr. Teicher had been invited to be a part of the proceedings.

Prior to the release of the February 1990 article, Eli Lilly, the manufacturer of Prozac, had dispatched several of its top experts to meet in Boston with Dr. Teicher and his colleague Dr. Cole in order to present statistical data that was based on clinical trials involving some 3,000 individuals, and that, supposedly, demonstrated there was no evidence correlating Prozac with suicidal behavior. In the light of clinical experiences with their own patients -- as well as based on the clinical experiences of some of their colleagues -- involving adverse reactions in patients taking Prozac, Dr. Teicher and Dr. Cole wanted Eli Lilly to fund a comparative study using Prozac and a placebo, but the company rejected the idea.

There was a strange dynamic taking place. On the one hand, Dr. Teicher and Dr. Cole had written an article indicating there might be some problems associated with the use of Prozac, and the prospect of

| Explorations |

that article had led Eli Lilly to send several scientists to Boston in an attempt to convince the doctors from McLean Hospital that their concerns were unfounded. Yet, when Eli Lilly was presented with an opportunity to acquire further proof that Prozac was safe and effective, the company appeared to be disinterested.

Of course, the company might have felt that its own clinical trial studies were so definitive that there was no need for further proof. Such additional testing might have been considered a waste of money.

Nonetheless, there were an increasing number of clinicians who were providing evidence that something of possible concern was taking place with their patients in relation to using Prozac. Moreover, such anomalous experiences seemed to indicate that Prozac might have something to do with whatever was taking place.

No matter how much Eli Lilly might have been committed to believing that its clinical trials had proven Prozac to be safe and effective, why would the company back away from an opportunity to further substantiate the correctness of its position and, in the process, help alleviate any doubts that clinicians might have concerning use of the drug? This question looms especially large given that all too many people taking Prozac were dying, and one of the primary suspects underlying those deaths was the drug itself.

Saving money by avoiding unnecessary testing is one thing, but the prospect of possibly saving lives raises the stakes to a whole different level. Of course, if one values money over life, then the nature of the calculus used to evaluate the situation will alter accordingly.

Interestingly, several organizations that fund research involving suicide, schizophrenia, and affective disorders also turned down the idea of providing a grant to support the aforementioned Prozac/placebo study. What is interesting is that those organizations received substantial funding from the pharmaceutical industry and, therefore, might have been reluctant to do anything that could jeopardize further funding of the organization by pharmaceuticals.

On September 21, 1991, the Psychopharmacological Drugs Advisory Committee of the FDA began hearings that supposedly were intended to explore the possible pros and cons of Prozac use. A number of people from the general public wanted to provide personal

| Explorations |

testimony concerning what they believed were possible negative dimensions of Prozac use and had traveled to the meeting at their own expense.

Following the foregoing sorts of personal testimony, much of the rest of the hearings turned to so-called scientific considerations. One of the speakers was Gary Tollefson, an Eli Lilly research scientist who provided an overview of the results of a variety of clinical trials involving Prozac.

After going through a number of slides with running commentary, he stipulated there was no evidence demonstrating any significant difference in the suicidal thoughts or actions of those individuals who were treated with Prozac during the trials relative to those subjects who had been administered a placebo. However, inadvertently or otherwise, Gary Tollefson had left out something of considerable importance from his presentation.

More specifically, he had neglected to point out that there actually had been a clinical trial held outside the Unites States showing a significant increase in the incidence of suicidal acts when one compared those subjects who had been placed on Prozac relative to those individuals who had been placed on a placebo during the clinical trials. The result of the foregoing trial had been sufficiently worrisome that the German government initially refused to grant approval for the drug, and only agreed to do so six years later when an appropriate warning accompanied the drug.

Earlier in the hearings, Dr. Paul Leber, who was head of the FDA's Division of Neuropharmacological Drug Products, had asserted that the only form of scientific assessment that was considered to be reliable – namely, randomized clinical trials – had provided no evidence indicating that the use of Prozac was associated with any increases in aggressiveness, violence, or suicidal behavior. Another speaker, Dr. Charles Nemeroff, who was a psychiatrist and a faculty member at Emory University School of Medicine, reiterated the position that no one had been able to establish a cause-and-effect relationship between Prozac use and increased suicidal thoughts or behavior, and in the process, claimed that the Prozac case studies discussed in the February 1990 edition of *The American Journal of Psychiatry* article, together with some other case studies along the

| Explorations |

97

same lines that had surfaced, could be attributed to various factors unrelated to Prozac. A third participant, Dr. Daniel Casey who was a psychiatrist with the Veterans Administration Medical Center and who was chairing the FDA session, also voiced his opinion that there was no credible evidence linking Prozac use with increased tendencies toward suicidal thoughts or behaviors.

At a certain point during the proceedings, Dr. Teicher was asked by someone in the audience to state his (Dr. Teicher's) views on the matter. Dr. Teicher began outlining some of his findings but was interrupted at different points by both Dr. Casey and Dr. Leber.

When asked to present evidence to back up his claims, Dr. Teicher offered to show some slides on the matter. Dr. Casey, who was chairing the session, discouraged Dr. Teicher from doing so despite the fact that other speakers had been permitted to do precisely that at some length.

Shortly thereafter, Dr. Casey called for a vote of the advisory committee with respect to whether, or not, the members believed there was any evidence to suggest that Prozac was associated with an increased likelihood of either suicidal thoughts or behavior. The nine member committee voted unanimously that there was no such evidence and, then, held a second vote, which carried 6-3, that there was no need to issue any sort of warning in conjunction with the use of Prozac.

Let's retrace our steps and reflect a little on what appeared to be transpiring at the advisory committee meeting. First, despite the fact that nearly 15,000 complaints had been received by the FDA concerning Prozac – far more than in relation to any other drug – and despite the fact that a number of people from the general public showed up at meeting to give testimony related to those complaints, those concerns were treated as non-evidence even though they were, supposedly, one of the primary reasons – if not the sole one – for the meeting being called in the first place. (A more cynical individual might suppose that the reason the meeting had been called was a strategic move by officials at the FDA to provide a pharmaceutical company with an opportunity to get out ahead of the mounting bad publicity and put a positive spin on things.)

Dr. Leber, Dr. Nemeroff, and Dr. Casey did not consider those complaints to constitute proof of any thing. In fact, during his presentation, Dr. Nemeroff claimed that such cases could be explained away by complicating factors of one kind or another.

However, providing a possible, alternative explanation for a given phenomenon is not really proof of much of anything. Indeed, why should anyone accept, at face value, a claim that only alludes to (and does not rigorously demonstrate) the possibility that there are alternative ways of accounting for the cases written about in *The American Journal of Psychiatry* article or in relation to any of the other 15,000 cases that had been reported to the FDA?

This is a very lazy person's way of doing research. Unless Dr. Leber, Dr. Nemeroff and Dr. Casey can prove that Prozac was not responsible for increases in suicidal ideation and/or behavior in the cases presented by Dr. Teicher or in the cases encompassed by the 15,000 other complaints, then their statements about science come to nothing.

The whole point of the Phase-IV portion of the drug approval process is to gather evidence concerning clinical experience involving drugs that have passed through Phase-III trials. If such evidence is considered to be scientifically useless, then why collect it ... especially given that it is precisely that sort of information which shapes the kind of warnings, contraindications, and so on that – moving forward -- will be associated with a given drug as a means of helping to protect the public?

Phase-IV information is important because it can provide data that cannot be provided by Phase-III testing. Randomized trials have a value, but they don't necessarily reveal the full story of what happens when drugs are released for public consumption and, therefore, are not being used by individuals who have been selected simply because they satisfy the conditions of certain protocols where many factors are controlled for in a way that does not occur in the 'wild'.

The 15,000 complaints registered with the FDA against Prozac were potential candidates to be mixed in with other Phase-IV data. The case studies being written up by Dr. Teicher and others were also potential candidates to be included in that data set.

Unfortunately, the foregoing information was being treated as if it automatically should be deemed to be of dubious pedigree and,

| Explorations |

99

consequently, should be rejected out of hand. However, there was never any proof put forward during the advisory meeting other than a series of summary judgments against considering such data to have any value, but proceeding in this manner does not constitute a proof of any kind.

When Dr. Teicher sought to present some evidence in support of his position through the use of a few slides, he was denied the opportunity to do so ... an opportunity, as noted earlier, that had been granted to other speakers. The proceedings of the FDA advisory committee bear more than a passing resemblance to the show trials that used to take place in Stalinist Russia where guilt and innocence were all arranged ahead of time and everyone went through the motions until the inevitable, pre-determined result is produced.

One might add to the foregoing considerations the fact that one of the speakers -- Gary Tollefson of Eli Lilly – was knowingly or unknowingly -- misleading everyone in the room. There was, in fact, randomized, clinical trial evidence indicating that Prozac could be linked to an increase in suicidal thoughts and behavior relative to a placebo control group.

There is a precautionary principle that often is mentioned in conjunction with ecological issues. More specifically the principle says that when there is doubt about whether, or not, some action will, or will not, result in harm being done to the environment, one should err on the side of caution and refrain from the action about which there is some doubt.

The members of the FDA advisory committee had a great deal of evidence in front of them (15,000 complaints-plus) indicating that Prozac might not be as safe as some of the clinical trials were suggesting was the case. However, those advisory committee members were prepared to accept only one kind of evidence – namely, clinical trials – not because this was the only scientifically justifiable way to proceed but because they couldn't be bothered to actually critically explore in a rigorous way the available evidence that ran contrary to their clinical trials.

Science is not just about conducting randomized trials. Science is, first and foremost, rooted in the process of observation.

| Explorations |

If the evidence arising from an array of observations runs contrary to the evidence arising from randomized trials, then, one needs to pursue the matter further. Among other things, this means that one should undertake further testing and exploration in order to address the questions and problems that are being suggested by those anomalies that are being observed independently of clinical trials.

Whenever evidence is available (and nearly 15,000 complaints, along with a number of case studies, do constitute evidence irrespective of whatever members of an advisory committee might say) and that evidence suggests the possibility there might be something in a drug -- or connected with its metabolism once ingested -- that induces violent or suicidal behavior, then one should be inclined to exercise caution ... perhaps even be willing to err on the side of caution because people's lives are at stake.

If someone has a product to sell, then, it is the responsibility of the manufacturer to prove that the product is safe. It is not the responsibility of a customer to do this.

The members of the advisory committee who unanimously voted that there was no scientific evidence to indicate that Prozac caused increased thoughts or behaviors involving suicide actually had failed in their fiduciary responsibility to the general public. There was empirical data indicating, at the very least, that caution should be exercised with respect to the use of Prozac, but the members of the advisory committee simply chose to discredit that data without providing -- or even being willing to entertain (e.g., none of them insisted on taking a look at Dr. Teicher's slides) -- any kind of evidence that was inconsistent with the sort of vote they seemed intent on taking.

There is a further set of problems surrounding the view of science that was being advocated by individuals such as the one being alluded to by Dr. Leber, Dr. Nemeroff, and Dr. Casey during the advisory committee meeting that had been convened by the FDA in conjunction with the safety of Prozac. More specifically, when such people speak about the absence of any cause-and-effect relationship between, on the one hand, the use of Prozac and, on the other hand, increased tendencies involving suicidal thoughts and/or behaviors, the aforementioned individuals tend to paint themselves into a corner.

More specifically, there is no evidence to prove that SSRIs have a cause and effect relationship with depression. The data is, at best, all correlational.

There is no cause-and-effect evidence to demonstrate that depression is caused by the absence of serotonin. There is no cause-and-effect evidence to demonstrate that the absence of serotonin is directly tied to the phenomenology of depression. There is no cause-and-effect evidence to demonstrate that the presence of extra serotonin in the synapses is responsible for changing the phenomenology of a person in a manner that removes all traces of depression.

As indicated earlier, whatever evidence exists between SSRIs and depression is correlational in nature – that is, there seems to be a positive relationship between the presence of an SSRI and a reduction in reported symptoms of depression. However, there is absolutely no biochemical mechanism that has been hypothesized (or proven to exist) which is capable of showing, in a step-by-step manner, that the absence or presence of serotonin is responsible for, respectively, the presence or absence of depression.

In other words, the members of the FDA advisory committee who were supposedly considering the possible merits and liabilities of Prozac were asking for a form of evidence and manner of proof from those who had their doubts about Prozac that the proponents of Prozac could not, themselves, supply. In addition, those members of the advisory committee seemed to have a very biased and limited view concerning the nature of science.

Because of their collective blind spots (and by referring to it as a 'blind spot', I am offering the benefit of a doubt that might not be deserved), the members of the FDA advisory committee – like the members of the clergy that Galileo invited to look through his telescope – were unwilling to take a look at anything that was not already a fixed and unchangeable part of their worldview. Furthermore, because of their collective "blind spots", unsuspecting people would continue to die as a result of Prozac being prescribed for them or administered to them.

Science does not necessarily exist simply because an alleged scientist says something. Science does not necessarily exist when a group of appropriately credentialed individuals makes a claim of some kind. Science does not necessarily exist just because certain people with technical credentials and political authority speak out about what they consider to be the sort of evidence that will, and will not, be acceptable to a given community of researchers.

Science only exists when there is a relentlessly rigorous and critically reflective attempt to establish the truth in a way that accounts for all the available data that bears upon a given situation and, in the process, provides a fully defensible account of whatever questions and problems have arisen during, or as a result, of the aforementioned attempt to establish the truth. What the FDA advisory committee was doing on September 21, 1991 in conjunction with the hearings on Prozac was not science because none of the individuals on that advisory committee exhibited any indication that they were committed to the process of trying to establish the truth in the manner outlined above.

The individuals on the advisory committee and some of the credentialed individuals who made presentations before them might have believed that everything they said gave expression to the scientific process. However, all they had to offer was a largely disingenuous set of words that had been salted here and there with traces of something that appeared to glitter with scientific value but was, in actuality, little more than fool's gold.

One might also raise the question of just how much homework the members of the advisory committee actually did in preparation for the hearing concerning Prozac. Did they go through the 15,000 complaints that had been filed with the FDA against Prozac? Had they read the article in *The American Journal of Psychiatry* written by Dr. Teicher and his colleagues? Were they familiar with the other case studies that had begun to appear indicating there might be a problem with Prozac? Had they gone through the clinical trial data with a fine-tooth comb?

To be sure, a representative of Eli Lilly (Gary Tollefson) gave a presentation during the hearing that summarized the clinical trial data. However, one cannot really understand the nuts and bolts of an experiment until one spends some time with that material, and the members of the advisory committee obviously had not done this because if they had, then, among other things, they would have come across the material that, for whatever reason, Gary Tollefson left out of his presentation on Prozac and that indicated there was, indeed, proof that use of Prozac was associated with a higher likelihood (nearly twice as much) of suicidal ideation and behavior when compared with the results of individuals who had been given a placebo.

Someone might try to argue that one couldn't possibly expect the very busy professionals on an advisory committee to take the time and make the effort required to do all the work that is being suggested in the foregoing several paragraphs. My response is: Why not?

What exactly are they advising about? What is the basis of such advising if those individuals aren't intimately familiar with all of the issues, problems, questions, and data that are entailed by the drug on which they are going to vote?

Without such knowledge and insight, the process of advising becomes a very macabre joke. After all, people were dying, and one might suppose that the individuals on an advisory committee might want to establish exactly why those people were dying and whether, or not, those deaths had anything to do with the drug for which they, subsequently, would be giving a vote of confidence.

Later on, following the September 1991 Prozac hearing that had been convened by the FDA, a few investigative journalists discovered that five of the nine members of the advisory committee had financial ties, of one kind or another, with pharmaceutical companies ... including one member – Dr. David Dunner -- who was a well-paid consultant for the pharmaceutical company that manufactured Prozac (i.e., Eli Lilly).

In addition, one of the speakers, Dr. Charles Nemeroff -- who had sought to discredit the case studies written up by Dr. Teicher and his colleagues that suggested there might be a problem involving Prozac -- not only was a paid consultant for Eli Lilly but owned stock in the company as well. Dr. Nemeroff waxed eloquently about the process of science and scientific proof, yet waned miserably when it came to being sufficiently honest to indicate to the audience that he had a conflict of interest on the topic about which he was speaking.

| Explorations |

The foregoing discussion was not really about Prozac, per se. Rather, that drug provided a concrete opportunity to further explore some of the issues surrounding not only the nature of science but, as well, to reflect on some of the problems with which each of us is confronted as we try to figure out 'the reality problem' and struggle toward our individual take on formulating a response to the final jeopardy challenge.

To begin with, we now know that the 'Burzynski Affair' -- which was explored in an earlier section of this chapter -- is not an isolated case involving a temporary, anomalous, and limited departure from the pursuit of truth. To that affair, one can add some data from a different sample set – namely, the case of SSRIs.

Those two samples provide evidence that people credentialed with degrees in technical subjects do not always have integrity. They are not always honest. They do not always exercise due diligence. They are not always tireless practitioners of something called science.

When individuals who are credentialed with some sort of technical expertise fall off the wagon and become intoxicated with their own delusional preoccupations, they do not deserve to be called scientists. Unfortunately, in the alleged name of science, such credentialed individuals are sometimes prepared to sacrifice other people on the altar of the former individuals' own professional, political and financial self-interest, and because this happens more frequently than many of us would like to imagine, a person cannot simply relax in an easy chair, kick up her or his feet, and claim that: Science tells us ... X, Y or Z.

In today's world, there is just as much of a willingness to blindly accept whatever comes out of the mouths of individuals who have degrees in the physical and biological sciences, as there is a willingness to blindly accept whatever comes out of the mouths of individuals who are credentialed in some theological or religious manner. However, the epistemological food chain has become compromised, and this places each of us in a very precarious position because none of us can be certain about the quality, or nutritional value, of the food for thought we are receiving through various channel ways of information.

| Explorations |

The Burzynski affair is not about just a few individuals. The Prozac/SSRI issue is not about just a few individuals.

Each of the foregoing sample sets give expression to the jagged components of an iceberg-like phenomenon whose surface features might seem relatively limited and innocuous but, in fact, is rooted in a depth of: practices, ideas, values, beliefs, understandings, emotions, motivations, and world views involving thousands of people that are collectively capable of scuttling the existential ships that we, as individuals, might have to sail in the vicinity of such potentially treacherous entities.

The Burzynski affair turned out the way it did because there is a whole system of thousands of credentialed individuals who were prepared to let it unfold as it did and who are prepared to let similar affairs happen in the future. Whatever their thoughts and feelings about science might be, they have been willing to permit those thoughts and feelings to be dominated and corrupted by considerations of: ignorance, bias, ambition, fear, jealousy, selfishness, greed, and indifference.

Furthermore, despite some relatively minor changes in the manner in which the legal drug business is conducted and despite the occurrence of a few, small legal and political victories over the last several decades that have resulted in some grudging, acknowledgement on the part of pharmaceutical companies and the FDA that, for example, there might be a link between the use of SSRIs and an increased incidence of suicidal thoughts and behaviors, and/or violent aggressiveness toward other people, things seem to be pretty much continuing along as they did back in 1991. Credentialed individuals today not only have little additional understanding of, or insight into, the functioning of psychoactive drugs in the brain than they did a quarter century ago, but, as well, there is a whole system of vested political, financial and ideological interests in place (made up, in large part, of individuals carrying technical credentials of one kind or another) that generate significant inertial drag with respect to trying to assist people to come to a better understanding of the problematic impact that a variety of FDA-approved drugs might be having on the human mind.

| Explorations |

For instance, you might want to reflect on the work of Dr. Peter Breggin, a psychiatrist, who has been attempting to sound a clarion call for more than thirty years. His concerns are directed toward the way in which psychoactive drugs – that is, commercial drugs that are intended, through their acting upon the brain, to alleviate psychological suffering – are used and understood by both the medical community as well as the general public.

According to Dr. Breggin there is a condition that he refers to as "medication madness" (to be discussed shortly) that sometimes afflicts individuals who have been prescribed one, or more, psychoactive drugs by their physicians or psychiatrists. However, there is also a condition of "medication madness", of a slightly different kind, that afflicts the understanding of the medical profession and scientific community when it comes to the issue of whether, or not, such credentialed individuals can put forth a coherent, consistent, provable theory concerning the nature of the relationship between the use of psychoactive drugs and various maladies of the mind.

Let's take a look at the first kind of medication madness noted above. That is, let's consider what happens to some people who are prescribed or administered various kinds of medically approved psychoactive drugs.

Dr. Breggin has engaged hundreds of cases involving the use of psychoactive drugs in a critically reflective manner. Some of those cases are a function of his practice as a psychiatrist, while other cases result from his work as a consultant for individuals who might have suffered some sort of debilitating problem due to the taking of psychoactive drugs that were prescribed by another doctor. Moreover, he also has accrued considerable experience due to his status as an expert witness in criminal cases in which medically prescribed psychoactive drugs might have played a significant role in inducing violent behavior in some individual who has consumed such drugs.

Dr. Breggin does not come to his conclusions concerning the potential relationship between certain psychoactive drugs and violent behavior through a non-rigorous methodology. His determinations are based on a fairly thorough process involving: Extensive interviews with a patient, client, or defendant in a criminal proceeding or civil trial, as well as conversations with family members, friends, neighbors, or other individuals who might have something of relevance to offer with respect to a given case.

In addition, the foregoing interviews are considered against a background of information that helps to provide something of a context for whatever has transpired. Included in the foregoing sort of information are: Educational records, medical files, employment reports, as well as whatever documents (e.g., toxicology tests, autopsies, etc.) that might be of assistance when trying to reach a thoughtful, evidence-based conclusion about matters.

Some people might not consider the foregoing methodology to be scientific. However, the use of case studies has had a long, productive presence in the annals of both the medical/psychiatric literature as well as in clinical practice.

The fact is: There are many facets of our lives that lie beyond the capacity of so-called scientific methodology (i.e., demonstrating the truth or falsity of a given hypothesis through means of experimental arrangements that are controlled to exclude any influences that might cloud the relationship between a hypothesis and data generated through the experimental process). Case studies give expression to a form of methodology that while not scientific in the experimental sense, nonetheless, can provide useful, often insightful clues concerning the nature of a given matter.

The goal is truth, not science per se. Good science is a multi-faceted set of protocols that are intended to probe for the truth from a variety of perspectives and via different methods that complement and supplement one another.

In his writing, Dr Breggin emphasizes that he is more concerned with the issue of the potential problems ensuing from legally prescribed psychoactive drugs than he is with trying to claim that medical doctors are the problem simply because they prescribe drugs that they consider to be safe and effective. I understand why Dr. Breggin might be taking such an approach because he really would like to enlist the support of the medical profession in his effort to institute the sort of precautionary principle that will help to responsibly regulate how medical doctors utilize and prescribe such drugs.

| Explorations |

Obviously, claiming that doctors are a fundamental part of the problem rather than attempting to narrow the focus to being just about the drugs might prove to be counterproductive as far as the main thrust of what he trying to accomplish is concerned. So, he tends to concentrate his attention on the effect of the drugs rather than the effect of the medical/academic/commercial mind set that ensures that such drugs will be prescribed.

Unfortunately, the fact of the matter is, the whole medical profession, along with the FDA, and an array of universities, pharmaceutical companies, researchers, and professional journals are responsible for, among other things, the current situation vis-à-vis the dark underside of psychoactive drugs. All of the foregoing players are spellbound by the delusion that they understand what is going on in the brain and mind when people suffer from some form of psychological disorder and, as a result, those professional individuals are inclined to recommend (or are in agreement with) the prescribing of various kinds of psychoactive drugs in order, allegedly, to engage those conditions constructively.

In any event, Dr. Breggin is convinced that psychiatric or psychoactive drugs can have a spellbinding impact on those individuals who take them. What he means by this is that individuals who are under the influence of psychiatric drugs and who subsequently become agitated, anxious, depressed, aggressive, violent, and/or suicidal tend to be oblivious to the possibility that their change in behavior and mental/emotional condition is a function of the drugs they are consuming rather than a reflection of personal pathology that supposedly exists within them independently of the psychoactive medicine being administered to them ... that is, the effect of the drugs are such that those people operate as if the thoughts, feelings, and behaviors arising within them are their own rather than a phenomenology that has been shaped, colored, framed, and organized by the presence of the psychoactive drugs in their bodies.

There is a related phenomenon going on in the minds of the medical doctors, researchers, psychiatrists, professors, and regulators who believe that such drugs have an important role to play in helping to alleviate – if not cure – the mental, emotional, and/or behavioral pathology of the individuals to whom the drugs are administered.

Those professional individuals are spellbound by their various conjectures concerning how they believe the universe operates with respect to psychological and biological phenomena ... that is, the effect of their ideas about the foregoing matters is such that they operate as if their thoughts, feelings, and behaviors were a function of the way the world is rather than merely being a function of the hermeneutical framework they are seeking to impose on reality and in the process completely obscure the latter.

According to Dr. Breggin, patients/clients who are prescribed or administered psychoactive drugs do not understand that their ideas, feelings, and behaviors are not necessarily rooted in reality but might be, in some way, artifacts of the drugs they are taking. Similarly, the doctors who prescribe such drugs do not seem to understand that their ideas, feelings, and behaviors concerning the efficacy of such drugs are not necessarily rooted in reality but might be artifacts of their delusions concerning how the mind operates and, more specifically, might be artifacts of their delusions concerning the way in which psychoactive drugs supposedly operate in the brain.

Earlier in this chapter, I explored, in a limited way, a few of the questions that swirled about Prozac back in the 1980s and early 1990s. Those same questions can be directed toward the pharmaceutical successors to Prozac – such as, Luvox (fluvoxamine), Zoloft (sertraline), Paxil (paroxetine), Celexa (citalopram), and Lexapro (escitalopram) – because all of those drugs are variations on an SSRI theme ... that is, they all revolve about a process of inhibiting the re-uptake of selected forms of serotonin back into the axon bulb of surrounding neurons, thereby keeping the concentration of serotonin high in the synaptic areas between neurons.

The aforementioned drugs all came after Prozac hit the markets. Nevertheless, none of the underlying, more up-to-date research in 'support' of those later drugs is any more capable of answering -- in a rigorously justifiable manner -- questions concerning the specific nature of the cause-and-effect dynamics that allegedly ties psychoactive drugs to various kinds of mental or emotional disorder than was the case in relation to Prozac.

In other words, we still don't know how the absence of a particular kind of serotonin causes a given form of psychological pathology.

Moreover, we still don't know how the presence of some specific form of serotonin brings about a change in the kinds of phenomenology that tend to be associated with such disorders.

Furthermore, there have been a number of studies that generated results indicating that SSRIs aren't necessarily any more effective than a placebo [a substance whose physical ingredient(s) is (are) considered to be inert with respect to brain functioning]. Double blind studies (neither the subjects nor the doctors know who is getting what) have been conducted which demonstrate that placebos are nearly as – if not as – effective in the treatment of conditions such as depression as is one, or another, brand of SSRI.

If substances that have no discernible impact on brain functioning – i.e., placebos – can operate as effectively as SSRIs can, then what does this say about the serotonin theory of depression? Conceivably, the administering of SSRIs work – to whatever extent they do – because of the placebo effect inherent in the patient's or client's expectation that they will be helped by the doctor and her/his prescribing of a drug in and of itself (that is, quite independently of whatever action the drug actually has on their brains).

At the very least, the waters of understanding are muddied by the presence of the placebo issue. No one really knows what is taking place, and, therefore, quite possibly, the presence or absence of serotonin might be completely irrelevant to the actual dynamics of either the presence or absence of depression.

The foregoing comments should not be construed in a manner that suggests I am trying to claim that SSRIs have no impact on the biochemistry of brain functioning. Rather, whatever effect(s) the presence of SSRIs has (have) in the brain is not because the etiology of depression has been discovered and worked out, and, as a result, serotonin has been proven to be at the heart of those dynamics.

Indeed, Dr. Breggin believes that psychoactive drugs like – but not restricted to – SSRIs can have a tremendously problematic impact on brain functioning. After all, his notion of medication madness -- or the manner in which a patient, subject or client can become spellbound by the effects of a given psychoactive drug – alludes to the kind of problematic effect he believes psychoactive drugs are capable of having on certain individuals.

SSRIs do affect brain functioning. They just don't necessarily affect that functioning in the way various clinicians, academics, and researchers have conjectured to be the case in relation to, say, the condition of depression.

Therefore, to whatever extent SSRIs have an impact on the phenomenology of depression, that impact might be entirely coincidental and indirect. For instance, if I have a pain in my arm and someone comes along and punches me in the jaw, knocking me out, the pain in my arm will, at least while I am unconscious, disappear.

Nonetheless, one cannot suppose that knocking people out should be considered to be a treatment for arm pain or that being knocked out addresses any of the possible causes underlying my arm pain. The process of being knocked out is entirely incidental to the issue of the arm pain.

Similarly, the presence of an SSRI might, like a blow to the head, mask certain symptoms of say, depression, just as the blow to the head brought about a cessation (at least temporarily) with respect to the pain in my arm. However, that process of masking is unrelated to the actual problem (depression), just as the blow to my head that masked the pain in my arm was unrelated to the underlying dynamics of my arm pain.

In short, the presence of the SSRI doesn't necessarily have any causal relationship with, nor does it necessarily address any of the underlying causes of, the condition of depression. Moreover, the impact of the activity of the SSRI in the brain might be purely coincidental as far as its relationship with depression is concerned.

According to Dr. Breggin, the use of a wide variety of medically prescribed psychoactive drugs, when taken in conjunction with various kinds of medical diagnoses, is capable of pushing individuals into a condition of neurological toxicity. There is an array of symptoms that might ensue from such toxicity – including: Delusions, hallucinations, agitated behavior (akathisia), dysfunctional memory, insomnia, anxiety, compulsive ideation, irrational thought processes, radical shifts in emotions, and so on.

There is a very sound basis for claiming that the foregoing symptoms can be attributed to the toxic effects of the psychoactive drugs being prescribed or administered. (1) Despite the relative absence of those problematic symptoms prior to taking the medically prescribed/administered drugs, nevertheless, those kinds of mental, emotional and behavioral symptoms tend to arise following the taking of such drugs (although it might be a matter of days, weeks, or months before the symptoms show up), and (2) when an individual is taken off those drugs, the problematic symptoms tend to disappear.

The technical terms for the foregoing processes are: 'challenge' and 'dechallenge'. Challenge and dechallenge tend to be followed by a third process known as: 'Re-challenge', which is designed to determine whether, or not, certain symptoms will reoccur once a person begins to take the drug at issue again.

Sometimes there is a complicating dimension associated with (2) above (i.e., being taken off a drug). More specifically, removing psychoactive drugs from a person's system might bring about another form of disorder known as 'discontinuation syndrome'.

Discontinuation syndrome is brought about in the following manner. First, a psychoactive drug initially causes a toxic, biochemical imbalance in an individual's brain/body for which a problematic, symptom-laden adjustment ensues (i.e., medication spellbinding). However, when that drug is removed (i.e., the person stops taking it), another symptom-laden biochemical adjustment occurs (i.e., discontinuation syndrome), and this tends to interfere with a person's being able to return to a condition of relative normalcy (that is, not having their thoughts and behavior being shaped by the toxic effects associated with taking, or going off, the psychoactive drugs that have been prescribed for, or administered to, an individual.

Putting aside the problems surrounding discontinuation syndrome, the primary point being made here is that taking the foregoing sorts of psychoactive drugs sometimes leads to a condition of involuntary intoxication in which a person becomes unable to exercise control over the thoughts, emotions, and behaviors that are being manifested through the individual. While in that condition, a person has difficulty: Distinguishing between right and wrong, or refraining from violent behavior (toward himself/herself and/or others), or reflecting on matters with any semblance of appropriate, ethical and rational deliberation.

Involuntary intoxication, as the term suggests, is not a case in which a person understands beforehand that he or she will become mentally spellbound after taking prescribed drugs or that she or he also might become engaged in problematic and/or violent behaviors as a result of taking those drugs. Rather, having been led to believe (by the medical establishment, the media, and one's doctor) that taking the prescribed drugs will help the person's mental/emotional condition, the drug or drugs is (are) taken in good faith ... with little, or no, understanding and appreciation that the prescribed drug(s) has (have) the potential to induce an individual to enter into a dysfunctional, impaired condition that was not of his or her personal choosing.

To add insult to injury, while under the undue influence of the psychoactive drug that has been prescribed or administered, a person believes there is nothing wrong with the problematic thinking and behavior that might be taking place while on the drug. The individual assumes – despite considerable evidence to the contrary -- that everything is normal and that she or he is functioning properly.

The aforementioned condition -- in which a person who has been prescribed or administered psychoactive drugs believes that he or she is doing fine even though, to varying degrees, the individual is dysfunctional emotionally, intellectually, and behaviorally -- is referred to by Dr. Breggin as "medication spellbinding". A person who is operating out of a condition of medication spellbinding suffers from impairment in her or his capacity to appreciate what is occurring in his or her life or such an individual is unable to observe himself or herself in any sort of objective, impartial, or self-critical manner. Such individuals tend to rationalize inconsistencies, and/or spin their situation in an attempt to justify what is going on, and/or they confabulate (make up stories) about events because they can't remember what has been taking place or can't make sense of what is transpiring.

For example, under the influence of a prescribed drug, an individual who is suffering from medication spellbinding might become apathetic about life but perceives or interprets that apathy (due to rationalization and confabulation) as an improvement in his or her life. A person in a condition of medication spellbinding might interpret life events in the foregoing way because the sadness, depression, and/or anxiety that had been present prior to taking psychoactive medication was difficult to deal with since, perhaps, the individual had no effective coping strategy through which to engage those feelings, or the persons did not have the ability to place those feelings in a manageable perspective.

In effect, by becoming indifferent or apathetic or removed from life's events through the condition of medication spellbinding, one's normal, existential concerns or emotions have become blunted. As a result, the psychoactive drug has taken away -- among other things -- an opportunity to try to work through those kinds of problematic experiences and come up with an effective way to deal with them.

The psychoactive drug hasn't cured anything. It merely has masked the presence of a problem while simultaneously leading an individual to believe that camouflaging a problem -- so that one won't recognize its presence or appreciate its significance -- is the same thing as addressing that problem.

A person might feel better about life. However, the feeling is illusory because there is nothing of substantive value connected to it.

One has been anesthetized, but one believes one is fully aware. One has been cognitively impaired, but one believes that one is functional and disregards, re-frames, or rationalizes, whatever facts are inconsistent with one's dysfunctional assessment of the situation.

In light of the foregoing considerations, one might ask the following question: Why do medical doctors and psychiatrists prescribe SSRIs when they actually don't have any idea about what is actually transpiring in the human beings to whom they are prescribing or administering such drugs? Naturally, if SSRIs had been proven to be completely safe, then one might argue that because there is no harm in providing such drugs, then, why not give those substances the opportunity to see what, if anything, of a constructive nature they might be able to accomplish?

Unfortunately, from the very beginning some warning signs concerning the safety – if not efficacy -- of those kinds of drugs had begun to emerge. For example, aside from some of the problems noted previously in this chapter, very early in the testing phase of Prozac, Eli Lilly, the manufacturer of Prozac, had discovered that when one uses

SSRIs to artificially maintain high levels of serotonin in the synapses, the brain will actually take steps to resist or counter that tendency by shutting down the production of serotonin and/or decreasing the number of serotonin receptors on the membranes of neurons.

The undermining of serotonergic functioning might continue on long after a given psychiatric drug has been discontinued. In other words, the presence of SSRIs brings about the very condition (the absence of serotonin) that those drugs were supposed to address or resolve.

Individuals such as Dr. Peter Breggin and Dr. Martin Teicher have tried to persuade people to critically reflect on an array of evidence (both experimental and clinical) that runs contrary to the way that medicine in America was, and is being, practiced. Since then, other researchers have added their voices of concern in relation to whether, or not, SSRIs are either safe or effective.

So, again, one needs to raise the question noted earlier. Why do medical doctors and psychiatrists prescribe drugs about which they really are almost completely ignorant?

Even Dr. Martin Teicher – who later sounded a warning about the possible adverse effects of SSRIs – was prepared to give SSRIs a try in the beginning despite the fact that there was no viable proof that depression was caused by the absence of serotonin. Moreover, even if one were willing to try to argue that the absence of serotonin was tied to the presence of depression, there was no plausible account about why levels of serotonin were depleted in the first place, and, therefore, it was quite possible that the absence of serotonin was, in some way, one of the residual effects of depression rather than being the cause of depression.

The degree to which medical doctors are apparently prepared to fool around with, and experiment on, the wellbeing of their patients, is deeply disturbing. Medical doctors and psychiatrists alike are completely ignorant about what, if anything, serotonin has to do with depression, and, yet, they readily buy into the idea that SSRIs are the key to the problem and are quite prepared to act on their speculations irrespective of the cost to their patients/clients.

| Explorations |

The actions of those medical doctors and psychiatrists are almost delusional – if not something worse. A delusion is when someone harbors a false belief about the nature of reality and resists evidence that runs contrary to that belief, and while no one has put forth definitive proof that depression is not a function of serotonin (so one could say that the serotonin hypothesis has been proven to be false), nonetheless, no one has provided any proof, either, that depression is a function of serotonin, and, yet, medical doctors and psychiatrists, on the basis of almost complete ignorance, have decided to either prescribe or administer a drug they knew little, or nothing, about (see pages 388-389 for a bit more on this issue).

Actions that are rooted in delusional thinking are bad enough. Actions that are rooted in an ignorance that credentialed people seek to pass off as if it is were based on knowledge when that is not the case seems, somehow, to be more problematic and dysfunctional than a delusion because such framing actions appear to be an intentional attempt to mislead people rather than just harboring a sincere belief in relation to a false premise or idea.

The professionals were intoxicated with their own ignorance concerning the nature of the relationship between a given drug and its effects on the human brain. In effect, the professionals were deeply ensconced in their own form of medication spellbinding or madness ... except the form of medication madness with which they were afflicted (i.e., the willingness to prescribe and administer drugs about which they knew almost nothing) was responsible for inducing another form of medication madness in their patients/clients ... and, therefore, constitutes an iatrogenic problem

The possible implications of the foregoing considerations for the reality problem and the Final Jeopardy challenge are pretty straightforward. Ideas are like drugs ... they affect the way we think, feel, and behave.

One might believe that the contents of one's thoughts, emotions, or actions are an expression of one's own critical, informed analysis of a given situation, when, in reality, everything might be the result of a process – such as occurs in medication spellbinding when a person undergoes involuntary intoxication by imbibing a psychoactive drug – that has been imposed on one through indoctrination, propaganda, or some other prescribed form of undue influence through which one loses the capacity to make free choices concerning the appropriateness or functional value of one's thoughts, emotions, or behaviors.

One should seek to avoid inducing other people to enter into the conceptual/spiritual counterpart to an involuntary condition of medication spellbinding, and, as well, one should seek to avoid any tendency that might lead to permitting one's own person to be so induced. All too many of the people with medical and technical credentials seem to be far too eager to impose on others a form of medication madness (world view spellbinding) concerning the nature of reality (or how one should respond to the Final Jeopardy challenge), despite considerable ignorance in this regard ... and there will be a great deal of discussion in the rest of the book about precisely this issue.

| Explorations |

HIV/AIDS Ambiguities

For more than thirty years, a mantra has been chanted around the world: -- namely, 'HIV causes AIDS'. 'HIV' stands for: "Human Immunodeficiency Virus", and 'AIDS" stands for: "Acquired Immune Deficiency Syndrome".

According to the theory underlying the foregoing mantra, there are two stages entailed by the disease process to which HIV and AIDS allude. In the first stage, a person somehow (e.g., infected needles, sexual activity) acquires the human immunodeficiency virus (i.e., HIV), and, in the second stage, HIV leads – in ways that are not currently understood -- to an array of diseases that, in one way or another, are expressions of a compromised immune system (i.e., AIDS).

A dim awareness of the problem first emerged in the early 1980s based on the clinical findings of Dr. Michael Gottlieb at the UCLA Medical Center. He had diagnosed a group of five men who were presenting symptoms of pneumocystis pneumonia as a result of immune systems that, for unknown reasons, seemed to be severely compromised.

The men were all gay. He coined the acronym: GRID (meaning: Gay Related Immune Deficiency), as a brief way of referring to people who were afflicted by such compromised immune systems.

A little later, evidence surfaced indicating that certain non-gay people also were exhibiting similar problems to the individuals that had been diagnosed by Dr. Gottlieb. As a result, the GRID acronym was transitioned into a more generic sounding: AIDS, that zeroed in on the underlying medical issue – that is, a compromised immune system – rather than containing any reference to sexual orientation.

Irrespective of the designation, Dr. Gottlieb had encountered evidence indicating that some unknown, new disease might be stalking humankind. As a result, in 1981 he compiled a case study on the men he had diagnosed with pneumocystis pneumonia and sent the information off to the CDC for consideration.

Not too long after receiving the material from Dr. Gottlieb, the CDC received a further 41 reports concerning a rare form of cancer, Kaposi sarcoma, that had surfaced in gay men. Once again, there was an indication that the immune systems of the individuals being described in these new cases had, for unknown reasons, become seriously dysfunctional.

Pneumocystis pneumonia and Kaposi sarcoma were indicator diseases. They were symptoms of some other underlying problem involving deficiencies in the immune system of affected individuals.

HIV had not, yet, entered the picture. However, a few years later (1983), Dr. Luc Montagnier and Dr. Françoise Barré-Sinoussi of the Pasteur Institut performed a series of experiments that, supposedly, not only demonstrated the existence of a new kind of virus but, as well, seemed to show that the virus they had discovered also caused AIDS. Furthermore, some twenty-five years later, the Nobel committee seemed to agree with them, and, as a result, in 2008 the French pair was awarded the Nobel Prize in physiology and medicine.

Dr. James Curran was Chief of the STD Division at the CDC when the case studies concerning a possible new infectious disease began to come in to the Center. He subsequently became the Director of the CDC AIDS division in 1982, and held that post until 1992 before eventually moving on to become Dean of RSPH at Emory University in 1995.

He maintained that the evidence for the idea that HIV causes AIDS is "incontrovertible". Let's reflect on this claim a little.

There are several forms of controversy surrounding the research of the two foregoing individuals (i.e., Montagnier and Barré-Sinoussi) who claimed to have discovered HIV and also allegedly found evidence indicating that HIV caused AIDS. First, Robert Gallo, an American medical doctor and researcher, also has laid some degree of claim concerning the discovery of the causal link between HIV and AIDS – a claim that has led to, among other things, litigation over issues involving discovery, priority, theft, and so on.

Whatever the nature of the foregoing controversy might be it pales in comparison with the second controversy swirling about the work of Montagnier and Barré-Sinoussi. More specifically, there might be considerable evidence to indicate that the French pair did not prove what they claimed to have done in their series of papers that were released beginning in 1983 – namely, that they had discovered a new virus, and, in addition, that this virus is the cause of AIDS.

| Explorations |

On the one hand, there are many medical doctors, research scientists, foundations, charities, academics, health/medical journals, and government agencies that have bought into, and religiously recite, the 'HIV causes AIDS' mantra. On the other hand, there are just a relatively few individuals who are claiming that not only is there no proof that HIV causes AIDS but, even more provocatively, that HIV might not exist at all.

And, then, of course, there is the little matter of the Nobel committee having awarded its prize to the two French researchers in recognition of their 'discovery' of HIV and its 'causal' role in AIDS. Surely, the Nobel committee couldn't have made such a fundamental mistake concerning the scientific significance of the research conducted by Montagnier and Barré-Sinoussi.

It might seem reasonable to suppose that the vast majority of credentialed individuals who have accepted the idea that 'HIV causes AIDS' are right, whereas the trifling group of people that seeks to argue against that theory is wrong. However, truth is not a democracy, and the majority does not necessarily get to arbitrarily determine what is, and is not, the truth ... although they often might try to accomplish precisely that objective.

The individuals who are challenging the link between HIV and AIDS are not necessarily claiming that AIDS does not exist. Their concerns tend to focus more on the alleged causal connection between HIV and AIDS.

Nevertheless, there are some very real problems and questions surrounding the meaning of AIDS. Among other things, there is a certain amount of vagueness or amorphousness permeating the idea of AIDS because it has become something of a catch-all umbrella designation under which 25, or more, clinical conditions have been placed, with no clear connection among any of these conditions except that they all involve problems, of one kind or another, with the effective functioning of the immune system.

Moreover, the idea of AIDS takes on different meanings as one travels from one country to the next. In addition, the term also has gone through a number of changes in the way that the 'professional' literature tends to define the acronym.

For example, in 1987 the CDC was responsible for several changes to the way in which AIDS was diagnosed. To begin with, a person could be given a diagnosis of AIDS without ever having had an HIV test, and, secondly, a person who had received a negative result on an HIV test could, nonetheless, still be diagnosed with AIDS if certain other conditions were present. Among other reasons, the changes were made because Alvin Friedman-Kien had come across 16 gay patients in New York City who were showing symptoms of Kaposi sarcoma and, yet, they did not show any evidence of having been infected with HIV.

In 1993, AIDS underwent a further significant change. A person could appear – at least on the surface -- quite healthy, but if that individual's CD4 count fell below 200, the person was diagnosed as having AIDS.

CD4 is a glycoprotein that is found on the membranes of cells such as macrophages and T helper cells (or white blood cells) within the immune system. These T4 cells are referred to as helper cells because they are involved with the communication of information about, and response to, threats of infection and alien invaders that might compromise the health of a human being.

Individuals with a CD4 count below 200 were believed to be vulnerable to succumbing to any number of opportunistic, infectious diseases. The CD4 count was considered to be a marker for, or indicator of, such a condition of vulnerability.

The issue, of course, was what caused the CD4 count to drop to such precarious levels. Presumably, this had something to do with the presence of an unknown – perhaps viral agent -- and the manner in which that agent compromised the immune system.

The title of the first paper (1983) by Montagnier and Barré-Sinoussi that purported to explicate the relationship between HIV and AIDS – the basis for, subsequently, being awarded a Nobel Prize – was: *'Isolation of a T-lymphotropic Retrovirus From a Patient at Risk for Acquired Immune Deficiency Syndrome (AIDS)'*. A retrovirus gets its name from the presence of the protein/enzyme reverse transcriptase that plays a key role – by transforming RNA to DNA -- in the ability of a virus to get itself multiplied using the machinery of whatever organism it is seeking to invade or infect, and, one of the key findings in the aforementioned paper was that the researchers supposedly had established the presence of reverse transcriptase proteins in the culture they were assaying using the T-lymphocyte cells of a patient who was thought to have been at risk for having AIDS.

Robert Gallo's experiments were roughly similar in general structure to those of Montagnier and Barré-Sinoussi except that he worked with a leukemic cell line known as H-9 -- rather than T-lymphocytes -- and H-9 is a clone of another cell line – namely, HUT-78, which came from a patient with T-4 leukemia – that might be caused by a retrovirus other than 'HIV' ... HTLV-I. Some researchers – such as Dr. Montagnier – believe the H-9 cell line contains a variety of different retroviruses that could muddy the waters of research. In any case, with respect to what follows, the work of Dr. Montagnier and Dr. Barré-Sinoussi will, for the most part, be featured since they are the ones who, according to a Nobel committee, first discovered HIV and its possible role in AIDS.

The two French researchers argued that the presence of the reverse transcriptase in their experimentally assayed cultures indicated the presence of a new retrovirus in their patient who was at risk for AIDS. They further hypothesized that the new retrovirus they believed they had discovered – based on the presence of reverse transcriptase -- was precisely what had put their patient at risk for developing AIDS.

However, before one can establish a causal connection between the putative retrovirus and AIDS, there are a number of issues that need to be settled in a clearly demarcated manner. For example, one must be able to demonstrate that a retrovirus is the only possible source for reverse transcriptase since if there are alternative sources for the presence of reverse transcriptase other than a retrovirus, then, one cannot be sure that the reverse transcriptase one has detected comes from a retrovirus.

As it turns out, reverse transcriptase is a common protein/enzyme that can be found in many, if not most, cells in human beings. For example, the ends of chromosomes are constructed via a process of reverse transcription, and, therefore, give expression to reverse transcriptase activity.

Furthermore, Dr. Robert Gallo (one of the alleged discoverers of the supposed link between HIV and AIDS) had indicated in a 1973 paper ('*On the Nature of the Nucleic Acids and RNA Dependent DNA Polymerase from RNA Tumor Viruses and Human Cells*') that one could induce reverse transcriptase activity in normal cells. More specifically, when one takes normal cells, places them in culture, and adds a growth agent such as PHA (phytohaemagglutinin, a mitogen derived from kidney beans that increases mitosis or cell division), then, one will be able to observe reverse transcriptase activity.

In their first experiment, the two French researchers cultured their sample from a patient who was said to be at risk for AIDS (to be precise, T-lymphocytes or T-cells were drawn from an enlarged lymph node that had been surgically removed from the neck of a gay man), and, then, they added a number of growth agents, including PHA. After 15 days, they examined the culture and found evidence of reverse transcriptase activity and attributed this to the presence of a retrovirus from the cultured blood of their patient, but their attribution was premature and, perhaps, erroneous.

The two French researchers might have detected reverse transcriptase in the cultures they were studying. Nonetheless, they had failed to demonstrate that the reverse transcriptase they found in those cultures was specific to, or caused by, the presence of a retrovirus rather than, say, the mitogenic action of the growth agent, PHA, or even the normal activity of a cell.

In a second experiment, the two French researchers placed cells from a normal donor – non-HIV/AIDS infected – together with cells from the same patient (said to be at risk for AIDS) into a culture that was augmented by various growth factors ... again, including PHA. Once more, after a period of time, the two researchers detected reverse transcriptase activity.

In this second experiment, Montagnier and Barré-Sinoussi concluded that the presence of the reverse transcriptase activity served as proof that the normal cells in the culture had become infected by the cells of their patient through the transmission of HIV. Unfortunately, the two researchers couldn't conclude what they did, with any degree of confidence, because, among other things, they had not shown that the reverse transcriptase activity they observed came from the presence of, or via the transmission of, a retrovirus.

| Explorations |

They assumed their patient had HIV because of the presence of reverse transcriptase activity. The presence of the reverse transcriptase activity was their marker for the presence of a retrovirus.

Consequently, when they mixed the allegedly infected cells with normal cells and observed reverse transcriptase activity, they assumed that this was proof that normal cells had become infected through the transmission of HIV. There were, however, problems inherent in their assumptions.

By assuming that the donor cells were normal, they believed this meant that there could be no reverse transcriptase activity that was taking place in those donor cells. Nonetheless, the two researchers were overlooking the well-established fact -- noted previously -- that normal cells also exhibit reverse transcriptase activity, and, therefore, observing reverse transcriptase activity in the mixed blood culture might mean nothing more than that the normal cells were doing what normal cells do, and this includes reverse transcriptase activity.

The baseline activity of a normal cell includes reverse transcriptase activity. The presence of PHA is also associated with the presence of reverse transcriptase activity in normal cells.

Therefore, there were two alternative explanations for the presence of reverse transcriptase activity in the mixed culture of the second experiment other than the possibility that the reverse transcriptase was due to the presence of a retrovirus. As a result, the French researchers were no more warranted in concluding that the reverse transcriptase activity observed in conjunction with the second experiment was due to the presence of HIV than they were warranted in concluding with respect to the first experiment that the presence of reverse transcriptase activity was proof of the presence of a new retrovirus in the cultured T-cell sample of their patient who was thought to be at risk of AIDS.

The whole idea of a good experiment is to rule out explanations other than one's hypothesis as the means to explain what is being observed. The foregoing two experiments did not do that.

In fact they did exactly the opposite. They introduced elements into their experimental design (e.g., the use of PHA) that compromised their belief (hypothesis) that a retrovirus was present in their cultured sample and that the retrovirus was the cause of their patient's compromised immune system.

In addition, the two French researchers had failed to establish a proper baseline that would permit them to unambiguously compare the activity of their sample culture from the patient against the activity of a normal cell. In other words, since it was known that reverse transcriptase activity is present in normal cells, the two French researchers had no way of proving that the reverse transcriptase they observed in the second experiment could only have come from a retrovirus since normal cells are capable of such activity on their own and because the growth agent, PHA, was also known to induce reverse transcriptase activity in normal cells.

Even if the two researchers had been able to establish that the only source of the reverse transcriptase in their first two experiments was the presence of a retrovirus, this would not have been sufficient to demonstrate that the retrovirus was the cause of the patient's compromised immune system. Under such contrafactual conditions, the researchers might have shown that their retrovirus had the capacity to infect normal, healthy cells, but it wouldn't necessarily follow that such a capacity was the cause of their patient's compromised immune system ... although such a finding might have been suggestive and provided direction for further research.

The third experiment described in the 1983, allegedly groundbreaking, Nobel-worthy paper by Montagnier and Barré-Sinoussi involved the use of umbilical chord lymphocytes. More specifically, the two researchers took the supernatant (liquid portion) from their second experiment and mixed it together with umbilical chord lymphocytes, and, after a set amount of time had elapsed, they once more observed evidence of reverse transcriptase activity.

They interpreted such activity as proof that material from their patient was infecting the lymphocytes from the umbilical chord. However, their interpretation failed to take into consideration some important data that already was known to the medical and scientific communities.

Umbilical chord lymphocytes originate from the placenta. Since the 1970s, researchers had known that extracellular virions – referred to as type-C particles -- are present in most, if not all, human placentas, and, in addition, there is reverse transcriptase activity associated with the presence of those kinds of particles. Consequently, the presence of viral-like particles and reverse transcriptase activity in the culture of their third experiment does not necessarily prove that both were the result of a retrovirus that had been transmitted from their patient's lymphocytes to the umbilical chord lymphocytes.

Moreover, the French researchers tended to undermine their own cause when they referred to the virus-like particles in the electron micrographs that were made in conjunction with their experiments as being typical type-C virus particles. Type-C virus particles are different from retroviruses.

If the two researchers were arguing that they had discovered a new kind of retrovirus and that this new retrovirus was the cause of AIDS, then the third experiment was inconsistent with their hypothesis. The third experiment showed the presence of type-C viral-like particles, and not necessarily the presence of a retrovirus. Furthermore, since type-C particles are associated with reverse transcriptase activity, the third experiment did not conclusively demonstrate that such activity came from a new retrovirus rather than from the normal, cellular activity of an umbilical chord lymphocyte.

Dr. Charles Dauguet -- who served as the electron microscopist in conjunction with the Montagnier and Barré-Sinoussi 1983 experiments at the Pasteur Institute -- claimed in a 2005 interview with Djamel Tahi that he did not observe any virus particles under the electron microscope when he was asked to prepare electron micrographs for the two French researchers in conjunction with their experiments. Instead, what he saw was just cellular debris.

In 1997 Dr. Hans Gelderblom, an electron microscopist (who later worked -- 1998-2004 -- at the Robert Koch Institute in Germany) was one of the authors of a paper entitled: '*Cell Membrane Vesicles Are A Major Contaminant of Gradient-Enriched Human Immunodeficiency Virus Type-1 Preparations.*' The authors had been attempting to purify HIV (i.e., nothing but HIV should be present) and discovered -- as the foregoing article title suggests -- that the membranes of the cells (the cells from which HIV was supposedly being drawn and purified) were a major contaminant in the process, and, as a result, the authors ended up with cellular debris rather than purified HIV.

The character of such cellular debris is identified through the generating of a gradient – based on molecular weight – with respect to the materials being assayed. More specifically, a centrifuge is used in the process of creating a sucrose gradient, and the spinning tends to tear cells apart, spilling their contents into the sucrose solution, and, as a result, if HIV is present, it cannot be differentiated from, and separated off from, that debris.

During an interview with Brent Leung, a Canadian documentary filmmaker, Dr. Gelderblom was asked about the electron micrographs that had been made in conjunction with the original Montagnier and Barré-Sinoussi experiment. Dr. Gelderblom indicated that one could not really clearly identify much from those electron micrographs because they were too small ... they were suggestive but they contained nothing of a definitive nature.

In the interview, Dr. Gelderblom also commented on some electron micrographs that accompanied a *Scientific American* article – '*AIDS in 1988*' -- by Dr. Robert Gallo. According to Dr. Gallo the electron micrographs displayed in his article proved the existence of HIV.

Dr. Gelderblom thought otherwise. He didn't feel the Gallo photographs were much, if at all, superior to the images he had seen in relation to the Montagnier and Barré-Sinoussi experiments, and, as a result, in his opinion, the Gallo photographs were no better able to prove the existence of HIV than the Montagnier/Barré-Sinoussi electron micrographs had been able to do.

Dr. Montagnier, himself, when interviewed by Djamel Tahi in 1997, clearly indicated that: "We found some particles, but they did not have the morphology typical of retroviruses." By "morphology" Dr. Montagnier was referring, among other things, to the knobs/spikes that supposedly were attached to the envelope surrounding the inner contents of the HIV virus and are considered to be the means through which infection is believed to be transmitted, and, yet, such knobs were not present in the viral-like particles Dr. Montagnier claimed to have observed in the electron micrographs associated with the series of experiments that he and Dr. Barré-Sinoussi had conducted in the early 1980s.

Furthermore -- although this is something of an afterthought as far as the 1983 paper by Montagnier and Barré-Sinoussi is concerned -- there was an article by Y.G. Kuznetsov ('*Atomic force microscopy investigation of human immunodeficiency virus (HIV) and HIV-infected lymphocytes*') that appeared in a 2006 edition of *Nature*, in which a possibility of some relevance to the Montagnier/Barré-Sinoussi "discovery" was advanced. More specifically, according to the 2006 *Nature* article by Kuznetsov, whatever spikes or knobs were observed via negative-staining microscopy could have been: "an artifact of the penetration of heavy metal stain between envelope proteins."

Making such a conjecture is not proof concerning the identity of what was observed. Nonetheless, the foregoing conjecture does indicate that there are a variety of lingering questions swirling about the problem of establishing the definitive nature of what had been seen in lymphocytes supposedly infected with HIV.

Another electron microscopy study by Ping Zhu et al (published in *Nature*) compared the knobs/spikes of SIV (simian – monkey -- immunodeficiency virus) with what was said to be an exemplar of the HIV retrovirus. While the electron micrographs of the SIV showed many knobs and spikes (the means through which a virus supposedly infects its target), the "evidence" for knobs/spikes on the alleged HIV retrovirus was so miniscule that the authors referred to them as "putative knobs" – that is, it was possible knobs/spikes were present in the alleged HIV retrovirus but, if present, they were hard to detect, and, in addition, similar "objects" could be seen in regions of the electron micrograph that were unconnected to virion particles.

No electron micrographs (pictures) appeared in the 1983 paper by Montagnier and Barré-Sinoussi. The foregoing admissions and considerations tend to indicate why this might have been the case since the electron micrograph evidence that did exist did not appear to support their hypothesis.

According to the HIV theory of AIDS, a virus begins to infect its target by first fusing with the membrane of the latter cell. Dr. Robert Gallo -- one of the alleged architects of the HIV causes AIDS theory -- said during an interview with Brent Leung that not only didn't he (Dr. Gallo) understand the nature of that fusion process, but, as well, he didn't think that anybody else really understood it either. But, if no one understands the nature of the process through which HIV supposedly infects a cell, then, how does one know that HIV causes AIDS?

According to the HIV theory of AIDS, HIV targets a population of lymphocytes called CD4 helper T-cells. By lowering the number of CD4 helper T-cells, HIV paves the way for AIDS to emerge.

Yet, in the September 2007 edition of the *Journal of Immunology*, a team of researchers at the Tulane National Primate Research Center presented evidence in an article that the onset of AIDS is not necessarily brought about by a loss of T-cells. If this is the case, then one of the essential components of the 'HIV causes AIDS' theory (at least as currently understood) has been removed from the equation.

There are many researchers and medical doctors who believe that the basic 'HIV causes AIDS' theory needs augmentation. In other words, they believe that while HIV does eliminate CD4 helper T-cells, and this set of events plays a role in the onset of AIDS, nonetheless, there need to be other co-factors that are present in order for the immune system to be severely compromised in a manner that is typical of AIDS.

In other words, they believe that by itself the loss of CD4 helper T-cells is not enough to trigger the onset of AIDS. Nevertheless, the identity of these other co-factors remains rather elusive.

Moreover, if the aforementioned 2007 *Journal of Immunology* article is correct and the loss of T-cells does not necessarily lead to the onset of AIDS, then, one might question whether, or not, one even needs the HIV component in a theory of AIDS. In fact, given that Montagnier and Barré-Sinoussi never actually demonstrated (and the previous discussion lays the basis for such a contention) they had isolated a new retrovirus or that their 'new' virus had the capacity to infect healthy, normal cells and destroy them, then, one wonders what the evidence is that proves that HIV causes AIDS.

Moreover, there is considerable evidence indicating that the 'HIV causes AIDS' theory might not be true. (1) The electron micrographs (from Montagnier/Barré-Sinoussi and Gallo) that allegedly depict the presence of HIV are inconclusive, if not suspect. (2) The three experiments that were carried out by Montagnier and Barré-Sinoussi and were described in their 1983 paper do not necessarily prove what

| Explorations |

the two French researchers claim with respect to those experiments. (3) Despite the attempts of Dr. Gelderblom and others, no one has been able to produce a purified form of HIV ... in other words the attempts at purification become contaminated by cellular debris generated during the process of attempted purification. (4) The loss of T-cells does not automatically lead to the onset of AIDS. (5) No one knows what combination of HIV – assuming that it actually exists -- and co-factors results in AIDS.

When Dr. David Baltimore -- a co-discoverer of the reverse transcriptase enzyme and a Nobel laureate in Physiology and Medicine -- was asked by Brent Leung about how he (the doctor) would isolate and generate electron micrographs in relation to HIV, Dr. Baltimore seemed to become irritated by the question. He indicated that Gallo already had done all of that and that he (Dr. Baltimore) didn't want to become someone's textbook concerning such matters.

Yet, Robert Gallo hadn't already done what Dr. Baltimore was alluding to, nor had Montagnier and Barré-Sinoussi. Nobody had.

What is troubling is that Dr. Baltimore – a Nobel laureate – didn't seem to understand this ... any more than the Nobel committee seemed to understand what was not actually understood about the 'HIV causes AIDS' theory, for which the committee awarded a prestigious prize concerning work that didn't really seem to deserve such recognition. Dr. Baltimore, like many other scientists and researchers in the HIV matter, were basing his judgments concerning HIV and AIDS on assumptions that weren't necessarily true.

There are a few other considerations that can be added to the foregoing ones indicating that HIV might not cause AIDS. First, as stated earlier in this section of the chapter, Alvin Friedman-Kien presented evidence in the 1980s that 16 men had been diagnosed with Kaposi sarcoma – a rare disease that, along with pneumocystis pneumonia, had been the first warning signs of a possible new infectious disease being reported to the CDC.

Yet, none of those 16 individuals were infected with HIV. If HIV were the cause of AIDS, then why didn't these patients show any signs of having been infected with HIV?

| Explorations |

Secondly, it turned out that the early cases of pneumocystis pneumonia and Kaposi sarcoma -- that had set off the warning bells at the CDC concerning the possibility of a new infectious disease -- were not necessarily the result of HIV. Rather, the culprit seemed to be linked to the excessive use of amyl nitrate (sometimes known as "poppers" because one popped open ampoules in order to sniff their contents) that were widely being used in the gay community.

Amyl Nitrate, when used extensively, had a toxic capacity to destroy the pulmonary immune system of an individual. Under such circumstances, individuals could become vulnerable to opportunistic diseases like pneumocystis pneumonia.

Moreover, there were reports that the incidence of Kaposi sarcoma apparently went down as the use of poppers and other sources of amyl nitrate declined. In addition, it was later discovered that Kaposi sarcoma is tied to a virus other than HIV – namely, human herpes virus, strain 8 -- so, again, one couldn't necessarily conclude that HIV led to such diseases as Kaposi sarcoma.

The drug being used to treat HIV/AIDS in the early stages of the "epidemic" also muddied the waters concerning the nature of the alleged link between HIV and AIDS. More specifically, AZT [3'-Azido-3'-Deoxythymidine (Azidothymidine)] was the drug of choice, but its activity was like a shotgun approach to treatment because it disrupted a lot of biological processes – both normal and otherwise. Peter Duesberg – who, almost from the very beginning, did not accept the idea that HIV causes AIDS (he believed that HIV was a harmless "passenger virus" linked, in some way, with the unknown cause of AIDS) – described AZT as "AIDS by prescription" since the impact of the drug on human beings compromised their immune systems.

When people tested positive for HIV, they were often prescribed AZT. Since the 'HIV causes AIDS' meme dominated the thinking of clinicians, when the patients who were taking AZT began to become progressively sicker and died, everyone attributed the downturn to the incredibly deadly and destructive nature of HIV/AIDS.

In point of fact, people were dying from the treatment and not necessarily because they had tested positive for HIV. Since everyone expected the immune systems of people who had tested positive for HIV to be compromised over time, clinicians mistook the effects of AZT for the effects of HIV ... erroneous beliefs about the latter masked the real-life impact of the former.

Christine Maggiore was tested for HIV in 1992. Her test came out positive.

Following her positive test, she began to work with a group called 'Woman At Risk'. She said there were 11 people, including her, who served on the board of directors for that organization.

Eight of those board members were taking AZT. Three of the women, including Christine Maggiore, were not taking AZT.

All of the women had tested positive for HIV. The people who were taking AZT died. The people who were not taking AZT lived.

If one is a believer in the 'HIV causes AIDS' theory, one probably could come up with all manner of ways to explain away the foregoing data. Nevertheless, such alternative explanations do not constitute proof of anything ... they are merely possibilities that would have to be more rigorously pursued to determine if there was any truth to such accounts with respect to the issue of what actually happened in the matter of the Women At Risk board members.

Moreover, when one juxtaposes Christine Maggiore's story next to the considerable evidence that brings the idea of 'HIV causes AIDS' into question, then attempts to rationalize or offer alternative accounts of what happened to the aforementioned board members can be seen for what they likely are. Those alternative accounts seem to give expression to the desire of true believers to hold on to their belief system in the face of evidence that strongly indicates those beliefs might be incorrect. Unfortunately, all too many true believers are quite prepared to fight to the death of their last patient in an attempt to avoid coming to appropriate conclusions concerning their worldview.

Dr. Daniel Kuritzkes (Associate Professor of Medicine, Harvard Medical School) said something that a lot of clinicians might have thought after the fact. He said: "I think in retrospect, the dosage that we began with ... with AZT was a dangerous and poorly tolerated dose."

However, the dosage issue might have only been a relatively small – though significant -- dimension of the problem. The real sin of the medical establishment might have been its hubris in assuming that it knew with what they were dealing when it came to AIDS and, nevertheless, prescribed a toxic drug to handle a situation that they did not necessarily understand.

A breakthrough, of sorts, in the treatment of HIV/AIDS seemed to emerge in the mid 1990s. For instance, *Time Magazine's* 'Man of the Year' in 1996 was Dr. David Ho.

Dr. Ho had helped put together a new form of retrovirus treatment – referred to as "the cocktail". The treatment combined various protease inhibitors (enzymes that inhibit the breakdown of proteins into smaller chains of polypeptides and/or amino acids) with traditional forms of chemotherapy, including AZT.

While individuals taking the cocktail seemed to fare better – at least for a short period – nonetheless, eventually, many of those individuals died, as well, due to various complications involving their immune systems. Moreover, there were a variety of side effects associated with long-term usage of 'the cocktail' that sometimes overshadowed whatever benefits might have ensued from its use.

Almost all, if not all, HIV/AIDS drugs carry a black box label. This is the FDA's way of informing potential users (whether through prescription or being administered such drugs) that a variety of serious side effects have been reported in conjunction with taking those drugs.

Notwithstanding the problems associated with the treatment of HIV/AIDS that were inducing people to mistake the destructive impact that those treatments had on human biology for the supposedly deadly nature of HIV/AIDS, there was other evidence that suggested researchers and clinicians might not have understood either HIV or AIDS – but especially HIV. For instance, *Life Magazine* shouted out from the cover of its July 1985 edition: '*Now No One is Safe From AIDS*', and, as indicated earlier, David Ho was Time Magazine's 'Man of the Year' for the role he played in developing new ways of treating HIV/AIDS. Yet, nonetheless, in June of 2008, The World Health Organization (WHO) issued a report that, among other things, claimed heterosexuals were not likely to become the victims of a worldwide HIV/AIDS pandemic.

| Explorations |

The timing of the report was somewhat ironic since a few months later, Montagnier and Barré-Sinoussi received the Nobel Prize for their discovery of HIV and its supposed causal role in AIDS. What is even more puzzling, is that eleven years earlier, in 1997, *The American Journal of Epidemiology* ran an article by a group of researchers, headed by Nancy Padian (who was the Director of International Research for the AIDS Research Institute at the San Francisco campus of the University of California) that, along with other research, pointed in the direction of the conclusions that were expressed in the aforementioned 2008 WHO report.

The study described in the 1997 article covered a period of ten years (and, therefore, started two years after the aforementioned shocking lead story on the cover of *Life* magazine) during which the HIV transmission rate of heterosexual individuals was quantified. To determine transmission rates, the researchers, first, recruited people who had tested positive for HIV, then next, the sexual partners of those recruits were asked to participate in the study, and, finally, the incidence of HIV in the partners was recorded over a ten-year period.

Surprisingly – perhaps shockingly – not one of the sexual partners of the individuals who had tested positive for HIV subsequently tested positive for HIV. This either suggested that HIV was a lot more difficult to transmit than previously had been believed to be the case (and this was the conclusion of Nancy Padian and her colleagues), or, perhaps, there were some other factors at play.

For example, testing positive for HIV might not mean what some people claimed it meant. In other words, a positive test does not necessarily constitute proof that the Human Immunodeficiency Virus is present in an individual.

HIV test kits are based on the premise that they are capable of detecting certain kinds of antibodies. However, the criteria used to determine what constitutes detection – as well as what exactly is being detected – tend to vary from manufacturer to manufacturer.

Antibodies are proteins that arise through the interaction of certain kinds of B-lymphocytes with some given antigen (foreign or otherwise) that induces an immune response (i.e., the interaction). The interaction causes the B-lymphocytes to differentiate into plasma cells

| Explorations |

that generate the proteins that become the antibodies for the foregoing response/interaction.

When a HIV test is conducted, the blood of the person being tested is introduced to (mixed with) certain proteins that are a key part of the testing protocol. The proteins contained in the kit are believed to be unique to HIV, so, if a person's blood reacts to those proteins via antibodies already present in that person's blood, then the detection of the antibodies (via a color change in the test kit), is interpreted as being an indication of the presence of HIV.

There are, at least, two problems with the foregoing perspective. Firstly, no one has demonstrated that the proteins contained in the kits are, indeed, unique to HIV – especially in the light of the fact that no one has been able to produce a purified version of HIV so that researchers could determine what components (enzymes, envelope proteins, RNA, etc.) actually make up HIV. Secondly, the fact that some of the antibodies in a person's blood responds to those proteins does not necessarily mean that HIV is present in the person being tested because antibodies are not always specific to a given antigen.

A given antibody might interact with a range of antigens (The term "antigen" is an abbreviated contraction of "antibody generating"). The fact that the presence of a given antigen – say the proteins in a HIV kit test tube or container – gives rise to a detectable response (e.g., color change), does not necessarily mean that the antibody (or antibodies) that are reacting with the proteins in the test kit is (are) an indication that those antibodies originally arose as a result of having interacted with HIV.

The type of antibody or antibodies that are reacting to the proteins in the HIV test kit might have been generated through any number of previous B-lymphocyte-antigen interactions Consequently, the reason why those antibodies are reacting to the test kit proteins is actually not necessarily known – even if one were to suppose that the test kit proteins had been proven to be unique to HIV (which is not the case).

Many people believe that HIV test kits prove the existence of HIV. After all, why would the proteins in the test kit – which, supposedly, are unique to HIV -- induce the antibodies in the person being tested to react to those test kit proteins if the antibodies had not originally arisen in connection with an encounter involving HIV?

The foregoing reasoning is circular, and, as well, it is predicated on faulty assumptions. The circularity of the reasoning is entailed by the fact that the test presupposes the existence of HIV and, therefore, it is believed that any change in the test kit indicator proves the existence of what has been presupposed by the test.

However, the presupposition on which such tests are based is, itself, suspect. More specifically, as previously indicated, there is no proof that the proteins contained in the test kit are unique to HIV, and, in addition, there is no proof that the antibodies in the blood that react to those test kit proteins originally arose as a result of having come in contact with HIV antigens or that the reason why the antibodies are reacting with the test kit proteins has anything to do with HIV.

According to people such as Dr. Robert Gallo – one of the earliest proponents of the 'HIV causes AIDS' theory – when the HIV test is done properly, there is a very low margin of error associated with the test. However, there is nothing to prove that what he is saying is true ... in other words, there is no independent means of establishing that the HIV tests do what people claim they do or that the HIV tests can serve as a reliable surrogate marker for the existence of HIV.

There are a variety of tests that allegedly screen for the presence of HIV. For instance, ELISA and Western blot are two standard HIV tests.

If one gets a positive result from ELISA, one, supposedly, is able to confirm the positive result by following up with a Western blot. Unfortunately, both tests are rooted in the same kind of circular thinking and problematic assumptions that have been outlined previously, and, consequently, the Western blot doesn't so much confirm the existence of HIV – if it does result in a positive result -- as it confirms the existence of the same sort of assumptions and biases that underlie both tests.

The Western blot test is not an independent confirmation of the presence of HIV because -- even if the test is somewhat different from ELISA -- it is, nonetheless, still based on the same underlying idea of antibody responses that ELISA is. Since antibody responses are not

| Explorations |

necessarily accurate indicators for the presence of HIV, neither ELISA nor the Western blot tests are necessarily reliable means for the detection, or proof, of HIV ... those tests might give expression to positive results, but the meaning of those results is cloaked with the mists of ambiguity that have been described over the last several pages.

In 1997, the journal, *Virology*, published an article written by, among others, Julian W. Bess. The title of the article was: '*Gel electrophoresis separation of proteins in non-infected and infected cultures.*'

The authors of the article concluded that the proteins they found in the assayed cultures -- which had been separated out and differentiated, through the process of gel electrophoresis (a voltage is applied to a gel and the electric field sends proteins through the gel at different speeds and, thereby, separates them out as a function of molecular weight) -- were essentially the same in both the allegedly infected cultures, as well as in the non-infected cultures. If the proteins in both cultures were the same, then there was no evidence (i.e., different proteins) to indicate that a new retrovirus of some kind – for example, HIV – was present.

However, one of the people who reviewed the article prior to its being accepted for publication suggested that the authors change the designation for a picture of some of the proteins they found in one of the separated bands generated by gel electrophoresis and label those proteins, instead, as HIV proteins. The authors complied with the suggestion and when the primary author Julian Bess was asked about the suggested change, he indicated that the reviewer had been right to make the suggestion.

The problem is that the researchers/authors already had stipulated in their article that they had come across no evidence in the experiment being described in the article to indicate that the re-labeled proteins in the separated band at issue were actually HIV proteins. So, one wonders on what basis the primary author was claiming that the reviewer had been right to indicate that the proteins in question were actually HIV proteins and, therefore, the labeling for the photograph of the band should be altered.

In a communication with the Perth Group in Australia -- who were, and are, of the opinion that there is no evidence that HIV caused AIDS and, therefore, were asking how the labeling of certain proteins as HIV proteins had come about in the 1997 *Virology* article -- Julian Bess said that the labeling had been at the suggestion of one of the article's reviewers who said he (the reviewer) "felt it would help orient readers when looking at the figure ...", and, then, Julian Bess went on to say in the same communication: "We did not determine the identities of the bands in this particular gel."

If the identities of the proteins in the bands had not been established, then, why refer to them as HIV proteins? Maybe those entities were HIV proteins and maybe they were not, but the truth of the matter is that according to the researchers of the experiment on which the article was based, their experiment had not generated any evidence to warrant referring to the proteins in the gradient bands as being HIV proteins.

Indeed, all of the proteins in the two cultures ("infected" and uninfected') were the same according to the Bess article. In order for there to have been evidence indicating the presence of a retrovirus, there would have had to have been some proteins in the "infected culture" that were not present in the uninfected cultures ... but the 1997 Bess experiment that was eventually published in *Virology* indicated this was not the case.

How does relabeling a figure help orient readers if the relabeling is not warranted on the basis of the evidence that was available to both the researchers and the reviewer? This is not helping to orient a reader, but is, instead, a process of framing things for the reader in a possibly distorted, if not incorrect manner.

I don't know which is more disturbing: (1) That a reviewer made a suggestion that would introduce something into an article despite the fact that the experiment on which the article was based had indicated there was no evidence that would justify such a suggestion, or (2) that the authors of the article were prepared to accept such a suggestion even though it flew in the face of the evidence generated by their own experiment. This seems like a 'lose-lose' situation.

The foregoing considerations aside, one might also point out that Jerome Bess conducted another experiment in which a number of the

| Explorations |

so-called HIV proteins were measured to be between 160 and 292 nanometers in size. Since the lentivirus (of which the retrovirus is a subfamily) tend to be between 100-120 nanometers (and possibly smaller), the morphological property of size alone tends to eliminate some of the particles in this second Bess study from being identified as HIV proteins because such relatively large proteins would not be able to fit into a lentivirus size virion.

Based on a variety of observations and experiments, a possible model of the hypothesized HIV retrovirus has been developed, consisting of a cone-shaped genome and nine proteins. However, the putative model is drawn from studying the remnants of gradient separation experiments in which particles are separated off from one another through a process that combines the action of a centrifuge with the capacity of a medium (e.g., sucrose) to 'capture' or differentially fix particles of various molecular weights in separate bands of the gradient medium.

The force of the centrifuge tends to lyse (i.e., to open up and break apart) the cells being spun. As a result the contents of the lysed cells spill into the medium being used to help establish or help generate a gradient based on differential molecular weights.

The nine remnants that have turned up from such gradient studies have been labeled: gp160, gp120, p66 (reverse transcriptase), p55, p51, gp41, p32, p24, and p18 (the designation "gp" in the foregoing list of particles stands for 'glycoprotein'). The numbers refer to the different, relative molecular weights of the particles that were found in the gradient solutions, but molecular weight, by itself, is not necessarily sufficient to identify what the foregoing particles are – e.g., proteins of roughly the same molecular weight can have very different properties, and, so, molecular weight, by itself, does not necessarily tell one with what protein one is dealing.

The Montagnier/Barré-Sinoussi experiments that were the basis of their 1983 paper involved the 'discovery' of only one of the foregoing particulates in their cultures – namely, p24 (it originally had been designated as p25 by Montagnier and Barré-Sinoussi, but was subsequently changed to p24 as a result of further measurement and research). Since 1983 most HIV/AIDS researchers have come to agree that p24 is not a reverse transcriptase protein, and, therefore, p24

| Explorations |

141

could not have been the source of whatever reverse transcriptase activity the two French authors had observed in their experimental cultures.

Moreover, there are a number of questions surrounding whether any of the aforementioned nine remnants actually give expression to HIV components in particular rather than merely constitute different kinds of cellular debris that arise from the process of being centrifuged that brings about lysis of the cultured cells. According to the experimental findings of Hans Gelderblom, Julian Bess, and others (previously cited), none of the foregoing nine remnants were definitively identified as having come from an HIV retrovirus rather than from cells that have been torn apart through centrifugal forces.

Furthermore, it is possible that p120 and p160 (two of the alleged proteins of the HIV retrovirus) are merely conglomerates of the smaller subunit gp41. According to Pinter, Honnen, Tilley, et al -- authors of a 1989 article (*'Oligomeric structure of gp41, the transmembrane protein of human immunodeficiency virus type I'*) appearing in the *Journal of Virology* -- p120 might consist of 3 p41 particles linked together, whereas p160 could be made up of 4 gp41 units.

Whether, or not, the foregoing considerations are correct, one is still left with the realization – previously noted -- that none of the alleged nine proteins of HIV have been conclusively identified as being components of an actual HIV retrovirus. In fact, the title of the foregoing article is somewhat misleading because an assumption is being made that what is being assayed is an HIV retrovirus rather than merely the cellular debris that had been created through the centrifuge portion of the experiment.

One gradient band of considerable interest to many people studying HIV and AIDS is found at 1.16 grams per milliliter because, among other things, Montagnier and Barré-Sinoussi had detected reverse transcriptase activity at that band. As a result, some researchers (Gallo, Montagnier, etc.) refer to the material found in that band as being HIV RNA.

However, some researchers (e.g., the Perth Group in Australia) believe that the material being referred to by, among others, Montagnier, Barré-Sinoussi, and Gallo as 'HIV RNA' is nothing more than a form of RNA called: "adenine rich RNA". As early as 1972, Dr. Robert Gallo had known from his own research that the RNA found in the 1.16 g/ml gradient band was not necessarily specific to retroviruses but could be a function of the activity of any cell that synthesizes proteins.

Furthermore, Hans Gelderblom, one of the foremost experts on the electron microscopy of retroviruses, referred to the electron micrographs of the density gradient material in the 1.16 g/ml bands as being 80% dirt (and this figure might understate the actual situation). It consisted largely of cellular microvesicles, and, as well, was devoid of any of the morphological properties one would expect to see in an infectious lentivirus (the subfamily to which retroviruses belong) such as knobs/spikes, lateral bodies, or a cone-shaped genome.

Neither Gallo nor Montagnier/Barré-Sinoussi was ever able to definitively identify the material found in the 1.16 g/ml band as being from HIV retroviruses. Moreover, as noted earlier, none of the putative 'proteins' found in various gradient bands could be identified conclusively as being from an HIV retrovirus, and, also, as indicated previously in conjunction with the Kuznetsov article, the so-called knobs/spikes on the envelopes observed by some researchers might only be artifacts of a staining process rather than the means through which the alleged virus would be able to infect cells.

Since the immune systems of various patients do become severely compromised, there is an evidential basis for talking about AIDS. The question, then, becomes: How was that immune deficiency syndrome acquired?

As outlined in the previous, extended discussion of HIV/AIDS, there is, on the one hand, actually very little reliable, conclusive evidence to prove that HIV is the means through which AIDS is acquired. On the other hand, there is considerable evidence that has been gathered which stands in opposition to the notion that HIV is the cause of AIDS.

A wide variety of people – professional and otherwise – talk about the AIDS pandemic that is said to have swept over Africa during the last 35 years. Now, while it might be the case that many people in Africa are dying from compromised immune system, there is at least

| Explorations |

one alternative account – other than HIV – that could explain those deaths – namely, poverty.

People who are poor often tend to be malnourished. Malnutrition has been demonstrated to be a major contributing factor to the compromising of an immune system since the bodies of poor people do not receive the nourishment needed to support a healthy immune system and, as a result, 'things fall apart'.

People who are poor often live in squalid conditions where open sewage, flies, and food intermingle. People who are poor often do not have access to clean drinking water. People who are poor usually do not have access to regular medical care.

People who are poor often die from contracting opportunistic diseases. Opportunistic diseases are those maladies that are able to infiltrate bodies through compromised immune system, establish themselves because compromised immune system can't properly resist them, and, in time – sometimes acutely and sometimes chronically -- wreak havoc on the bodies of the unfortunate.

People who are poor might be diagnosed with AIDS. However, such a diagnosis does not necessarily mean that those individuals have arrived at their condition of AIDS via HIV infections.

Poor people in Africa might present symptoms of: (1) significant weight loss (at least 10% of body weight); chronic diarrhea (lasting for a month or more); (3) coughs that persisted for a month, or more; and/or (4) long lasting fevers of either a persistent or recurrent nature. After the early 1980s, such individuals often were diagnosed with AIDS.

While the assumption was frequently made in the post-1983 era that such cases of AIDS were the result of a previous HIV infection, the condition of AIDS in those patients might have come about in any number of ways that were rooted in, among other things, poverty rather than HIV. Indeed, there was absolutely no independent proof that any of the people in Africa who were being diagnosed with AIDS had been infected with HIV.

The 'HIV causes AIDS' meme became the focus of a huge, worldwide public relations campaign that, over time, became nurtured with the added growth factor of hundreds of billions of dollars of

| Explorations |

funding from government agencies (both national and international), charitable foundations, and pharmaceutical companies. However, it was a campaign rooted in an unsubstantiated ideology that was seeking to infect those whose critical faculties suffered from their own species of immune deficiency syndrome in the form of an inability to fight off an opportunistic and toxic belief system in which the issue of truth didn't seem to matter at all.

If someone came along today and was able to definitively prove not only that HIV existed, but, as well, that it caused AIDS, this would not alter the character of what has happened over the past 30-plus years. During that period of time, thousands of credentialed individuals have used advanced technologies and various sophisticated protocols to engage in a process that is not really so much science as it is a counterfeit of science ... and, therefore, not science at all.

To be sure, there have been some individuals who pursued the scientific process in a rigorous, critical fashion and were prepared to go wherever the evidence permitted them to go. Such individuals did care about the truth, but, unfortunately, there were all too many so-called 'professional' researchers, clinicians, academics, government officials, and journalists who were interested in conforming to a set of standards that were not really scientific in any meaningful sense. Such individuals might have referred to themselves -- and been referred to -- as "scientists," but, in truth, they were just empty lab coats.

If Montagnier, Barré-Sinoussi, and Gallo were all suddenly vindicated by someone who actually did some real science with respect to the conjectures of those three individuals that HIV caused AIDS, this wouldn't alter the fact that the processes the aforementioned individuals described through their articles back in period between 1983-1985 were sloppy, poorly conceived experiments that did not necessarily support the conclusions they were drawing. Their 'hunches' or intuitions concerning the relationship between HIV and AIDS eventually might be proven to be correct [the best (??) case scenario], but those individuals did not prove this was the case through scientific means back in the early-to-mid-1980s.

Those three individuals did some experiments, and they wrote some articles. However, science was largely absent from the technical character of the details that gave expression to what they were doing.

Science was also missing in action with respect to the thousands of credentialed individuals who uncritically accepted the claims of the foregoing three individuals. There might have been many reasons for such credentialed individuals proceeding as they did, but little of it was based on science as a process of being able to uncover, establish, and substantiate the truth concerning some given conjecture, hypothesis, or theory.

In the introduction to this book, I mentioned the lecture given by C.P. Snow that gave rise to the notion of the 'two cultures' issue – science and humanities – in which neither culture seemed to understand the other one. As I indicated in the introduction, I believe the only culture that matters is the one in which concern for the truth is pre-eminent.

The exploration of the Burzynski affair earlier in this chapter, together with the critical reflection on the issue of SSRIs that took place in the following section, along with the present section's commentary concerning the relation, if any, between HIV and AIDS all provide evidence indicating that credentialed individuals are capable of allowing their thinking processes to be corrupted in a variety of ways and, as a result, they permit themselves to wander away from the principles and methods of real science. However, more important than the issue of whether, or not, one should label certain activities as scientific, is whether, or not, one can label those activities as being essentially truth-seeking in nature because there are many things done in the name of science that have little, or nothing, to do with the truth.

The culture of science is as rife with ideologues as is the culture of humanities. The culture of science is as corruptible as is the culture of humanities.

The nature of reality is neither a function of science nor of the humanities but is, instead, a function of whatever set of experiences help lead to discovering the truth. The challenge of Final Jeopardy is about trying to establish the best means of seeking and, to whatever extent is possible, realizing such truth.

Observation is not enough ... the data is not enough ... experiment is not enough. One has to have insight into what is being observed. One has to be able to listen to the data and understand what it is actually saying. One has to be able to interpret experience correctly. One has to be able to ask the right questions. One has to be able to grasp the logical and structural character of relationships. One has to be willing to acknowledge the shortcomings of one's hermeneutic and develop a sense for what needs to be done to improve the extent to which one's understanding is in compliance with, or reflective of, experiential data.

Science doesn't necessarily lead one to the truth ... but it can help place one in a position to have an opportunity to grasp parts of the truth if one is able to understand what the results of scientific methodology are telling one about the nature of experience. On the other hand, all experience has the potential to put one in a position to provide opportunities for grasping aspects of the truth if one can manage to have understanding and reality merge horizons with one another.

Understanding must reflect reality – not just in terms of surface features, but in deeper ways as well. To whatever extent the mirror of understanding reflects the nature of reality, then, one might be in a good position to write down one's response to the Final Jeopardy challenge of life.

However, we often are in a better position to say what reality is not than what it is. In fact, our response to the Final Jeopardy challenge might be stated more in terms of removing things that are likely to obscure or distort the process of trying to mirror reality than the Final Jeopardy response is a matter of being able to assert, in some definitive fashion, what the nature of reality is.

The Final Jeopardy challenge is not necessarily about establishing what the nature of reality ultimately is. Rather, that challenge is about discovering what the available evidence permits one to justifiably say about what makes the phenomenology of experience have the character or properties that it does.

Responding to the Final Jeopardy challenge might be a bit like the way Michelangelo reportedly described his method for generating the sculpture of David. Michelangelo indicated that he took away whatever didn't belong.

| Explorations |

Trying to understand the nature of reality is a lot like trying to produce a sculpture in Michelangelo's sense. We try to remove whatever does not belong – the falsehoods – in order to attempt to better grasp the form that remains.

Of course, we might never be in a position to remove everything that needs to be removed from the process of sculpting our understanding. However, at the end of our lives, we hope that the hermeneutical sculpture with which we end up is capable of being a reasonable facsimile for the nature of reality.

Part of the problem with the whole enterprise of trying to learn how to sculpt understanding in the foregoing fashion is that there are all too many people who are prepared to try to impose the ideologies of science on people (as was illustrated through the Burzynski, SSRI, and HIV/AIDS discussions of this chapter) rather than assist individuals to become active, constructively functioning participants in the culture of truth. The present book is directed toward – hopefully -- the latter possibility and not the former one.

One's response to the Final Jeopardy challenge should be one's own. However, that response also should be rooted in truth – to whatever extent this is possible – but the truth cannot always be found through the cultures of science or the humanities.

The culture of truth requires something different, something more, even if, at certain points, there might be some degree of overlap with various dimensions entailed by the cultures of science and the humanities. In many, if not most, respects, the nature of reality lies beyond both the cultures of science and the humanities, and to the extent that this is the case, one's Final Jeopardy response needs to be somewhat of an interstitial character ... found – perhaps -- within the cracks and shadows that lie outside, and beneath, and between both the cultures of science and the humanities.

| Explorations |

| Explorations |

Chapter 2: The Evolutionary Landscape

Setting the Stage

Perhaps, nothing is uttered by most scientists and many non-scientists with a greater sense of certainty these days than that life is a function of, and arose due to, the process of evolution. However, like the meme that "HIV causes AIDS", the meme that "life is caused by evolution" might not be the slam-dunk that so many people appear to suppose is the case, and, furthermore, as with the "HIV causes AIDS" meme, such certainty is often rooted in ignorance about the underlying nature of what is being said with such alleged certitude.

More than 150 years ago, Charles Darwin conjectured that every modality of life that exists, or has existed, or will come to exist on (and in) the Earth has descended from one primordial life form. Approximately 113 years later Theodosius Dobzhansky, an evolutionary geneticist, wrote an essay for the March 1973 edition of the *American Biology Teacher* that bore the title: 'Nothing in Biology Makes Sense Except in the Light of Evolution."

A similar statement had surfaced nine years earlier in another piece by Dobzhansky that appeared in the 1964 edition of *The American Zoologist*. The title of that article was *'Biology – Molecular and Organismic.'*

Although Dobzhansky was a Christian in the tradition of Russian Orthodoxy, he also became a world-renowned evolutionary biologist who advocated a form of theistic evolution that he believed should be developed through the principles of science rather than received through the pages of scripture. According to him, the Bible, the Qur'an and other books of sacred teachings were very useful when it came to exploring the relationship between human beings and God, but those same works should not be, and -- according to him -- were never intended to be, treatises on science.

Echoing Darwin, Dobzhansky was committed to the idea that life arises via an evolutionary process that depends on the woof and warp of (a) unified principles of biological dynamics being intermingled with (b) different patterns of diversity. He believed that the Divine juxtaposing of biological principles of unity and diversity were what enabled evolution to make sense of the vast array of biological data that, otherwise, would remain as, apparently, disparate pieces of information.

One could point out in passing, however, that the property of being 'disparate pieces of information' is a rather relative notion. The biological information that Dobzhansky believes would be disparate if the theory of evolution were not true could still make a great deal of sense if it were considered from some other perspective, and the fact Dobzhansky has not grasped the nature of such a perspective doesn't mean that unity and diversity couldn't give expression to a mode of reality other than the evolutionary one championed by Dobzhansky.

In the aforementioned *American Biology Teacher* article, Dobzhansky stated: "I am a creationist and an evolutionist. Evolution is God's, or Nature's, method of creation. Creation is not an event that happened in 4004 BC; it is a process that began some 10 billion years ago and is still under way." As Dobzhansky pointed out in his article, it was not scripture (either Biblical or Quranic) that put forth the figure of 4004 BC as fixing the beginning of life on Earth but, rather, a 17th century figure, Bishop James Ussher, who, apparently for good measure, also specified in a 1658 publication that the great event of Creation took place between the night of October 22nd and the following day of October 23rd ... possibly feeling that specificity might be construed as an indication that his pronouncement was giving expression to the 'gospel truth'.

A contemporary of Bishop Ussher, Sir John Lightfoot -- Vice-Chancellor of Cambridge University – came to the same general conclusions as Ussher did but added that the time of the Creation event was 9:00 A.M. Moreover, Sir John apparently came to those conclusions 14 years earlier than Bishop Ussher had been able to do.

Now, as preposterous, amusing, or amazing (take your pick) as the foregoing calculations might seem, one cannot necessarily attribute the attempt to come up with precise answers to difficult questions as a function of the ignorance of 17th century scholars. After all, in an exercise of calculation that is an attempt to be even more precise than Ussher and Lightfoot had been, Nobel Laureate, Steven Weinberg, had a book published in 1977 entitled: *The First Three Minutes* in which he sought to explain what was transpiring in the universe from about 10⁻

^{32} seconds (the end of the Planck epoch) through the next 2 minutes, 59 seconds-plus seconds following the Big Bang.

What happened prior to the 10^{-32} second mark is said to be something of a mystery because, according to many modern scientists, the laws of physics apparently were in disarray during that period of time. The idea that the laws of physics were in some sort of chaotic, broken down state in the time before the 10^{-32} mark is a long-winded euphemism for ignorance.

If we don't know what the status of the universe was prior to 10^{-32} seconds ... if we don't know what laws of physics, if any, were operable prior to that time ... if we don't know how the laws of physics suddenly became operational in the transitional period leading up to the 10^{-32} second mark, then, in some ways, the intriguing calculations of Steven Weinberg are every bit as contentious as are the calculations of Bishop Ussher and Sir John Lightfoot. All three of the foregoing individuals were trying to provide something of a temporal timeline or perspective according to what was considered to be the 'best' evidence available to each of them, but all three accounts leave much to be desired.

While the alleged nature of the unfolding of the universe within the first three minutes of the universe's existence is certainly an evolutionary theory of sorts, in the present chapter I would like to concentrate on the issue of biological evolution. However, I will return to the theory of 'The Big Bang' in a subsequent chapter.

Among other things Darwin's *Origins of Species* (The original title was longer – namely, *The Origins of Species by Means of Natural Selection or the Preservation of Favored Races in the Struggle for Life* – but the book's title was shortened for the 1872 6th edition) put forth data and arguments to support his belief that species or populations of organisms undergo a process of change, or evolution, in accordance with the principles of natural selection to which the environments in which such species exist give expression. This central notion of changes in a species brought about forces of natural selection is really not all that extraordinary although, as ensuing history has shown in dramatic fashion, Darwin's idea was interpreted as being in conflict with a variety of theological positions, and, as a result, there was considerable resistance to the foregoing theme in Darwin's initial, written foray into the issue of origins.

Slightly more controversial was Darwin's belief that new species could arise (the process of speciation) through the action of natural selection on a given population of organisms (i.e., a specific species). To claim that the conditions of natural selection might bring about changes in what properties of a population were most likely to be passed on to future generations is one thing (and breeder's of plants and animals had been demonstrating this for centuries prior to the time of Darwin), but to argue that entirely new species could arise through such a process seemed to be pushing the envelope of credulity, and this was especially the case since quite a few theological positions that were prominent during Darwin's time presupposed that species had been fixed at the time of creation.

More controversial still was Darwin's contention that all species in existence or that had been in existence at some point in the past were derived from a common, primordial form or ancestor. For example, maybe, given the right conditions of natural selection, it might be possible for different subsets of a specific population of organisms to biologically drift apart from each other to a point where the members of those subsets could no longer interbreed with the members of the other subsets (or with the remaining members of the "mainstream" population) and, in addition, drift apart to the point where various characteristics of the larger, mainstream population might disappear altogether from one, or both, of those subsets – pushing those subsets in a different evolutionary direction and, in the process, generating new species. However, to try to maintain that all life forms evolved from a common, primordial form of life seemed – at least for many people – to push the matter of evolution beyond the pale of reasonable, plausible discussion.

Darwin's books, based on extensive years of meticulous research, were collectively quite suggestive with respect to the idea that all current life forms might possibly have arisen from a common primordial form of life. Nonetheless, not only did his books fail to definitively prove what was being suggested (this task fell to his successors), but, in addition, Darwin had no explanation for how the first primordial form of life came into being.

| Explorations |

Although Darwin rarely wrote or spoke about the issue of primordial origins, he did, on occasion, speculate about such a possibility. For example, in a February 1st 1871 letter to his friend Joseph Hooker he wrote:

"It is often said that all the conditions for the first production of a living organism are now present, that could ever have been present. But if (& oh what a big if) we could conceive in some warm little pond with all sorts of ammonia & phosphoric salts — light, heat, electricity etc. -- present, that a protein compound was chemically formed, ready to undergo still more complex changes ... ."

Obviously, the implication of Darwin's foregoing conjecture was that a collection of the right sort of chemical elements might, somehow, come together under the right sort of environmental conditions and, somehow, form a complex compound that was, somehow, capable of undergoing still more changes until, eventually, somehow, life emerged. It would take another 60-70 years before various individuals began to try to fill in the details of the "somehows" that were left unanswered by Darwin even as the nature of those possible 'somehows' were being alluded to by him in his letter to Hooker.

There is a similar set of lacunae inherent in Darwin's contention that once a primordial form of life somehow came into being, then, all subsequent life forms would descend from that point of origin. More specifically, even if were to accept the idea that new species might arise through one, or another, collection of forces of natural selection acting on the original population of primordial organisms (assuming, of course, that such a population could, somehow, arise from a single primordial form of life), there is nothing to guarantee that the capacity to give rise to the emergence of <u>some</u> new species necessarily would lead to the rise of <u>all</u> subsequent species.

In other words, one needs to distinguish between: (1) speciation as a function of natural selection whose capacity to produce new forms of life constitutes a potential of unknown parameters, and (2) the idea of common descent from a primordial form of life. More specifically, the three-four billion history of life on Earth consists of millions, if not billions and trillions, of changes – some minor and some major -- in the forms, functions, capacities, biological components, and metabolic pathways of living organisms, and the fact that one might be able to account for some of these changes through the processes of speciation does not necessarily mean that one can plausibly account for all such changes through the kinds of speciation process that were being proposed by Darwin and that are being explored by modern evolutionary biologists.

Darwin believes (as do most, if not all, evolutionary biologists) that speciation tends to generate further speciation. Darwin also believes (as do most, if not all, evolutionary biologists) that if one were able to add up the entire set of instances of speciation that have arisen over billions of years as a result of the forces of natural selection (although, for practical empirical and methodological reasons, one might not be able to succeed in completely accomplishing such a project), then one will be able to account for all branches of the tree of life ... in other words, one will have demonstrated (or so the claim goes) that one can trace an unbroken path extending from a primordial form or species of life that, subsequently, transitioned seamlessly into other species, that, in turn and over vast swaths of time, led seamlessly to the successive generation of every single life form that ever existed in conjunction with the planet Earth.

Even if we limit our discussion to just the considerations introduced in the last several pages, it is obvious that the term "evolution" can have a variety of meanings. For instance, 'evolution' might refer to the process in which a given population of organisms (a specific species) gives expression to changes over time with respect to which set of physical and biological properties will come to enjoy the most success as a function of a given set of conditions of natural selection. Moreover, this way of rendering the notion of evolution also would include the belief that as the conditions of natural selection change, then, so too, will the character of the set of properties that are able to take advantage of the changes occurring with respect to various forces of natural selection.

A second sense of 'evolution' has to do with the process of speciation in a limited sense. In other words as environmental conditions and a given population of organisms (a specific species) engage one another, the dynamic of that engagement might lead to the generation of subsets of the population that, in time, become, among other things, reproductively isolated from one another and in the process give rise to modified or descended form(s) of the original species population that constitute the beginning of a new branch that is growing on the tree of life.

However, the extent to which such a process of speciation is capable of proceeding might be limited. In other words, while speciation does occur, there might be limits to how far it can proceed and on what 'new' possibilities might arise in conjunction with that sort of process.

A third meaning of 'evolution' concerns the limits, if any, in relation to the potential for speciation. That is, there are those who believe (and Darwin was one of these individuals) that the potential inherent in the process of speciation is, for all practical purposes, indefinitely great and, as a result, such a process has the capacity, sooner or later, to generate every form of life that has arisen since the first primordial organism arose on Earth … assuming, of course, that the forces of natural selection co-operate with, and lend support to, such changes in speciation.

Finally, a fourth notion of 'evolution' concerns the origins of life. More specifically, this sense of the word has to do with accounts of how the first primordial form of life – the first species – emerged.

Returning to the ideas of Dobzhansky, he seems to have had some strange ideas about what making sense entails with respect to the relationship among God, evolution and biology. For instance, Dobzhansky raises some rather arbitrary issues in his *American Biology Teacher* article about what God might and might not do in conjunction with the human task of trying to figure out what is going on in the universe.

More specifically, Dobzhansky seems to be of the opinion that God would not perpetrate hoaxes on, or try to deceive, or seek to fool human beings by fabricating evidence in an effort to mislead human beings concerning the origins of life or the laws governing life. While Dobzhansky might well be correct in his beliefs, his manner of reasoning doesn't eliminate the possibility that human beings can perpetrate hoaxes on themselves (e.g., the Piltdown man), as well as deceive and fool themselves, without any assistance from God, about any manner of things … including the issue of evolution.

| Explorations |

In any event, after putting forth additional arguments, Dobzhansky comes to the conclusion that the unity and diversity of life can be explained best as a function of evolutionary processes that are shaped and molded by forces of natural selection. According to Dobzhansky, this is how God proceeded with respect to the act of creation.

I can't say that I know what God would and wouldn't do in the case of human beings, and I have my doubts about whether Dobzhansky knew such things either. I do have an intuitive feeling that I cannot expect God to operate in accordance with principles that conform to what does and doesn't make sense to me, and while I appreciate that what made sense to Dobzhansky was a function of what he believed to be the case concerning how things (such as evolution) worked in the universe, I don't necessarily have a lot of confidence in certain aspects of what made sense to him with respect to such issues.

Maybe the position outlined in the '*Nothing in Biology Makes Sense Except in the Light of Evolution*' article by Dobzhansky is correct. Indeed, I pointed out in the Introduction to this book, that if so inclined – which I am not – I could accept much of what evolutionary biologists have to say about the origins of life or its descent across time, and all this acknowledgment would mean to me is that I might have to rework certain aspects of my worldview so that those features of my understanding reflected necessary "truths".

The fundamental issue is to seek and determine the nature of truth. Our belief systems need to adapt to whatever that truth turns out to be.

Nonetheless, the ideas of Dobzhansky notwithstanding, there might be other ways to account for the principles of unity and diversity to which life gives expression that need not depend on the physical principles of evolution. Moreover, just because we might not know what those ways are does not necessarily mean that the process of life on Earth is without sense ... rather, the nature of life – on a number of levels -- just might have a sense that we do not, yet, grasp ... and, perhaps, we never will.

The fact an idea helps one to make sense of things is not proof that one's sense of things is true. Truth (and proof) requires something more than meaningfulness.

For example, Dobzhansky points out in his *American Biology Article* that the idea of evolution is able to make sense out of the fact that extinction is the fate of most species that have appeared in Earth's history since environmental conditions have changed during that time and, yet, only a relatively few species have been able to successfully adapt to those changes and continue the process of descent. He goes on to assert: "but what a senseless operation it would have been, on God's part, to fabricate a multitude of species ex nihilo and then let most of them die out."

In effect, Dobzhansky is saying that if something does not make sense to him, then, it couldn't possibly make sense to God. Apparently, Dobzhansky believes that what makes sense to God should be a function of what makes sense to Dobzhansky.

The fact of the matter is -- and let us accept Dobzhansky's assumptions: That God exists, that God created life ex nihilo (whatever this means), and that God permitted most life forms to become extinct – Dobzhansky is engaged in an exercise of speculation concerning how God 'thinks' about things or how God goes about making sense of Creation. Conceivably -- and, like Dobzhansky, I am just speculating here -- God permitted so many life forms to become extinct because (a) this constituted a heuristically valuable theme on which human beings needed to reflect or meditate, and (b) perhaps the nature of creation is about constantly giving expression to new forms of manifestation while letting the old forms of manifestation become extinct after they run their course with respect to whatever role the latter played in the Divine scheme of things … a scheme that I am not claiming to understand and a scheme that I suspect Dobzhansky did not necessarily understand either.

Evolution might be an idea that helps people like Dobzhansky to organize a vast array of biological data in order to try to make sense of that material. However, perhaps, one needs to engage in a process of critical reflection with respect to whether, or not, evolution's manner of organizing such data makes as much sense as Dobzhansky and other evolutionary biologists seem to believe.

For instance, I believe that many facets of biology make sense in the light of evolution in both of the first two senses noted previously. In other words, when one considers the changes that a given population or species undergoes across changing environmental circumstances, or when one considers the possibility of speciation as an expression of a relatively limited set of combinations and permutations that are inherent in such a population's gene pool (i.e., there are various kinds of forces and factors that place constraints on how far speciation can proceed with respect to the possible subsets of a given population), then evolution in the foregoing two senses does tend to give a unified sense to a great deal of diverse biological data.

Essentially, both of the foregoing senses of the idea of evolution are entailed by the principles of population biology. Moreover, I believe there is a great deal of evidence to support many of the principles of population biology.

However, I believe many things in biology do not make sense in the light of a sense of evolution that shines forth from the second and third meanings of evolution noted earlier. In other words, first, I have a lot of questions concerning the tenability of the idea that the potential of speciation is so indefinitely great that, given appropriate conditions of natural selection, it can account for the diversity of all life forms that have appeared over the last 3-4 billion years with respect to Earth. Secondly, I question the tenability of claims that the origins of the initial, primordial life form can be explained (as Darwin hinted might be the case in his February 1, 1871 letter to Joseph Hooker) in terms of known principles of physics and chemistry.

According to Dobzhansky's article in the *American Biology Teacher*: "Evolution as a process that has always gone on in the history of the earth can be doubted only by those who are ignorant of the evidence or are resistant to evidence, owing to emotional blocks or to plain bigotry." Dobzhansky's 'my way or the highway' sort of mentality is fairly dogmatic and resonates with the way many so-called experts propagandized the meme of: "HIV causes AIDS" or the myth that there is a chemical cure – e.g., SSRIs -- for mental illness.

Such intransigence in understanding is also reflected in Dobzhansky's subsequent contention that evolution: "…is a general postulate to which all theories, all hypotheses, all systems must henceforward bow and that they must satisfy in order to be thinkable and true." Well, I suppose it is not that much of a leap to go from -- as pointed out earlier – telling God what must make sense to Divinity, to telling human beings what must make sense to them.

Evolutionary biologists often switch between referring to evolution as a fact, and/or a hypothesis, and/or a theory. However, let's reflect on this a little.

For example, currently, there is no plausible evolutionary account for the origins of life (and there will be more on this issue a little bit later in the present chapter). Consequently, one is not necessarily entitled to refer to evolution as being a fact when it comes to the origins of life issue.

Moreover, evolution is not, really, even a hypothesis when considered in conjunction with the task of trying to explain the origins of life. To formulate a meaningful hypothesis one has to have a way of testing that hypothesis, yet, in many, if not most, respects, one can never recreate the conditions of early Earth because we do not know precisely what those conditions were, and, consequently, any hypotheses that might be postulated in this regard are entirely arbitrary and predicated on some presumed scenario concerning the conditions of early Earth.

The foregoing comments should not be construed to mean that nothing is known about whatever conditions might have been present some four-to-five billion years ago. Rather, what is being alluded to is that we don't currently possess sufficient, specific knowledge to be able to construct a reliable picture of what was taking place in any given location on early Earth.

We might know some of the <u>general</u> things that likely might have been happening in and on early Earth from a geological, hydrological, meteorological, and/or chemical perspective. Nonetheless, we do not know enough about how those forces were <u>specifically</u> interacting with one another from place to place on early Earth to be able to generate a reliable model or simulation of how protocells supposedly came into existence.

To be sure, individuals (such as Darwin in his previously cited letter to Joseph Hooker) have speculated about what the conditions on primordial Earth might have been. Furthermore, various researchers have run experiments (there will be more discussion on this later on) that were based on what those individuals believed might have been realistic conditions out of which components of the first protocell could have emerged, but there is no independent way of demonstrating that such proposed conditions are, in fact, realistic representations or models of what was the case on early Earth.

If one likes, one can formulate any number of arbitrary hypotheses rooted in speculations about the conditions of early Earth (and the prebiotic literature is replete with these sorts of arbitrary speculations). However, all one is testing are the conditions set forth in those speculations ... speculations that might have little, or nothing, to do with the realities of actual conditions 4-5 billion years ago.

We just really don't know all that much about such matters. Furthermore, so-called "educated guesses" are, first and foremost, just that – namely, guesses. In addition, 'educated guesses' leave open the question of whether, or not, one should accept all the biases, assumptions, and philosophical understandings that frame someone's notion of what it means to be "educated".

For example, as noted previously, Dobzhansky was of the opinion that individuals who did not accept the theory of evolution are "ignorant of the evidence or are resistant to evidence, owing to emotional blocks or to plain bigotry" ... and, therefore, he had a rather self-serving view of what it means to be educated. One can throw in for good measure the theory of education that was given expression by the anthropology teacher I mentioned in the introduction to this book who responded so contemptuously toward me when I had the audacity to raise a few questions in conjunction with the tenability of evolutionary theory.

All too frequently, scientists are all for skepticism, open discussion, and critical inquiry except when it comes to questioning the theories that they hold dear. It is difficult for education in any meaningful and heuristically valuable sense to take place in such an oppressive atmosphere.

So, if one cannot refer to evolution as a 'fact' or a 'hypothesis' when it comes to accounting for, among other things, the origins of life, can one refer to evolution as a theory that attempts to make sense of that issue? A theory is said to be a coherent collection of interconnected claims that are given expression through, and shaped

| Explorations |

by, an array of reasoned arguments and empirical data that have the potential capacity to account for a variety of phenomena.

Given the foregoing characterization of the notion of a theory, then, certainly, evolution is a theory. However, saying that something is a theory is not necessarily coextensive with saying that such a theory is either true or that it is necessarily even scientific.

To be sure, the theory of evolution (however one might wish to parse the term "evolution") is a relatively coherent body of interconnected claims. Furthermore, the theory of evolution does consist of a set of reasoned arguments concerning a body of empirical data. And, finally, the theory of evolution does offer an account of – although not necessarily the truth about -- why certain phenomena might have the character they do.

All theories – whether philosophical, religious, psychological, historical, or technical – consist of a relatively coherent body of interconnected claims. What makes evolutionary claims either true or scientific?

All theories – whether philosophical, religious, psychological, historical, or technical – consist of a set of reasoned arguments concerning some aspect or aspects of the empirical data of lived experience. What makes evolutionary arguments true or scientific, and what are the criteria for considering whether, or not, something has been effectively reasoned?

All theories – whether philosophical, religious, psychological, historical, or technical – purport to offer an explanation of why something is the way it is. What makes an evolutionary explanation true or scientific?

Furthermore, is it possible for something to be true but not scientific? Alternatively, is it possible for something to be scientific but not necessarily true?

The first chapter of this book used a fair amount of space, time and words to point out that people who refer to themselves as scientists, or who are referred to by others in this manner, don't necessarily always know what they are talking about. Cancer treatments based on the use of Antineoplastons were – and still are – opposed by a majority of the cancer research and medical communities around the world despite

| Explorations |

162

the fact that Antineoplastons have been proven to be non-toxic, effective, and have successfully met the challenge of Phase III, randomized trials. In addition, SSRIs are almost universally endorsed by psychiatrists, medical doctors, and researchers despite the fact there is no proven, specific, underlying theory about what role serotonin plays in the dynamics of depression (or its treatment), and despite the fact there is considerable evidence to indicate that SSRIs are extremely toxic and, as a result, are capable of inducing various forms of 'medication madness' and discontinuation syndrome in those individuals to whom it is prescribed or administered. Furthermore, despite the existence of a significant amount of evidence supporting the idea that HIV does <u>not</u> cause AIDS -- as well as the existence of very little evidence which demonstrates that HIV does cause AIDS – the vast majority of clinicians and researchers continue to maintain that HIV causes AIDS.

The thirty-plus year campaign <u>against</u> Antineoplastons claimed to be rooted in science, but it wasn't. The thirty-plus year marketing campaign to promote SSRIs as a chemical cure for depression (and a growing assortment of other maladies) was based, supposedly on science, but this was not, and is not, the case. The thirty-plus year attempt to claim that HIV causes AIDS had its origins in an allegedly Nobel-worthy series of experiments performed in the early 1980s, and, yet, none of those experiments -- along with the hype that surrounded and permeated them -- seemed to have little to do with anything that could meaningfully be described as scientific because 'bad science' is not really science at all despite the presence of labs, experiments, technical gadgetry, and people who have credentials of one kind or another.

Science cannot exist in the absence of critical reflection. Whatever other trappings of science might be used and applied, if rigorous critical reflection is not in evidence, then, the activities taking place in the midst of such trappings is something other than science … at best they might be referred to as being pre-scientific.

Mathematics and quantification might be necessary for science to be possible, but they are not sufficient conditions to guarantee that science will take place. Observations, hypotheses, and experiments tend to constitute necessary conditions for the existence of science, but those activities do not necessarily constitute sufficient conditions for the possibility of science to be manifested. The use of instrumentation plays a useful, if not crucial, role in the activity of science, but the presence of instrumentation is not necessarily sufficient to ensure that science will take place. Having individuals who have the credentials and/or the experience that enable those people to have facility with: Mathematics, measurement, observation, generating testable hypotheses, experimentation, and instrumentation are all necessary – but not sufficient -- conditions for the practice of science.

The Antineoplastons issue, the SSRI matter, and the 'HIV causes AIDS' affair all entailed substantial elements of mathematics, quantification, observation, hypotheses, experiments, instrumentation, and credentialed, experienced individuals. Yet, most of the people involved in those controversies were not doing science because they refused -- for whatever reasons (e.g., fear, greed, ego, power, jealousy, corruption, etc.) -- to critically engage the issues at the heart of those discussions.

Only a small number of people were actually doing science in any of those three areas of research (i.e., Antineoplastons, SSRIs, and HIV/AIDS). This is the case because only a relatively few people engaged in those areas of research were employing the necessary qualities of critical reflection to be able to ask the right kinds of questions concerning the tenability of the uses to which various modalities of mathematics, measurement, observation, hypothesis, experimentation, instrumentation, and expertise were being put.

Although skepticism plays a role in the process of critical reflection, the latter process involves much more than being willing to maintain a stance of caution concerning the veracity of various claims about the nature of the universe. One must be willing to ask questions that are intended to be something more than expressions of resistant doubt but, instead, are intended to seek out and realize the truth of an issue ... at least to whatever extent such truth can be sought out and realized.

The individual who spends his or her life committed to nothing except the practice of skepticism is not really a scientist. If there is no intention to try to ferret out whatever dimensions of truth are possible to grasp in some set of circumstances, then one is a philosophical skeptic, not a scientist.

There might be any number of questions surrounding whether, or not, one actually has grasped some sort of truth in a given situation. Nevertheless, asking questions in an attempt to be able to root one's claims in the truth in some demonstrable, substantive, fashion is a very different sort of activity than just raising questions and stating objections as ends in themselves.

The questions that are asked during the process of critical reflection should be directed toward establishing a form of understanding that is capable of engaging, and withstanding, rigorous forms of challenge concerning the quality and reliability of whatever modes of mathematics, observation, hypothesizing, experimentation, instrumentation, and expertise are employed in a given research project. With important exceptions, there is a fatal absence of the right kinds of questions, understandings, and critical reflections that is all too evident – as I feel has been demonstrated in Chapter 1 – with respect to the controversies involving Antineoplastons, SSRIs, and HIV/AIDS, and I believe there is a similar fatal absence of the right kinds of questions, understandings, and critical reflections evident with respect to certain dimensions of the evolution issue.

The theory of evolution is often said to be true because a group of scientists have come to agree on the general form of the nature of the coherency that lends sense to the set of interconnected claims and statements that give expression to a coherent hermeneutic of experience with respect to, among other things, an array of biological phenomena. However, how does agreement concerning the nature of coherency in the foregoing manner make such a theory either true or scientific since there have been many occasions during the history of scientifically oriented endeavors in which a coherent sense of things was discovered not to be true or was considered to be scientific only to be shown later to be quite unscientific as well as false?

Eliminating falsehoods is part of the process of science. Nonetheless, does advocating a theory that turns out to be false make such a theory scientific in any way other than that some individuals referred to as scientists once believed the theory to be true, or, is it the

| Explorations |

case that even though some people called scientists subscribed to the theory, it might be said that such a theory was never really scientific?

Is a hypothesis that is proven to be false, a scientific hypothesis? Aren't the waters of clarity muddied by the ambiguity that is created when someone refers to hypotheses as being scientific when, later on, they are demonstrated to be false?

Forming a hypothesis is not necessarily a scientific process. On the other hand, demonstrating that such a hypothesis is either true or false might be an expression of science ... depending on the character and quality of the demonstration.

If a group of people who are referred to as, or who refer to themselves as, scientists put forth a set of reasoned arguments concerning some set of empirical data, does their claim that the arguments are reasoned make them reasoned? Or, does their agreement that the arguments are reasoned just – possibly – a matter of unjustifiably labeling those arguments as being reasoned?

Furthermore, even if those arguments were considered to be well reasoned, does this necessarily make such arguments true or scientific? And, if those arguments are not true, then, can those arguments legitimately be described as being scientific no matter how well-reasoned they might be?

If a group of people referring to themselves as scientists – or who are referred to in that manner by others – cite a theory as the explanation for why things are the way they are, does such a claim make the theory a true explanation or even necessarily make such an explanation scientific? For example, as part of the arguments put forth in his *American Biology Teacher* article, Dobzhansky provides an explanatory account concerning what, apparently, should make sense to God.

Was such an explanation scientific? And, if so, in what sense was it scientific?

Was the argument he used to substantiate his sense of things with respect to the foregoing account well reasoned? Without really giving a great deal of serious effort to critically analyzing Dobzhansky's argument, I put forth several suggestions earlier in this chapter indicating that, perhaps, his reasoning wasn't as conclusive or as well-conceived as he seemed to believe.

His way of understanding the matter made sense to him. However, wasn't the coherency to which his sense of things gave expression really anything more than a circular function of his belief system and for which he had no independent evidence to advance in support of his claim?

Many people claim that evolution is the best scientific theory to account for an array of biological data. While evolution might well be a theory, it might not really be a scientific theory except when it comes to the principles of population biology (more on this later).

However, many individuals (some of whom are scientists) want evolution to encompass more than the dynamics of population biology. Such individuals want to be able to claim that evolution is a scientific explanation for the origins and subsequent descent of all life forms.

While evolution might be a theory in the aforementioned generic sense of constituting a coherent set of interconnected statements that entail a group of reasoned arguments concerning a body of empirical data that collectively serve as a meaningful account for various biological phenomena, nevertheless, none of this makes the theory of evolution either true or scientific when it comes to both the origins of life issue or when it comes to proving that speciation is capable of accounting for all changes that can be observed (either directly in living organisms or indirectly via fossils) across the millions of species that make up the tree of life. In fact, I believe it is possible to demonstrate that the theory of evolution falls far short of having proven to be either a true theory or even a scientific theory when it comes to issues such as the origin of life.

The purpose of this chapter is not to advance a creationist perspective or an intelligent design worldview as an alternative to the theory of evolution. Rather, this chapter is about exploring the possibility that the theory of evolution does not actually constitute a viable account of anything in relation to either the origins of life issue or the idea that speciation, in conjunction with natural selection, is sufficient to explain the multiple branches that make up the tree of life.

| Explorations |

Some people seem to think that providing an account of the origin (s) of life is an either/or issue. That is, either one must accept some version of the theory of evolution or one must accept a theory of creation or intelligent design.

However, it might be the case that neither theories of evolution nor theories of creation -- as currently conceived -- are necessarily correct or the only plausible possibilities. Perhaps Hamlet was right when he said: "There are more things in heaven and earth, Horatio, then are dreamt of in your philosophy."

By pointing out problems with the theory of evolution, this exercise in critical reflection does not automatically make me a card-carrying member of some philosophy club involving one, or another, version of creationism or intelligent design. Moreover, pointing out problems with the theory of evolution does not automatically require me to commit to any particular alternative to the theory of evolution or to a specific theory of creationism or intelligent design.

If we return to the Michelangelo approach to sculpting a statute that I alluded to earlier, sometimes it is more important to remove what doesn't belong in a given situation than it is to try to fashion a structure and, in the process, impose an arbitrary design on the materials with which one is working. Continuing to search for and, where possible, realize the truth of things is the appropriate alternative to accepting theories (such as a theory of evolution or a given theory of creation) that might be problematic in important ways.

If a given theory is problematic in the foregoing sense, then one cannot automatically assume that such a theory necessarily gives expression to a scientific theory (best or otherwise) simply because it is the only one currently available that is alluded to in those terms (i.e., as being scientific) by people who refer to themselves as scientists (or who are referred to as such by others) and, as a result, should (as Dobzhansky's previously quoted comments seem to suggest) become everyone's default position. If a given theory is problematic in important ways, then the existence of those kinds of problems is the very issue that stands in the way of the theory being considered to be scientific in any substantial, rigorous, and plausible sense.

A theory entails problems in "important ways" if one can demonstrate the existence of themes that undermine the essence or heart of a theory's sense of coherency, modes of reasoning/arguments, and/or explanations concerning the nature of the universe, or some aspect thereof. The theory of evolution is a theory that is problematic in important ways – or so it will be argued in the following pages – and, consequently, that theory is not really scientific in any substantial, rigorous, plausible, or definitive sense.

When it comes to issues like the origins of life, evolution is a theory. However, it is not necessarily a scientific theory despite the fact that it emerges in a context that has many of the trappings of a science-like process with respect to the use of observation, hypothesis generation, experimentation, measurement, instrumentation, and credentialed individuals.

The Final Jeopardy challenge doesn't necessarily require one to identify the full extent of the truth of the reality problem. Rather, the challenge is for an individual to be able to give the best response possible, and part of that sort of response is to eliminate as many questionable claims to truth as one can ... such as in the case of the theory of evolution when applied to certain topics involving the origin of life or involving the nature of, and possible limits entailed by, the process of speciation.

Critique of An Abbreviated Textbook Perspective

In most, if not all, textbooks that provide an introductory overview concerning the theory of evolution -- along with many of the specifics that the authors of those books believe are in support of, or entailed by, the theory of evolution -- a person is likely to find chapters dealing with a variety of issues. The following discussion constitutes, I feel, a fairly typical synopsis from which chapter themes are often derived, developed and expanded upon according to the inclinations of the author(s).

First and foremost, the idea of evolutionary change is rooted in the dynamics of the changes taking place within a population of organisms that are collectively referred to as a species. Such a population can be described in terms of a combination of both phenotypic and genotypic properties.

A phenotype refers to a particular, observable physical trait – such as size, weight, color, anatomical features, and so on – that is given expression in an individual exemplar for the species being considered ... traits that tend to be exhibited, by most, if not all, members of a species population. Not every member of the population will necessarily manifest phenotypic properties to the same quantitative extent or in the same qualitative manner, but for the most part -- and despite the presence of some exemplars or properties in members of a population that might be phenotypically anomalous in some way – nonetheless, a set of phenotypic properties exists that tends to be characteristic of a given species and helps differentiate the members of one species from the members of other kinds of species who manifest their own unique set of phenotypic traits.

Genotype refers to the genetic capacities that help to make possible and give expression to phenotypic traits, and, as well, that have the potential of being transmitted to subsequent generations (if any) via the coding, transcription, and translation that occur in conjunction with DNA and RNA molecules. Although the genotype for a given individual tends to be fixed, the expression of different dimensions of that genotype tends to vary with changing conditions both within and without such an individual.

The gene pool (the collective set of genotypes) for the population to which an individual belongs might contain phenotypic potentials that are not necessarily included in the genotype of a given individual exemplar of that species population. Among other things, this means there might be more than one version of a given gene (known as alleles) that have the capacity to underwrite which variant of a certain phenotypic trait will be expressed in a given individual.

A particular phenotype can be the result of the gene expression that is either simple or complex. In the case of simple forms of genotypic expression, usually only one gene underlies a given phenotypic trait, while in more complex forms of gene expression, a number of genes might interact to produce a specific phenotypic trait.

Phenotypic expression also can be shaped by more than genotypic considerations. In other words, the environment in which an individual's set of phenotypic and genotypic potential is rooted can affect the way in which genotypic potentials unfold and give rise to observed phenotypic characteristics of one kind rather than another.

Generally speaking, although the environment can affect the way genotypes and phenotypes are expressed in a given organism, the environment does not usually have any impact on the nature of the properties of the genotype that are passed on. In other words, phenotypic characteristics that are acquired during the life of an organism's life cycle usually are not passed on to subsequent generations.

However, there is a growing amount of evidence indicating that the foregoing position might not be as set in stone as once thought. More specifically, there are dynamics at work involving, for example, methyl groups – referred to as epigenetic tags -- that have the capacity to affect whether, or not, certain genes will be expressed.

Histones are proteins that form the structural spools around which DNA winds itself. Depending on now tightly or loosely DNA is wound around the histone core, the expression of the genes present in such wound DNA might be easier or more difficult to express.

Each and every cell of the human body is believed to possess a unique pattern of histone and methylation activity. Consequently, methyl groups interact with DNA and can have a determinate effect on whether, or not, a given stretch of DNA will be expressed.

Changes in epigenetic tagging can be acquired during the life of an organism. For example, a poor diet might lead to methyl groups binding to DNA in ways that tend to switch off the expression of one, or more, genes.

Such epigenetic changes can be passed on to, or inherited by, offspring. Consequently, there is a sense – i.e., the epigenetic tagging of DNA by methyl groups -- in which acquired characteristics could be inherited by subsequent generations, and "epigenetics" is the field of study through which the nature and impact of such changes are explored.

The evolutionary change that occurs in a given population is a function of the transition in frequencies and proportions of genotypes and phenotypes that are brought about by the way genes are transmitted in that population and, as well, by the way in which the forces of natural selection act on those patterns of transmission over time. As the frequency and proportion of certain genotypes change, the phenotypic characteristics of that population also are likely to undergo transition.

For the most part, evolutionary change is a function of what takes place within a population (or its subsets) in relation to a given species. Among other things, this means that evolutionary change is not generally measured by what happens to individual members of a population but only by what happens over time to the frequencies and proportions of different kinds of phenotypes and genotypes that characterize a given population or its subsets.

Obviously, the potential for evolutionary change begins when certain kinds of changes occur in relation to individual members of a population. However, unless those changes lead, eventually, to transitions in the proportions and frequencies of such genotypic and phenotypic traits in the population as a whole (or subsets thereof), then, change of an evolutionary nature has not really occurred.

Changes in genotype frequencies and proportions are believed to come about through two primary forms of dynamic. These two modalities are known as 'genetic drift' and 'natural selection'.

| Explorations |

Genetic drift refers to those kinds of fluctuations in the frequencies and proportions of genotypes within a small population that are brought about by what is described as a random dynamic involving various environmental forces and circumstances that result in the removal of certain genes due to either the death of individuals or the inability (for whatever reason) of those individuals to reproduce and leave offspring containing the genes in question. The disappearance of such genes is not because they, in some way, lack adaptive capacity but because the luck of the draw (i.e., random events ... including mutations, a perfect storm of circumstances that are disadvantageous, "freak" accidents, etc.) did not permit them to continue.

The idea of genetic drift is intertwined with the neutral theory of molecular evolution. This latter theory contends that: (1) while a relatively small minority of mutations result in some form of advantage with respect to the prevailing conditions of natural selection and, therefore, are fixed or favored by those conditions, and (2) while other mutations result in some form of disadvantage and, as a result, are eliminated by the forces of natural selection, nonetheless, (3) the vast majority of mutations are relatively neutral in character – that is, such mutations are neither more advantageous nor less advantageous than other genetic possibilities – and are fixed or eliminated by the vagaries of genetic drift.

Natural selection is a determinate process in which given subsets of a population exhibit a superior capacity, relative to other members of the population, to, in general, survive, and, in particular, to successfully pass on those kinds of capacities to their offspring. Adaptation gives expression to the interaction between individual organisms and their environments that results in the natural selection of those organisms that have best adjusted to existing circumstances and, in the process, both survive and reproduce at rates and in ways that allow a particular set of genotypes and phenotypes to continue on in subsequent generations.

Evolutionary biologists maintain that natural selection has the capacity to alter the characteristics of an existing population through changing the frequencies and proportions of various genes that might affect the way a given phenotypic and/or genotypic property is manifested. For example as genes are combined and recombined with one another during the process of reproduction, new genotypes and phenotypes might arise, and those new phenotypes and genotypes will be acted upon by the forces of natural selection that, in turn, provide the new kids in town with the opportunity to spread through the population, and, in time, possibly alter the genotypic and phenotypic properties of the population.

Members of the same species might respond differently to different geographical conditions. Those conditions will tend to induce various dimensions of the underlying genotype to express itself in different ways over time as a result of changes in the nature of competition, together with changes in the kinds of opportunities and challenges that exist with respect to changes in geographic conditions.

Genetic differences also arise in subsets of a given species through changes in one or several genes. Many of those changes have phenotypic consequences of one kind or another, and such phenotypic consequences are acted upon by natural selection.

As a result, populations possess genetic and phenotypic variability. That variability engages changes in environmental circumstances in different ways, and under the appropriate conditions of natural selection, certain dimensions of that variability might change more quickly than other dimensions of that same variability.

Speciation refers to the process in which two or more subsets of a ancestral population arise through processes that entail sufficient genetic differentiation and/or geographic separation to bring about a genotypic and phenotypic break with, or branching from, the ancestral population. Over time, the frequency and proportion of such changes move through the newly formed subsets of the ancestral population. Moreover, those changes occur in such a way (due in large part to the existence of relative, geographic segregation) that occasional or sporadic instances of interbreeding with members of the ancestral population do not prevent the transition in genotype and phenotype frequencies/proportions from continuing to move away, to varying degrees, from the set of genotypic and phenotypic traits that characterized the ancestral population.

The processes that lead to gradations in phenotypic and genotypic differences generating speciation tend to continue across hundreds of millions of years. Eventually, out of the foregoing continuous processes, the collective series of instances of speciation will lead to the emergence of new kinds of genera, families, orders, classes, phyla, and kingdoms ... that is, taxonomic categories.

The foregoing several pages of discussion highlight the essential themes of most textbooks that deal with the theory of evolution. Those themes are: natural selection (sexual selection, kin selection, and group selection are just variations on this theme), adaptation, population dynamics, genetic drift, modalities of geographic segregation, transitions in phenotypic traits, recombinant DNA/gene shuffling, mutation, biodiversity, and speciation.

The textbooks that are being alluded to in the foregoing several pages will develop the aforementioned themes in different ways. While the vocabulary that is used to accomplish such augmentation will introduce topics involving: historical considerations, various discoveries, fossil records, modes of classification, methods of quantification, and a plethora of details based on observations, experiments, studies, and disagreements, nonetheless, all of the new vocabulary being introduced into such textbooks tends to be directed toward expanding and lending specificity to the ten, or so, central themes that give expression to the theory of evolution and that previously have been outlined (however briefly) in the present chapter.

Unfortunately, although attempts are made in those textbooks to explain various topics – for example, the diversity of life, together with the biological principles that unify such diversity, as well as the origin(s) of life -- by weaving together, in different combinations, various elements from the ten, or so, central themes of evolutionary theory, nevertheless, there are key junctures in those explanations that repeatedly disappear into an omnipresent mist of assumptions. As result, those elements are never verified or substantiated.

For example, earlier, in conjunction with providing a brief overview involving the ideas of genetic drift and the neutral theory of molecular evolution, the notion of randomness was mentioned. Genetic drift was described as being the result of some combination of chance, random events that had nothing to do with the evolutionary fitness of an organism but were just a matter of the slings and arrows of outrageous fortune that impacted on whether, or not, an organism survived or reproduced and whether, or not, a given gene survived in order to be passed on to the next generation.

What does it mean for an event to be random? There are several possibilities.

One characterization of the idea of randomness is that we do not possess (at least currently) the methods, means, or understanding to be able to trace the ultimate causes of certain terminal events – including, for example, the occurrence of what are referred to as instances of genetic drift and/or mutations. The causes of those events are indeterminate in nature, and by referring to those kinds of causes as random, we really are saying we don't know why the events occurred in the way they did.

Of course, although we don't know how a given event came to be, nonetheless, there might be a possible explanation that does account for such an event, but, at the present time, we just don't know what that kind of an explanation looks like. However, one of the <u>possible</u> explanations for this or that event has to do with another sense of the meaning of randomness.

More specifically, this alternative approach is rooted in a philosophical orientation that claims there is no ultimate purpose to the universe. As a result, events merely give expression to the dynamic interaction of a chain of forces and factors that happen to come together – for no overarching rhyme nor reason -- and give expression to this or that phenomenon.

The foregoing philosophical mode of engaging the issue of randomness comes in at least two flavors. (a) There is no determinate set of principles and forces that required a given event to have occurred but, rather, <u>independent</u> forces and principles arbitrarily engaged one another and, in the process, became entangled in such a manner that, among other things, an event or phenomenon of a certain kind took place. However, the nature of the entangled dynamic of forces and principles that did take place might have turned out otherwise if slightly different kinds of interaction had taken place at certain points along the way ... slightly different kinds of interaction that might easily have occurred but, inexplicably, did not. (b) There is an <u>interdependent</u> and determinate set of principles and forces that led to the occurrence of a given event, but there is no reason or purpose underlying why such a particular set of principles and forces exists or gives expression to the universe rather than some other set of principles and forces ... this is just the way things are.

Consequently, from one perspective, randomness is just another term for ignorance. From another perspective, randomness gives expression to a philosophy concerning the ontological nature of the universe and how it supposedly operates.

Are mutations random? If so, in what sense is that the case?

Are mutations random in the sense that we do not necessarily know how they came about? Or, are mutations random in the sense that they merely constitute the outcome of a long chain of interacting dynamics that, ultimately, are arbitrary in nature and just happen.

Whether one construes the idea of randomness as a way of alluding to one's ignorance or one construes the idea of randomness as a way of referring to how one believes the universe operates, in neither case does one actually <u>know</u> what, ultimately, is transpiring in the universe ... although, obviously, one might have <u>beliefs</u> concerning those matters. On the one hand, ignorance concerning the nature of how an event came to occur is a confession that one does not know what is going on, and, on the other hand, those who advocate randomness as an inherent property of the universe are not in any position to prove that this is the case and, therefore, really have no knowledge about whether, or not, the universe is random in any sense at all and have no knowledge concerning the manner in which random events conspired to generate one set of events rather than some other set of events.

I remember reading (nearly four decades ago) a May 1975 *Scientific American* article by Gregory Chaitin entitled '*Randomness and Mathematical Proof*'. One of the central themes of the article was that while one might be able to define randomness and measure it, one could not always prove – except in certain, special cases -- that a given sequence of numbers was random.

The general ideas underlying, and associated with, Chaitin's algorithmic approach to the issue of randomness will surface again later on in the book when various issues are explored in conjunction

| Explorations |

with: black holes, thermodynamics, and mathematics. So, for present purposes, I will restrict my comments concerning the foregoing *Scientific American* article.

Chaitin maintained that one of the key differences between random and non-random sequences had to do with the issue of compressibility. More specifically, on the one hand, non-random sequences could be represented by an algorithm that provided one with a set of instructions or a formula that permitted one to generate the sequence in question but that algorithm came in a compressed form which was smaller (contained less information) than the sequence that it generated, whereas, on the other hand, a random sequence could not be compressed into an algorithm that contained less information than the sequence itself.

Conceivably, a sequence of numbers might appear to be random because one hadn't found any algorithm capable of compressing the information so that the algorithm could be expressed using less information than the sequence it generated. However, what if an algorithm were subsequently discovered that could compress the information contained in the sequence in the desired way ... that is, into a specifiable, relatively short (compared to the sequence) algorithm?

One of the reasons why a sequence might not be capable of being proven to be random is because any proof that one advanced in this respect could not eliminate the possibility that the right kind of algorithm might emerge at some later point in time. As a result, there would be a certain amount of uncertainty or incompleteness concerning such proofs.

Chaitin makes a similar-sounding point in the aforementioned article by tying his definition of randomness to Kurt Gödel's work. However, I am going to construe the idea of uncertainty/incompleteness in a slightly different direction.

For example, I can think of at least one sequence of numbers (and there are many others that are similar to it) that might prove very difficult to predict what came next in the sequence unless one knew the algorithm for producing such a sequence. That sequence of numbers belongs to π.

| Explorations |

To some, the sequence of numbers in π might appear to be random. However, there is a determinate method for producing each succeeding number in the sequence even though the number itself is said to be infinite in character.

What happens if one uses the notion of randomness in conjunction with a theory – such as evolution -- that is said to be scientific in nature? In what way is the notion of randomness scientific?

If something actually were random (whatever this might mean), we could never prove that this was the case. If there is no possibility of proof, then in what sense is science present?

Furthermore, if one were to talk about mutations in terms of what was, or was not, compressible algorithmically, this still would leave open the possibility that someone, at some later point in time, might be able to come up with an algorithm that could account for such a mutation that was expressible as a function of some compressible, algorithmic form capable of describing the dynamics underlying a mutation that, initially, appeared to be random (e.g., as might be the case if someone discovered -- after the fact -- that a given, known chemical was a mutagen or had carcinogenic properties and played a prominent role in causing a given mutation).

Alternatively, some individuals might like to argue that the idea of randomness is one of the assumptions or postulates that one takes as given, and, then, science proceeds from there. The issue, then becomes, one of trying to account for how events of a provably determinate and functional nature arise out of phenomena that are, ultimately, said to be random in character.

For instance, one might ask: How do random events lead to determinate and functional metabolic pathways, genetic systems, or viable organisms? The modern answer -- from an allegedly "scientific" perspective -- is that the processes of natural selection and genetic drift -- along with the other set of usual suspects or central themes of evolutionary theory -- tend to shape which series of random elements will be fixed or eliminated.

However, both natural selection and genetic drift presuppose the existence of a functional system or organism upon which to operate.

Therefore, neither natural selection nor genetic drift can explain the origins of the functionality or order that they are said to fix.

The neutral theory of molecular evolution maintains that most changes at the molecular level are random events that confer no advantage or disadvantage (i.e., are neutral) with respect to fitness. Consequently, such molecular changes cannot necessarily be described as the source of new modes of functionality

Of course, the foregoing sorts of changes might affect whatever genetic and phenotypic properties are present, but they cannot do so in any way that compromises the evolutionary fitness of existing, biological functionality. Furthermore, in order to be able to provide a scientific account concerning the emergence of such new functionality, one would have to be able to show how that new kind of genotypic and/or phenotypic functionality arose through a given set of neutral changes that, on the one hand, were random and, on the other hand, did not confer any advantage or disadvantage in the process of coming together as a new kind of functional unit.

Mutations -- alleged to be random -- that are disadvantageous tend not to survive. Forces of natural selection generally (but not always or not always right away) eliminate organisms containing traits that don't function properly or capacities that do not adapt well to existing, environmental conditions.

Therefore, while disadvantageous or lethal mutations are a source of newness in a biological system or population, that modality constitutes a form of 'newness' that is destined to disappear in either the short run or the long haul. As a result, no new forms of constructive, lasting functionality arise out of those kinds of mutation.

So, the only source of constructive newness must be in the form of mutations – said to be random – that lead to a sequence of events that inexplicably acquires the capacity to function in a way that can be endorsed, reinforced, or fixed by the forces of natural selection. However, in effect, one has assumed one's conclusions by arguing that functionality arises out of random events without ever demonstrating the truth of one's claims (e.g., that the events are truly random), and this is little more than argument by assertion.

| Explorations |

Previously, I spoke about the idea that one could not prove that a sequence of numbers was random. One could only demonstrate that one did not currently know whether, or not, there was an algorithm capable of generating that sort of sequence.

Now, it seems that one cannot prove that a new form of functionality in an organism is a product of random events. One can only acknowledge that one does not currently possess an understanding capable of explaining how functionality arose out of randomness but, instead, one must assume (due to ignorance and/or philosophical inclination) that this is the case.

The randomness of something cannot be proven. Furthermore, the idea that randomness is capable of generating order cannot be proven if something cannot be shown to be random in the first place.

After all, what one is assuming to be a random phenomenon might not be. Instead, that phenomenon might just be the result of some determinate process for which one does not, yet, know the underlying algorithm.

By making randomness a fundamental postulate for a theory alleged to be scientific, what is one actually doing? One is muddying the waters as far as being able to clearly demarcate between science and philosophy is concerned.

If one has arranged one's postulates or assumptions in such a way that one either cannot know how things have come to be the way they are, or, one must allude to unproven philosophies concerning the manner in which the universe supposedly operates, then how can one be said to be doing science? If one cannot prove the likelihood of one of the most basic assumptions underlying the theory of evolution – namely, randomness – then while one might have a theory of evolution, the theory is not a scientific one because the ultimate 'explanation' for the origins of everything in biology that has a novel, functional character rests on something other than what can be shown to be true or accurate in a scientific manner.

Sometimes, the idea of randomness plays a central role in the formation of models that might reflect the possible nature of how things work. In other words, one develops a quantitative framework for what one might expect if events were described as being of a

| Explorations |

181

random nature, and, then, one compares what is observed against that model. However, most, if not all, quantitative models of randomness tend to be rooted in a theory about what constitutes the criteria of being random ... criteria that tend to entail arbitrary considerations.

For instance, consider the tossing of a coin. Supposedly, there are two possible outcomes to such a tossing process.

In actuality, there are more than two possibilities. For example, a coin could be lost when it lands ... perhaps, disappearing down a hole in the ground or down a heating duct in the floor. Or, a coin might fall in a way that it ends up landing on an edge and, perhaps with the help of some object against which it leans, stays that way.

There are an indefinite variety of ways that a tossed coin might become lost or land on an edge. Nonetheless, such possibilities are ignored, and a simplifying assumption is made that limits those possibilities down to just two.

The coin can turn up heads, or it can land tails up. The likelihood that either a heads or a tails will show up on any given toss of the coin is calculated to have a probability of ½ or .5.

Tests have been carried out, and the long-term distribution of coin tosses tends to match the foregoing probability. The more tosses that take place, then the closer the statistical distribution of those coin tosses approach the indicated probability calculation.

Does such a probability calculation capture something of the dynamic of randomness? To be sure, there is an element of randomness in the sense that we don't know which side of the coin will show up on any given toss.

If we bet on the outcome, we are taking a chance that we could be wrong in with respect to the character of our guess. However, ignorance concerning an outcome doesn't necessarily make the outcome an ontologically random event.

On the other hand, the nature of the collective sequence from one coin toss to the next might be considered to form a random sequence of an epistemological character. Nevertheless, aside from the previously mentioned issue of not being able to prove that a given sequence is random in an ontological sense because of the possibility that there might be some unknown algorithm capable of producing such a sequence, there is another consideration that impinges on the judgment of randomness with respect to such a sequence.

If the sequence is truly random, why does it generate a long-term distribution pattern of ½? The law of large numbers indicates that the more trials of the coin toss that are conducted, the closer the average of those trials should come to the expected distribution value of – in the case of coin tosses -- .5, but no one has ever explained why the law of large numbers works.

If that law were explained, perhaps we would know how order comes out of randomness. Unfortunately, the law of large numbers doesn't really explain anything ... it merely describes the determinate character of the average, expected outcome of a series of events.

In other words, the law of large numbers talks about how the expected outcomes -- based on the calculation of probabilities in a given situation – tend to approach what is actually observed if enough trials are completed. That law says nothing about how, or why, the dynamics of events that seem to give expression to a so-called random sequence are able to generate a determinate result.

Why assume that the expected outcome for a coin toss is 50-50 or .5? Why couldn't it be 70-30 or 20-80?

As indicated earlier, experiments have shown that the statistical distribution for heads and tails will approach the .5 figure given enough trials. Moreover, if there were a departure from such a distribution profile, one might begin to suspect there was some force or factor that was skewing the results away from an outcome for which there seems to be no obvious reason why it should be other than it is – that is, .5.

The law of large numbers resonates with the idea introduced earlier that indicated one isn't able to prove that a sequence is random because there might be an unknown algorithm capable of generating such a sequence. The law of large numbers alludes to the existence of such an algorithm, and, in fact, indicates – at least in the case of coin tossing -- that the nature of the algorithm consists in the flipping of the same coin in roughly the same fashion for a large number of trials or times, and one will be able to produce a long-term determinate outcome with respect to the distribution of heads and tails.

| Explorations |

The foregoing algorithm is shorter than the sequence of heads and tails that it produces – assuming, of course, that the process of tossing the coins goes on for a sufficiently long enough period of time. Thus, the coin-tossing sequence is compressible (it can be represented by an algorithm) and, therefore, is not random in nature.

So, in a sense, we know the nature of the algorithm underlying the production of a sequence of events that appears to be random and, yet, is not random because that sequence leads to a determinate result or outcome that displays an average distribution sequence that is close to that which had been expected or predicted on the basis of a probability model developed in relation to a given set of conditions. Indeed, we might argue that one can repeat the experiment as often as one likes, and although the sequence from one experiment to the next is likely to be different and will appear to be random, nonetheless, the outcome of those experiments will always end by approaching a determinate result if the sample of experiments or trials is sufficiently large.

Nevertheless, despite what we might know about the probabilities of average outcomes, we still don't know what is going on. Does a sequence of events -- that are described as being random -- produce predictable, determinate results, or is that sequence of events only apparently random but, in actuality, gives expression to a determinate set of forces that – at least for the moment -- has escaped our understanding or ability to grasp what is transpiring?

Models of probability do not necessarily describe random events. Those models are about constructing methods for calculating outcomes based on the perceived number of degrees of freedom in a given set of circumstances. When it comes to coin tosses, there are two degrees of freedom ... in the case of dice, there are six degrees of freedom (and more degrees of freedom if one uses a pair of dice) ... in the case of playing cards, there are – if one excludes jokers -- 52 degrees of freedom (or 13 degrees of freedom if one only considers the members of a given suit, or 12 degrees of freedom associated with face cards, or 36 degrees of freedom for numbered cards, or 4 degrees of freedom for aces) ... and so on.

The degrees of freedom with respect to coins, dice, cards, and the like constitute <u>framed limits</u> that are <u>determinate</u> in terms of the kind of possibilities that they allow, but the manner in which those degrees of freedom will be manifested is unknown in terms of how that dimension of being determinant will play out in any given instance, Not just anything happens, but, rather, what happens, happens in terms of the nature of the phenomenon being considered.

In addition, models of probability are predicated on the principle that there is no force or set of forces that is capable of affecting how those degrees of freedom will normally manifest themselves in a given set of circumstances. For instance, dice should not be weighted in any manner that could render some results as being more likely than other possibilities, or cards cannot be shuffled in ways that lead to a stacked deck or they cannot carry identifying marks that reveal their identity in a manner that would skew the degrees of freedom that normally govern what can occur in conjunction with a deck of 52 cards.

Probability models constitute <u>descriptions</u> of how certain phenomena manifest themselves over time. Probability models will try to accurately reflect the degrees of freedom present in such phenomena in order to be able to construct reliable methods for quantifying what will happen in conjunction with such a set of degrees of freedom in the long run.

If the law of large numbers holds in relation to those sorts of phenomena, then – given a sufficiently large number of trials -- there will be a correlation between observed outcomes and predicted outcomes. However, probability models do not constitute an <u>explanation</u> for how or why a series of seemingly random events – that is characterized by some given number of degrees of freedom -- is able to end up as a determinate result.

Now, let's shift gears a little and consider the issue of mutations. Mutations might have x-number of degrees of freedom associated with the parameters of possibility to which those mutations are capable of giving expression. Moreover, the mutations that occur in conjunction with any of those degrees of freedom might prove to be advantageous, disadvantageous, or neutral.

However, on what basis would one claim that such mutations are random in nature? If one has developed a probability model to describe and predict the possible outcomes for what might happen in relation to the degrees of freedom entailed by the process of mutation, none of those degrees of freedom necessarily constitute <u>random</u>

variables, per se, and to label them as such is an exercise in arbitrariness.

On the one hand, if we <u>don't know</u> what brings a given mutation about, then, one is not in any position to claim that the mutation is a function of random events in any ontological sense that gives expression to a provable theory about how the universe operates in accordance with allegedly random forces. On the other hand, if we <u>do know</u> what causes a given mutation, then, an individual has his or her work cut out with respect to proving that the known proximate cause of the mutation is, actually, the end result of a random conjoining of a long chain of previously unrelated events.

Neither the idea of natural selection nor the ideas of adaptation, genetic drift, geographic segregation, or speciation can, in and of themselves, account for how new functional capacities arise. All those ideas presuppose biological functionality, and the forces to which those terms allude operate in conjunction with existing biological functionality.

Speciation occurs under two broad sets of general conditions. Those conditions involve: Either some modality of geographical segregation, or the emergence of new forms of genetic variation, or a mixture of both sets of conditions.

If one, or more subsets, of an ancestral population becomes geographically segregated from that population, the physical character of the segregation might, in and of itself, induce the genotype of members of the segregated subset to manifest different phenotypic properties as a result of the: New opportunities, decreased competition, and different challenges that might be associated with the formation of an environmental niche that is brought about by the process of segregation.

Any speciation that occurs in relation to the foregoing set of circumstances does not necessarily require, or depend on, the existence of entirely new capacities. Rather, new dimensions of already existing capacities are brought into play as a function of the changed character of the dynamic between the members of the subset of the original ancestral population and the new geographical circumstances that segregates them – temporarily, partially, or permanently – from the original population.

The question, then, becomes, what are the limits, if any, on the potential for manifesting different capacities as a result of the possibilities inherent in the gene pool that constitutes the collective potential for the members of a given subset of the ancestral population? Can one suppose there are no limits and, therefore, the potential for continued speciation is indefinitely large? Or, are there determinate limits on what is possible with respect to the shuffling of genes within any given gene pool as far as the emergence of further subsets is concerned that take place in conjunction with additional instances of geographical segregation that might tap into previously unexpressed genetic dimensions of new subsets that are drawn from the subset that, in turn, had been drawn from the original, ancestral population?

The boundary conditions of speciation are shrouded in uncertainty. We often do not know what the capacity for speciation of any given gene pool is ... that is, we do not know how many previously unexpressed dimensions (capacities) of a gene pool (or its descendent gene pools) are capable of being induced to express themselves under the right circumstances of geographical segregation, and, in the process, lead to further instances of speciation.

There is nothing that is currently known which justifies assuming that the capacity for speciation with respect to any given population, or descendant subsets, is indefinitely large. At the same time, we cannot necessarily establish or determine what the precise limits are in relation to the capacity for speciation with respect to a given population or its descendant subsets.

There are several ways in which it can be said that we don't know what the capacity for speciation is with respect to any given population -- together with descendant subsets. First, we do not know what the capacity is for the process of geographical segregation to be able to induce a given gene pool to manifest the sort of genotypic and phenotypic differences over time that would generate a new species. Secondly, we do not know what the capacity of a given gene pool is with respect to generating the sort of genotypic variation (via conjugation, recombinant DNA, mutations, and/or gene shuffling) that would be capable of leading to continuous speciation given the right opportunities (such as certain kinds of geographical segregation).

| Explorations |

Is the process of speciation capable of leading to the formation of all the species, genera, families, orders, classes, phyla, and kingdoms that make up the known tree of life? We don't know, because, as indicated earlier, we don't know what the capacity for speciation is with respect to any given population or descendant subsets.

Many textbooks on evolution provide an array of specific instances -- steeped in considerable detail -- that explore the issue of how certain kinds of speciation might have occurred. Nonetheless, one cannot use an individual case – or even a series of them – to prove that all cases of speciation, in general, must have come about in a similar fashion.

Specific, documented cases of speciation certainly are suggestive with respect to what might have gone on in relation to undocumented instances of speciation. However, the former cases do not necessarily constitute any sort of proof as far as what can, or can't be said, with respect to the process of speciation in general.

Since the tree of life first set down roots on the planet Earth, it has sprouted millions, if not billions, of branches. Every branch entails some form of speciation that carries implications for issues involving the possible origins of genera, families, orders, classes, phyla, and kingdoms.

Speciation leads to what might be termed the branching problem. Although evolutionary biologists assume that all the branches on the tree of life have been generated through the known dynamics underlying speciation (e.g., natural selection, genetic drift, geographical segregation, biodiversity), there is really very little, if any, proof concerning any of this.

The movement from branch to branch is largely a function of assumption. Speciation occurs at the branching points, but what exactly is involved in such a process is not necessarily known.

This is especially the case when it comes to the appearance of new capacities and new functions that cannot necessarily be shown to have been possible in the context of a given gene pool ... even when conjugation or gene shuffling is taking into consideration. While some new genotypic and phenotypic capacities can be accounted for by the manner in which geographic segregation induces previously untapped

| Explorations |

dimensions of a gene pool to become manifest, one cannot necessarily demonstrate that the emergence of all new phenotypic and genotypic capacities came about in that fashion.

For example, Darwin's finches give expression to the sort of speciation potential that might be contained in an ancestral population from which different subsets break off and become geographically separated from one another. Over time, and given different geographical/ecological niches, one might anticipate that different subsets of the original ancestral population of finches might eventually show up with, among other things, longer beaks, or more curved beaks, or shorter beaks, and so on.

However, one would not expect those finches to show up as giraffes, kangaroos, or T-Rexes. The potential for speciation in a given population might not be precisely known, but there are certain types of limitations that seem to circumscribe that potential.

The members of the population for a given species give expression to an array of possibilities. Nevertheless, that array of possibilities cannot give expression to just any characteristic one likes but, instead, the set of possibilities for a species (its potential for speciation) tends to fall within a range of variations on particular themes that typify such a species.

The potential for speciation of a given population is intertwined with the branching problem. If one does not know what the potential for speciation is for a given population, then, one will have difficulty accounting for how a new species arose – if it did – from such a population.

There are all manner of questions entangled with the aforementioned branching problem and the related issue concerning the indeterminate character of a given species' potential for speciation. For example, we don't know how the first protocell(s) branched off from inorganic and organic chemical reactions, and among the reasons why we don't know the foregoing, is because we don't know what the speciation potential is -- if anything -- for prebiotic interactions.

Similarly, due to the indeterminate nature of the speciation potential for the relevant population, we don't know how the capacity for DNA coding branched off from life forms with no capacity for

| Explorations |

coding DNA? In addition, we don't know how organisms with the capacity for photosynthesis branched off from organisms without such a capacity. We don't know how the capacity to generate and use adenosine triphosphate to provide energy for metabolic pathways branched off from organisms that did not possess that capacity. We don't know how active forms of membrane transport branched off from non-active forms of membrane transport. We don't know how optical handedness in the molecules of life consisting of sugars (D – Dextrorotation – optical isomers) and amino acids (L – Levorotation -- optical isomers) branched off from life forms whose sugar and amino acid molecules might have consisted of racemic mixtures as far as their optical activity is concerned with respect to the way in which such molecules polarize light. We don't know how organisms with the capacity for meiosis and mitosis branched off from organisms without such capacities. We don't know how bacteria branched off from protocells. We don't know how aerobic life forms branched off from anaerobic life forms. We don't know how multicellular organisms branched off from single cell organisms. We don't know how the Eucarya, Archaea and Bacteria Kingdoms branched off from one another? We don't know how organisms with the capacity for motility branched off from organisms without motility. We don't know how animals and plants branched off from one another. We don't know how organisms with immune systems branched off from organisms without immune systems. We don't know how flowering plants branched off from non-flowering life forms? We don't know how organisms with skeletal systems branched off from organisms without a skeletal system. We don't know how organisms with a developmental life cycle rooted in specialized cell functioning branched off from organisms without such developmental life cycle that is rooted in cell specialization. We don't know how organisms with the capacity to form hearts, kidneys, livers, lungs, pancreases, stomachs, and circulatory systems branched off from organisms without such capacities. We don't know how neurons and glial cells branched off from other kinds of cells. We don't know how organisms with the capacity for memory branched off from organisms without a capacity for memory. We don't know how organisms with endocrine systems branched off from organisms without endocrine systems. Finally, one needs to add to the foregoing considerations, the array of branching problems that arise in conjunction with issues of how consciousness, intelligence, emotion, language, and creativity arose from organisms not possessing those sorts of capabilities.

Evolutionary biologists <u>always</u> assume that the speciation potential for the relevant population in all of the foregoing cases is capable of accounting for the branching problem associated with each of the challenges noted above. However, as far as the cases cited in the previous paragraph are concerned, evolutionary biologists have not brought forth any conclusive evidence about how any of the foregoing branching problems would have been bridged by the population that is, supposedly, giving rise to the new species ... a species that has capacities not present in the previous population.

As a result, allegedly random events that, supposedly, are helping to account for speciation -- or the branching problem -- are shrouded in the mists of the unknown and, perhaps, the unknowable. Moreover, the process of speciation – along with the issue of speciation potential for any relevant population linked to the branching problems outlined in the last several pages – also are shrouded in mists of the unknown and, perhaps, the unknowable.

The branching problem encompasses both of the foregoing dimensions of the unknown – and, possibly, the unknowable. In other words, neither known forms of speciation, nor allegedly random events – considered separately or together -- can necessarily account – in any reasonable or scientific manner -- for how the transition from one branch of the tree of life to another one actually takes place, but, instead, the transitions are often bridged by assumptions that are not capable of being proven.

Conjectures abound. Unfortunately, proof concerning the truth of any of those conjectures is largely, if not entirely, absent.

The extended dynamics of population biology are capable of plausibly accounting for <u>some forms</u> of speciation, but not necessarily <u>all forms</u> of speciation (and one should keep in mind that a plausible account is not necessarily the same thing as a true account). Many of the theories that describe the dynamics of population biology can justifiably be referred to as scientific ... but only to the extent that the claims entailed by those theories can be rooted in the rigorous practices of scientific method.

| Explorations |

The theory of evolution might well be a theory. However, it cannot necessarily be justifiably referred to as a scientific theory because the dimension of science is often missing from its conjectures concerning its proposed solutions to the branching problem that has been outlined in the last several pages.

Aside from the dynamics of population biology considered in rather narrow terms (i.e., minus conjectures, speculations, and assumptions), the theory of evolution is largely a narrative, rather than a scientific theory. That narrative is glued together with assumption upon assumption inserted at critical junctures in relation to all of the foregoing sorts of branching problems (and millions more) involving speciation and, as well, is glued together with assumption upon assumption inserted at critical junctures in relation to the idea that so many evolutionary events are supposedly of a random nature ... but a randomness that cannot be proven as such.

Theodosius Dobzhansky claims that 'nothing makes sense in biology except in the light of evolution' because the latter theory is capable of tying together a large set of what, otherwise, would be isolated, disparate pieces of biological information and showing how that theory provides a unified framework for understanding diversity. However, that sense of unity is largely a function of assumptions involving the roles that speciation and randomness are conjectured to play in the grand philosophy to which evolution gives expression.

As far as Dobzhansky is concerned, nothing makes sense in biology because he – and anyone else who thinks in the same way – was not prepared to take a sufficiently, rigorous critical look at all the ways in which evolution is not capable of making scientific sense of anything in biology unless one buys into a litany of assumptions concerning speciation and randomness ... assumptions that have not been proven and might never be able to be proven. Stated in another way, for Dobzhansky, the nature of biology is largely bereft of meaning unless one subscribes to the philosophical assumptions that subsidize the theory of evolution and render it meaningful.

Whatever science exists in conjunction with the theory of evolution is a function of what is required to establish the truth concerning the disparate observations, measurements, and experiments that Dobzhansky seems to find so devoid of meaning.

| Explorations |

Consequently, up to a point, the framework of population biology is able to make sense of many of those variable instances of observation, measurement, and experiment, precisely because it gives expression to a methodologically rigorous way of tying together many observations, measurements, and experiments that, otherwise, would be isolated pieces of information.

The framework of population biology is not necessarily co-extensive with evolutionary theory. In fact, population biology only gives expression to one relatively small dimension of evolutionary theory.

Population biology – which, among other things, studies changes in the phenotypic and genotypic frequencies/proportions that characterize a given population over time and, as well, explores how such changes tend to hinder or help 'fitness' with respect to a given set of environmental conditions -- entails a considerable amount of science. Technical areas of study such as: Statistics, mathematics, genetics, molecular biology, and ecology are all part of the mix when it comes to exploring and developing the science of population biology.

Evolutionary theory attempts to bask in the glow of the foregoing sorts of scientific features. In the process, evolutionary theory seeks to illicitly borrow some degree of credibility from the science that takes place in conjunction with the study of population biology and, then tries to transfer that illegitimately acquired credibility to the philosophical narrative that falls beyond the horizons of population biology but lies at the very heart of evolutionary theory.

Population biology does not try to – nor does it have to -- solve the branching problem outlined earlier because population biology does not concern itself with explaining how speciation occurs. Rather, population biology takes the existence of a species as a given, and, then, seeks to explore what happens, over time, with respect to changes in the frequencies/proportions of phenotypic and genotypic properties of a species under different environmental circumstances and genetic conditions.

The theory of evolution does not make a whole lot of sense unless one can demonstrate that all the branches of the tree of life are a function of the processes of speciation that operate in collaboration with a lengthy series of allegedly random events. If there is no detailed, coherent account of speciation that demonstrates how each and every branch of the tree of life arose, then, one really doesn't have a scientific theory, but, instead, one has a philosophical narrative that is posing as a scientific theory.

| Explorations |

| Explorations |

A Few Lessons Related to Archaea

Some scientists never seem to learn. They are like a more sophisticated version of those times when Charlie Brown believes that he has Lucy all figured out and has come up with satisfactory answers for his anxieties about whether, or not, Lucy will pull the football back just as Charlie is trying to kick the ball.

Unfortunately, Charlie's calculations and predictions in this respect invariably turn out to be wrong. There are some relatively simple reasons for why things consistently turn out the way they do for Charlie as far as the football kicking (euphemistically speaking) issue is concerned.

Firstly, Charlie doesn't seem to have much insight into how Lucy's mind works. Secondly, Charlie is inclined to extend the benefit of a doubt (involving his own assessment of the situation) to someone that he shouldn't trust.

Similarly, many scientists don't necessarily have much insight into how the universe works and, as a result, they keep deluding themselves concerning the nature of reality through one conjecture or another. Moreover, many scientists often give the benefit of a doubt to other individuals – scientists who believe they know when they don't – and toward whom the former individuals ought to harbor a more critical perspective.

Approximately 39 years ago, a revolution began with respect to the way in which evolutionary biologists and microbiologists, among others, understood the nature of reality. As is the case with so many revolutions in science, the upheaval in understanding that began to emerge nearly four decades ago was in opposition to the biases and beliefs of an array of scientific experts and leaders who, in certain respects, conflated their ignorance with whatever knowledge they actually had.

Unfortunately, there were a lot of researchers and academics that, like Charlie Brown, placed their conceptual trust in individuals who didn't necessarily deserve that sort of consideration. At least part of the reason for such misplaced trust is that many of those researchers didn't necessarily have all that much insight into the issue under consideration, and, as a result, they permitted scientific reputations to lead them around by the nose instead of critically engaging the topic for themselves.

Up until approximately 1975, the world of living organisms had been divided into two broad Kingdoms – prokaryotes and eukaryotes. The differences between the two categories of life are fairly extensive.

Prokaryotes do not have a true nucleus (that is, there is no permeable membrane surrounding, among other things, the genetic instructions for a cell), but eukaryotes do exhibit a true nucleus. Eukaryotic cells wrap their DNA around histones (a certain kind of protein), whereas prokaryotes wind their genetic material around histone-like proteins. Eukaryotes possess multiple chromosomes, whereas prokaryotes tend to have one plasmid (often consisting in a circular strand of DNA). Mitochondria -- where biochemical processes involving energy production and respiration take place -- exist in eukaryotes but do not exist in prokaryotes. The ribosomes -- functional units that bind messenger RNA and transfer RNA in order to generate (synthesize) polypeptides and proteins -- in prokaryotes are significantly smaller than their counterparts in eukaryotes. When chlorophyll is present in prokaryotes it tends to circulate freely in the cytoplasm of the cell, but in eukaryotes, chlorophyll is contained within organelles known as chloroplasts. Organelles such as: the Golgi apparatus (which has various functions including intracellular transport), the endoplasmic reticulum (a network of membranous-like structures connected to the nucleus that plays a role in the synthesis of lipids and proteins), and lysosomes (contains enzymes that can break down various kinds of molecular structures) exist in eukaryotes, but not in prokaryotes.

There are a variety of other potential differences between prokaryotes and eukaryotes. However, the foregoing set of comparisons is adequate with respect to the current discussion.

Beginning in the early-to-mid 1970s, research by Carl Woese, a molecular biologist, strongly suggested that a third realm of life forms should be added to the previously established bi-modal classification scheme that divided up life forms into prokaryotic and eukaryotic kinds of organisms. Although the name eventually given to these newly discovered life forms was "Archaea", there was a time between 1977 and 1990 when Woese referred to them as archaebacteria.

| Explorations |

The latter terminology might have misled some people. More specifically, the name seemed to suggest that the newly discovered life forms were some species of bacteria, but this was not the case (more on this shortly).

Around 1990, Woese began to refer to three domains of life: namely, eukaryotes, bacteria, and archaea. The designation "prokaryote" had disappeared from his manner of classifying the different kingdoms of life.

For quite a few years -- beginning in the early 1960s and before his discovery of archaea -- Woese had been trying to come up with a molecular taxonomy for life forms that would help connect known organisms to their molecular origins in relation to the formation of the first, primitive protocells. If – as evolutionary biologists maintained – inorganic and organic chemistry somehow led to the appearance of semi-functional and/or functional protocells, then all subsequent life forms should be solidly rooted in the formation of the specialized molecules that arose out of various kinds of inorganic and organic reactions that, eventually, led to the emergence of a variety of life forms.

Thus, one of the major reasons for organizing life forms into the aforementioned tripartite scheme of classification was rooted in Woese's interest in drawing the attention of scientists to some of the differences in molecular biology among various life forms. In other words, Woese wanted to develop a taxonomy for certain kinds of life forms that was based on molecular differences and that might be capable of linking life forms (both current and extinct) to their molecular past in relation to the advent of the first protocells since protocells were thought of as a set of interconnected molecular pathways that, somehow, had acquired the capacity to organize the synthesizing and degrading of various molecules in ways that helped make life possible.

Prior to the time when Woese began his project concerning the development of a system of molecular taxonomy, microbiologists and evolutionary biologists had invested considerable time in trying to discover some principle or set of principles that might point the way to arranging the bewildering array of microorganisms in an ordered, understandable manner. They had considered all kinds of physical, chemical, and metabolic properties in the search for a theme or themes that might help structure the multitude of microorganisms in an intelligible way ... but to no avail.

As a result, many microbiologists and evolutionary biologists seemed to have become disillusioned with the possibility of ever being able to make sense of the history underlying the evolution of different kinds of microorganisms and how they might have branched off from one another. The discovery of archaea might provide the sort of conceptual foothold needed to begin to make progress in the development of a molecular-based taxonomic system.

Quite a few scientists seemed to think that once the structural character of the code for DNA had been established, everything else was merely derivative detail. Woese, on the other hand, believed that more was needed in order to be able to get a better grasp of how things might have developed over evolutionary history, and, for Woese, part of the 'more' that was needed revolved around the problems involved in coming to understand how DNA coding was translated into components that could give expression to biological activity.

Ribosomes consist of an integrated set of proteins and RNA molecules that are responsible for stringing together an array of amino acids to form various kinds of polypeptides and proteins. Given the significance of the role played by ribosomes, Woese felt that these entities might cast an illuminating light on some of the possible ways in which the capacity to synthesize (to translate) polypeptides and proteins might have arisen over the course of evolutionary history.

In other words, differences in the structural character of ribosomes might imply differences with respect to evolutionary history. In this respect, Woese believed that an important key to unlocking at least part of the character of evolutionary history might come through identifying the structural character of ribosomes that were intimately involved in the process of translating DNA coding into proteins ... proteins that, in turn, could be used to lay down metabolic pathways through which an array of other kinds of biological activity might arise.

Woese concentrated on sequencing the 16s rRNA (ribosomal RNA) gene that occurs in microorganisms. These units consist of just

| Explorations |

1,542 nucleotide bases, and, yet, they became the royal road to differentiating microorganisms from one another because each species of organism had an oligonucleotide 'fingerprint' – that is, a relatively small subsection of the nucleotide bases that constituted a unique sequence of coding for any given species of microorganism.

Woese knew from his own research that the nucleotide base pairings that underwrote 16s ribosomal RNA tended to be highly conserved in various species. Consequently, when one came across significant differences in those base pairings, one had found something that might be of considerable importance with respect to being able to develop a method for tracing or mapping the changes in various kinds of microorganisms that occurred over time.

Woese believed that the more similar the 16s rRNA oligonucleotide sequences were in relation to different species, then, the more closely (in terms of evolutionary history) their branches might be connected to one another. Alternatively, the more dissimilar the 16s rRNA oligonucleotide sequences for different organisms were, then, the more distantly related – in evolutionary terms – those organisms were considered to be with respect to one another.

While identifying unique oligonucleotide sequences might be able to help one to classify and differentiate microorganisms from one another, this capacity doesn't necessarily permit one to resolve the branching problem discussed the previous section of this chapter. In other words, establishing the fact (as Woese did) that microorganisms carried oligonucleotide signatures or markers that enabled one to classify different species of microorganisms, this mode of classification didn't necessarily account for: How any given oligonucleotide signature/marker arose in the first place, or how the transition was made from one kind of signature/marker to another.

Some of those transitions might be accounted for in a reasonable manner by means of the dynamics of speciation as understood by evolutionary biologists. However, possible transition scenarios might not always be plausible, and, consequently, one would have to go on a case-by-case basis as to whether, or not, any given proposed transition of oligonucleotide sequences made sense or, instead, began to stretch one's willingness to extend the benefit of a doubt concerning the credibility of such proposed transitions.

| Explorations |

In any event, as Woese's catalog of oligonucleotide sequences began to grow, one of Woese's colleagues – Ralph Wolfe – began to wonder about where some of the microorganisms he (Wolfe) had been studying might fit into the molecular taxonomy that Woese was constructing, and, as well, Wolfe began to wonder where some other interesting, but little studied, microorganisms might be placed in such a taxonomy.

More specifically, Wolfe had acquired some expertise in being able to culture or grow anaerobic (environmental conditions involving no free oxygen), methane-producing microorganism (known as methanogens). Establishing such cultures was a finicky affair involving, among other things, the right combinations and amounts of nutrients.

In nature, methanogens were found in some rather unsavory environments – or so it might seem to some individuals -- such as sewage sludge and the rumens (the first stomach) of cows. Later on, it was discovered that methanogens could also flourish in the high temperatures of volcanic vents.

Wolfe also knew about the existence of other microorganisms that were found in environments of a rather inhospitable nature. For example, some microorganisms had been discovered basking in extreme conditions involving both elevated temperatures (thermophiles) and high sulfur content, while other organisms had been found in conditions characterized by high salt content (halophiles).

When the 16s rRNA oligonucleotide genetic sections of such organisms were sequenced, the foregoing organisms, along with methanogens, seemed to exhibit oligonucleotide signatures that were very different from any of the other microorganisms (mostly bacteria) that had been catalogued by Woese. In addition, these particular life forms seemed to share other characteristics that were not found in bacteria.

For example, the organisms that appeared to be un-bacteria-like displayed lipid linkages -- as well as a form of chirality with respect to the central carbon atoms in glycerol units -- that were different from what one encountered in most bacterial lipid molecules (which play important roles in the membranes of bacterial and archaea cells).

Furthermore, these apparently non-bacterial forms of life used a different kind of RNA polymerase – the enzyme that is used to convert DNA into messenger RNA – than bacteria do, and, as well, they shared a resistance to certain antibiotics (e.g., rifampicin ... which disrupts bacterial transcription – the process of instantiating DNA information in the form of RNA sequences).

The newly discovered life forms seemed to be neither fish nor fowl. That is, they didn't seem to belong to either prokaryotic or eukaryotic categories of classification.

In 1977, Carl Woese, along with George Fox (a post-doctoral student), wrote a paper that appeared in the November edition of the *Proceedings for the National Academy of Science*. Their paper discussed some of the evidence that supported their ideas about a new way of classifying life, and the two authors of the article argued that the newly discovered, non-bacterial and non-eukaryotic forms of life to which they were alluding in their paper should form a domain of their own.

The new domain of life subsequently was described by NASA, NSF (National Science Foundation), and *Newsweek* magazine as being a more ancient form of life than either prokaryotes or eukaryotes. However, such descriptions seemed to be devoid of any explanation with respect to how the transition in speciation from the new domain of life forms -- archaebacteria -- to prokaryotes was made.

After all, as indicated previously, the differences between archaebacteria and bacteria went beyond their respective oligonucleotide signatures, but encompassed, as well, major differences in, among other things, RNA polymerase enzymes, antibiotic sensitivity, and lipid formation. Consequently, there were a lot of changes for which to account before someone might plausibly claim that she or he could explain how bacteria branched off from archaebacteria ... if that is how things actually took place.

Notwithstanding the foregoing considerations, many scientists – including at least one Nobel laureate -- ridiculed the idea that a new domain of life needed to be added to the already established domains of prokaryotes and eukaryotes. However – and most unfortunately -- the criticisms directed toward Woese and Fox did not revolve around meticulously crafted scientific arguments that were rooted in observation, experiments and critical analysis.

| Explorations |

Rather, those attacks were rooted in the stasis of entrenched ways of thinking about things. Inertial conceptual forces had been set in motion as a reaction to the Woese/Fox paper, and those forces were trying to prevent the light of a different and promising way of looking at data from gaining traction in the hallowed halls of research and academia.

People that shouldn't have been trusted on the issue -- because, at least for a time, they forgot what science actually involves -- were trusted. Furthermore, individuals who weren't willing to critically engage the evidence concerning archaebacteria on its own terms were prepared to act like lemmings and follow the nominal 'leaders' over the cliff of scientific propriety.

One giant figure in the annals of evolutionary biology – Ernst Mayr – appeared to support the work being done in conjunction with archaebacteria ... at least this seemed to be the case in the early years of that research. However, Mayr became opposed to things when Woese started to treat species of archaea as part of a formal, taxonomic system of classification that divided life forms up into three domains.

As a result, Mayr went to his grave maintaining that archaea did not form a separate domain of life forms. He felt that Woese had gone too far in relation to the molecular approach to taxonomy that was being thrown into the fray, and, yet, the criteria for what constituted going 'too far' seemed rather arbitrary and tied to unproven, pet theories about how the universe of evolution was believed to operate.

Arthur Schopenhauer once indicated that all truth goes through three stages. "First, it is ridiculed. Second, it is violently opposed. Third, it is accepted as being self-evident."

For years certainly, Woese's research was ridiculed. In addition, it was opposed ... adamantly and unpleasantly perhaps, rather than violently so. And, finally, it was accepted as being – if not self-evident – at least true.

J. Craig Venter sequenced the genome of a methanogen and compared it with both the sequenced genome of a bacterium as well as with certain oligonucleotide sections that had been derived from eukaryotic organisms. On August 25, 1996, Venter, together with some

| Explorations |

editorial personnel from the prestigious magazine *Science*, organized a press conference at the National Press Club in Washington, D.C. in order to announce the results of Venter's comparison study.

Venter had come to the conclusion that there should no longer be any doubt concerning whether, or not, Archaea constituted a different taxonomic domain of its own. There were, in fact, significant differences among the sequences for the three life forms that were being compared in his study.

Indeed, during the press conference, Venter noted that at least two-thirds of the genes sequenced in the methanogen did not resemble anything that had been observed in conjunction with either bacterial or eukaryotic life forms. Venter was confirming -- and rather emphatically expanding upon -- the research that Woese had been carrying out for more than a quarter of a century.

Unsuspectingly, Venter also was contributing to the branching problem outlined in the previous section of this chapter. More specifically, how does one account for the emergence or origin of so many genes that are unlike anything previously seen in either bacterial or eukaryotic life forms? How does one account for the transition from such a different set of genes in archaea to the ones that are observed in bacterial and eukaryotic life forms?

Woese has indicated that it might not be possible to sort out such questions and issues. The reason for this has to do with something called "horizontal" or "lateral" gene transfer.

Horizontal gene transfer does not operate in accordance with the normal mode of gene transfer – referred to as "vertical gene transfer" – in which genes are passed down to progeny via some form of reproductive process (asexual or sexual). Horizontal gene transfer involves the exchange of genes via conjugation or via the transfer of genes in conjunction with some sort of viral agent or via jumping genes (mobile segments of DNA).

Ever the maverick and original thinker, Woese had developed a perspective that ran counter to the more traditional or Darwinian idea in which all subsequent life forms (including all three domains or kingdoms) arose from a common ancestor. Instead, Woese believed that 'in the beginning' there might have been three sorts of protocells or protocell-like organisms that were immersed in a medium consisting of, among other things, many kinds of genes.

Moreover, it is even possible that the starting points for life might have been some sort of network of metabolic pathway that could have served as precursors to the emergence of protocells. In either case, genes flowed into and out of metabolic networks and/or protocells via horizontal gene transfer.

According to Woese, horizontal gene transfers, operating in conjunction with whatever protocells or networks of metabolic pathways existed in the early days of evolution, eventually led to the rise of the three domains of life forms that are known today. Nevertheless, in whatever way Woese wishes to describe his ideas, they still leave unanswered or unaddressed the issue of how functional genes of any kind arose in the first place.

Proposing that a medium existed at some point on early Earth that was replete with sequences of DNA that are referred to as "genes, is neither here nor there. Unless those 'genes' have some sort of functionality of their own and/or have a functionality in the context of a network of metabolic pathways that is capable of synthesizing one, or more, components that leads to the establishment of biological functioning of some kind, then one could exchange as many 'genes' as one likes through horizontal gene transfer, and nothing of much interest will necessarily take place.

Not just any sequence of DNA or RNA will suffice. As indicated in the foregoing paragraph, sequences must have, in some sense of the term, "functional potential", and, therefore, there needs to be an account of how functionality arises in the sea of genes that Woese is envisioning.

If one likes, one can assume that metabolic pathways made up of an interlocking set of functional genes somehow emerged. Nonetheless, one still needs to scientifically demonstrate how any of this is possible ... if not plausible.

One can assume as many things as one likes. However, at some point, the inclination to rely almost exclusively on assumptions as a means of bridging whatever seems inexplicable or problematic takes one beyond the horizons of science and into the realm of philosophy.

| Explorations |

205

The issue of functionality is related to, but not necessarily coextensive with, the branching problem discussed earlier. To be sure, the branching problem requires one to explain how one moves from one kind of biologically functioning system (i.e., species) to another – somewhat different – kind of biologically functioning system (i.e., the new species that gives expression to the process of speciation).

Nevertheless, one encounters a different set of problems when one is faced with the task of trying to account for the emergence of functionality in the first operational protocell or network of metabolic pathways. In other words, accounting for how the very first species – along with the archetypal prototypic capacity for speciation – came into being entails a slightly different set of explanatory problems than does trying to account for how subsequent species arise <u>given</u> the existence of an already functional life form ... although, admittedly, there is a certain amount of overlap between the two kinds of problems.

Similarly, accounting for how a protein with an entirely new kind of functional capacity arises is a different kind of problem than trying to account for how a certain protein might have transitioned into a slightly different protein that possesses a marginally different function than did the former protein. Furthermore, trying to explain how a new metabolic pathway first became established is a different issue than trying to explain how an existing metabolic pathway might have acquired certain differences over a period of time, and, in the process, led to the formation of a new species.

For example, consider the archaea life form known as Nanoarchaeum equitans. This organism was discovered at a depth of approximately 350 feet within a volcanic vent of the Kolbeinsey Ridge, north of Iceland.

The foregoing organism is attached to the outer membrane of a variety of archaea species. Many, if not most or all, of these latter species belong to groups known as thermophiles (able to flourish in conditions of high heat ranging from 150 to 170 degrees Fahrenheit) and hyperthermophiles (flourishing in temperatures up to, at least, 235 degrees Fahrenheit) ... if not beyond.

| Explorations |

Nanoarchaeum exists in a number of different forms. These differences seem to be a function, at least in part, of the kind of hyperthermophiles to which they are attached.

In a variety of ways, Nanoarchaeum constitute a rather strange form of organism. On the one hand, it operates without a complete set of genetic instructions.

Therefore, like a virus, it must borrow a certain amount of metabolic machinery from its host ... machinery that is needed for the synthesis of, among other things, amino acids, certain co-factors, and lipids. Furthermore, like a virus, it apparently remains dormant when not attached to a host.

Yet, Nanoarchaeum has not been classified as a virus. Instead, Nanoarchaeum is considered to belong to the domain of Archaea ... although -- since it appears to be either a symbiont or a parasite -- it is a form of archaea that had not been encountered previously.

Relatively recently, various kinds of megaviruses have been discovered ... some of which have roughly four times (2300 genes) the number of genes (563 genes) contained by Nanoarchaeum. In addition, relative to other non-viral entities, Nanoarchaeum is quite small, and, in fact, it is one of the smallest -- if not the smallest – life form ever discovered.

Based on an analysis of the amino acid sequences found in a number of its ribosomal proteins, Nanoarchaeum turns out to be quite different from many other species in the domain of Archaea. Indeed, some of its properties are so different that various microbiologists believe – but not everyone agrees -- that Nanoarchaeum might form a separate branch of life within the domain of Archaea.

On the other hand, whatever disagreements might exist in conjunction with whether, or not, Nanoarchaeum gives expression to a new branch of Archaea, there seems to be a general consensus that this species of Archaea constitutes a very ancient form of life. Some individuals believe that it might even have made up part of the root of the tree of life from which subsequent species sprang.

The foregoing possibility leads to a variety of questions. For example, if Nanoarchaeum is closely affiliated with, or is an instance of, some of the primitive precursors of later life forms, and if

Nanoarchaeum consists of a system of genes that cannot function on its own, and if Nanoarchaeum tends to remain dormant without the presence of an appropriate host, then how did Nanoarchaeum – along with the other species of archaea on which it depends -- come into existence.

By being one of the smallest -- if not the smallest -- life forms known to humankind, Nanoarchaeum might only possess an incomplete set of 563 genes, but, nevertheless, they are functional genes. The origin of that sort of functionality needs to be explained, and this amounts not to one question, but 563 of them … in fact, additional questions (at least 490, 885 of them) will arise and lead beyond the foregoing number (563) as one tries to account for how the hundreds, if not thousands, of nucleotide base pairs that make up each of those 563 genes came to have sequences that, when translated and transcribed, formed functional units.

The foregoing issues, problems, and questions are not inconsequential. This is because the aforementioned figure – 563 genes – is close to what some evolutionary biologists consider to be around the minimal number of genes needed for life to be self-sustaining and, therefore, might, or might not, be intimately caught up with the origin of life issue.

Aside from the considerations noted during the last several paragraphs, there are other sorts of questions and problems that tend to emerge. For example, if Nanoarchaeum life forms came into existence before, say, the aforementioned hyperthermophiles, and, as such, constitute some sort of predecessor to the latter species, then, how did the hyperthermophiles arise? On the other hand, if the hyperthermophiles were first up on the tree of life, then one must try to account for a form of life that has many more genes than Nanoarchaeum does (and, consequently, is capable of generating many more questions) and, as well, there will be an additional litany of questions about how Nanoarchaeum evolved subsequent to the hyperthermophiles.

Earlier, in passing, entities referred to as megaviruses were mentioned. The size of some of these megaviruses – in terms of the number of genes and the number of base pairs they encompass, as well as in terms of the fact that they are big enough to be seen with a light

| Explorations |

(rather than with an electron) microscope – dwarfs the size of Nanoarchaeum and are even are larger than some forms of bacteria.

The genome of the larger of two megaviruses found in the ocean near Chile and in a fresh-water lake in Australia contained as many as 2.6 million base pairs. The genome of Nanoarchaeum contained less than one-fifth (490, 885) the number of base pairs carried by the larger of the two aforementioned viruses.

When the base pairs of the megaviruses (referred to as Pandoraviruses) were sequenced, something very intriguing was discovered. More specifically, only between 7 and 15 percent of the base pairs matched up with anything in the databases that catalogued sequenced base pairings.

Since, for the most part, the foregoing base pairing sequences didn't match up with known base pairing sequences this means there are millions of questions surrounding how such differences arose. Those questions have to do with trying to figure out how millions of base pairings came together to form 2300 functional genes ... and why certain genes necessary to make the megavirus into an autonomous, self-perpetuating life form were missing.

One of the smallest -- yet fully autonomous -- species of bacteria that exists is quite common in the oceans of the world. Its name is Pelagibacter ubique.

It consists of 1,389 genes and 1,308,759 base pairs. This makes it more than twice as large as Nanoarchaeum, but only half the size of some Pandoraviruses.

Having a substantial number of functional genes doesn't, in and of itself, necessarily confer life. Pandoraviruses have more genes and more base pairs than Pelagibacter, but the former is not considered a form of life – at least not of an autonomous kind – while Pelagibacter is classified as a bacterial life form.

Nanoarchaeum has less than half the genetic material (both in terms of the number of genes and the number of base pairs) that is contained in the bacterium, Pelagibacter ubique. In addition, Nanoarchaeum does not carry the full complement of genes needed to code for proteins, lipids, co-factors, and so on, and, yet, unlike

| Explorations |

Pandoraviruses, Nanoarchaeum is still considered a life form belonging to the domain of archaea.

Where and how one draws the line that separates the living from the non-living does not seem to be a straightforward function of either the number of genes, the number of base pairs, and whether, or not, a given entity is fully autonomous. Nonetheless, no matter how one defines the line of demarcation between life and non-life, one still has to account for how genes with some degree of functionality arose out of thousands, if not millions, of base pairs ... because although functional genes obviously exist in species from the domains of archaea and bacteria – both of which are described as being made up of living species -- nevertheless, functional genes also exist in megaviruses such as Pandoraviruses that are considered to be non-living entities.

How does functional order arise out of an ocean of 'genes' that are not necessarily functional to begin with ... unless, of course, one arbitrarily – and, therefore, without proof -- supposes that at least some of those 'genes' have a functional capacity? Even given an ocean of at least some genes with a degree of functional capacity, how does the horizontal transfer of genes bring about ordered systems of biological functionality?

Various microbiologists seem to feel that the discovery and study of Archaea – and, perhaps, megaviruses -- gets us all closer to arriving at an understanding concerning the origin(s) of life. However, evolutionary biologists don't seem to have any means of separating the wheat from the chaff when it comes to trying to answer any of the foregoing sorts of questions in a rigorous and a reliable fashion.

Saying -- as Woese does -- that protocells or networks of metabolic pathways arose in an ocean of "genes" -- where horizontal gene transfer was common -- doesn't address any of a variety of basic questions in a very specific manner. Instead, 'explanations' – if one can call them that -- are so saturated with assumptions of one kind or another that trying to claim that any such network of assumptions gets us closer to understanding the origin of life is a lot like trying to claim that landing on Pluto gets us closer to reaching the Andromeda galaxy ... which in a sense might be true, but not in any way that makes much of a difference as far as reaching Andromeda is concerned.

| Explorations |

A reader should not infer from the foregoing comments that I believe horizontal gene transfer doesn't occur in 'real' life or that such transfers don't play important roles in the lives of microorganisms. For example, one might note that since 1988 the Hawaii Ocean Time-series research project (HOT) – together with related research projects elsewhere in the world – acquired microorganisms and viruses from ocean samples collected at depths ranging 40 to 13,000 feet.

The researchers have sequenced the genomes of those samples. Among the millions and millions of base pairs that have been catalogued in relation to those samples, a multitude of new genes (extending into the thousands) have been discovered.

More importantly, at least for present purposes, those researchers uncovered a great deal of evidence supporting, if not proving, the idea that an extensive amount of horizontal gene transfer occurs among the microorganisms and viruses that made up the samples collected. However, demonstrating that horizontal gene transfer currently occurs in viruses and microorganisms – and, as well, has occurred in the past – does not really explain how the capacity for horizontal gene transfer arose originally, nor does it account for how the genes that are being horizontally transferred acquired their initial functionality millions – perhaps billions -- of years ago ... nor does the current existence of horizontal gene transfer explain how the functional genes that have been horizontally transferred became incorporated into the genetic programming of the entity to which the genes have been transferred ... nor does it account for how the capacity to incorporate genes from other organisms came into being so that those transferred genes could become appropriately modified to become adaptive, functional units within the cellular ecology of the latter organisms.

The foregoing issues point in the direction of something that, potentially, has considerable importance. More specifically, those considerations suggest – as do many other considerations in this chapter -- that the theory of evolution is not a scientific theory missing a few, inessential details. Rather, it is a theory that is missing almost all of the foundational components needed to explain and demonstrate the specific character of the dynamics that, supposedly, are at the heart of evolutionary change.

| Explorations |

The theory of evolution pretends to be a scientific theory. However, when it matters most, that worldview, again and again, resorts to the use of unproven – and, perhaps, unprovable -- assumptions, speculations, or conjectures in an attempt to provide the underpinnings for purported explanations concerning a vast array of questions and problems that the theory should be able to address in a plausible manner if were truly scientific in character ... but does not do so.

One of the features that typify philosophical activity has to do with the inability of such a process to be able to demonstrate – in an independent and rigorous manner -- the truth of many, if not most, of its claims concerning the nature of reality. Yet, when the theory of evolution manifests the same sort of inability to prove its essential claims, nevertheless – and, perhaps (given the nature of philosophical bias), not so mysteriously -- that theory retains its alleged scientific status.

Consider the following. At the heart of the dynamics of many extremophiles (organisms capable of surviving and flourishing in extreme physical conditions), are proteins with specialized properties of functionality. These proteins have the capacity to assist organisms to adapt to extremes of, among other things, acidity, alkalinity, salinity, radiation, heat, cold, and pressure.

For instance, thermophiles and hyperthermophiles possess certain kinds of proteins that exhibit enhanced hydrophobic (water resistant/avoidant) properties along with an elevated capacity for a variety of electrostatic interactions that are needed to help lend stability (through, among other things, packing and folding activities) to the metabolic pathways that must operate in the midst of conditions involving high temperatures (up to, at least, 235 degrees Fahrenheit). Now, since proteins with a certain amount of hydrophobic properties and capacity for electrostatic interactions exist in most cells, the problem becomes one of explaining how thermophiles and hyperthermophiles acquired the ability to push – in a functional manner -- the cellular envelope with respect to such properties and capacities.

The general issue being alluded to in the foregoing paragraph also applies to halophiles ... that is, organisms which have the capacity to survive and flourish in conditions involving high saline content. In other words, while the specialized proteins that help make halophiles possible tend to exhibit a high negative surface charge -- as a result of: The presence of an increased number of acidic amino acids, together with the insertion of certain kinds of peptide linkages at appropriate junctures -- nonetheless, other cells that cannot tolerate conditions of high salinity also possess proteins with some degree of acidic amino acid content, and, so, one wonders how the right set of specialized proteins (or the underlying base pairing) arose in halophiles that enabled them to deal with conditions of extreme osmotic stress brought about by the presence of a high saline content in the environment in which the halophiles exist.

Similarly, psychrophilic organisms – ones that survive and flourish in temperatures near, or below, freezing – possess certain proteins that exhibit reduced hydrophobic properties, as well as display a reduced electrostatic charge on the surface of those proteins, and, in the process, helps such organisms to adapt to cold temperatures. How did proteins with these kinds of characteristics arise?

The specialized proteins that are key to thermophilic adaptation are different (in terms of hydrophobic properties, acidic amino acid content, electrostatic interaction on their surfaces, as well as properties of folding and packing) from the specialized proteins that are key to halophiles and psychrophiles. Indeed, they are all different from one another in various ways.

Similar sorts of differences extend to other kinds of extremophiles that inhabit conditions of high pressure, radiation, acidity, and alkalinity. In certain cases, however, there is some degree of overlap with respect to various amino acid sequences and base pairings since some organisms that can exist in, say, conditions of high saline content also exhibit the capacity to survive in conditions of high alkalinity, or organisms capable of existing in conditions of low temperatures also often tend to display an ability to deal with conditions of high salinity.

Areas of overlap notwithstanding, there still are different kinds of specialized proteins that play various kinds of roles in all of the foregoing cases ... although in certain instances involving multiple conditions of extreme environments (e.g. low temperatures and high saline content, or high temperatures as well as a high acidity), some of

| Explorations |

these proteins might play a secondary role rather than a primary one. Consequently, at some point the existence of proteins with the foregoing sorts of specialized functions and capabilities have to be accounted for as far as questions involving the origins of those proteins are concerned.

There are many conjectures that might be offered with respect to such matters. Maybe, for instance, the transition to proteins with a specialized capacity for functioning was gradual (Many, if not all, of the following comments also could be directed toward the idea of non-gradual transitions as well.).

If the transitions were relatively gradual, there are many pathways that might have been made such transitions possible. Nonetheless, if a person advances a theory of transition concerning the origin of a given form of extremophilic protein, then, one would like to know not only the precise route that was taken to make the transition from some kind of non-extremophilic protein to an extremophilic one, but, as well, one would like to know the nature of the dynamics at each step along that route.

In addition, one would like to know how the ancestral proteins emerged that, allegedly, predated the appearance of the specialized, extremophilic proteins. One can point, if one likes, to any number of possible transitions from the base pairings underlying one kind of protein to the base pairings underlying some kind of subsequent, specialized, extremophilic protein, but, at some point one is going to have to explain how the first protein arose that was part of the original branch that, eventually, led to the evolutionary branches on which specialized, extremophilic proteins are found.

Moreover, one cannot suppose that the functionality which might arise from the fact that some given sequence of thousands of nucleotide base pairings came together in just the right way to be selected by natural selection is capable of accounting for why one such sequence, rather than some other sequence, occurred. Natural selection acts upon such sequences after the fact and not before the fact.

In other words, natural selection might be able to help explain why a given set of genes -- with certain capabilities – survives or flourishes in a given set of environmental circumstances. However, natural selection cannot necessarily explain how those genes or a sequence of base pairings came to exist in the first place.

Therefore, when one engages issues such as trying to account for the origins of specialized, extremophilic proteins (or their supporting metabolic pathways) an individual is always engaged in matters that tend to transcend the horizons of the idea of natural selection. One is engaged in a rather mysterious realm that the theory of evolution attempts to explain away through, among other conceptual devices, use of the notion of random mutations (see the following 'Deep Solutions ...' section of this chapter for a discussion concerning some of these other conceptual devices being alluded to in the foregoing).

If mutations constitute the ideational bridge that is intended to 'explain' the movement and dynamics along some proposed pathway of gradualness, then, what caused which mutations to happen at what points and in which sequence? If someone objects that such questions cannot be answered, then, to whatever extent they cannot be answered, then, to that extent one does not have a scientific theory.

Moreover, if someone claims that the mutations were random – and, therefore, inexplicable in character -- then, one should be ready to acknowledge that this sort of claim doesn't really explain much of anything. Instead -- as pointed out earlier in this chapter during the brief discussion that revolved about the idea of randomness -- such an account tends, at best, to presuppose its own truth ... something that, scientifically speaking, is not really an appropriate thing to do.

How does one prove or demonstrate what the nature of the sequence of events was that made a protein with specialized, extremophilic capabilities possible? How did the requisite kinds of nucleotide sequences come together to underwrite such a capability, and how did the requisite base pairing coding for the associated metabolic pathways come about in a manner that would be able to arrange for supplying the right kinds of specialized proteins at the right times and in the right amounts and in the right places?

One could imagine many scenarios for how such a complex, integrated set of events might have come about. Imagination is capable of many things.

Nonetheless, imagination does not always give expression to, or lead one toward, the truth of things. In fact, we often can image what is false much more readily that we can imagine what is true.

Many so-called scientific journals, books, and academics are often filled with conjectural imaginings of all kinds as a way of alluding to the possible significance of a given set of observations or experiments. Yet, most of those imaginings disappear as quickly as they arose because they lack the necessary, substantive properties that can tie them to reality in anything more than what ultimately proves to be a tangential -- if not asymptotic -- manner.

The process of conjecturing and speculating about the nature of reality can be a useful exercise because it helps to stimulate further research and critical reflection. However, the content of those conjectures and speculations does not become scientific until one can rigorously demonstrate that such content gives expression to the truth or can play a substantial role in helping to lead one to the truth.

| Explorations |

Deep Solutions for the Problem of Biological Origins

In addition to the notion of random mutations (and, some of the problems surrounding this notion have been touched upon previously), there are a variety of other terms that appear in some of the literature that seeks to outline and explore the theory of evolution. Like the idea of "random mutations", these other terms are used in ways that create the impression that something is understood when this is not necessarily the case.

For instance, some people refer to the chaotic properties of various kinds of biological or chemical systems in which small changes in initial conditions can lead to unpredictable results. One could accept such a statement without necessarily being any closer to understanding – in specific, provable ways -- how, say, non-living systems turn into living systems, or how non-extremophilic proteins transition into extremophilic proteins, or how metabolic pathways come into existence.

The earlier reference to chaotic properties can be replaced by an array of other terms such as: 'spontaneous', 'self-organizing', 'far from equilibrium conditions', 'self-criticality', and 'emergence'. In each case, a term is used that is intended to serve as a means of explaining how some given structure, property, activity, network, or capacity arose in a given set of circumstances that didn't contain such structures, properties, activities, networks or capacities prior to a certain point in time ... or prior to some given threshold being reached.

Thus, far from equilibrium conditions generate dissipative structures. The properties of such structures could not have been predicted on the basis of the existence of far from equilibrium conditions on their own.

Or, interacting components of the right kind spontaneously lead to self-organizing systems. The possibility of systems with those sorts of capacities could not have been predicted knowing just the nature of the properties of the individual components involved prior to the point of being brought into an interactive dynamic with one another.

Or, complex systems give rise to emergent properties. The nature of these latter properties could not have been predicted before the

| Explorations |

conditions necessary for such complex systems occurred and attained a certain level of self-criticality.

No one who has any degree of familiarity with what has been taking place in science over the last 50 years, or so, would deny that there are an array of circumstances in which far from equilibrium conditions are capable of generating unanticipated forms of dissipative structures ... or, in which certain kinds of systems do organize themselves -- seemingly spontaneously – in unexpected ways as a function of the forces and elements present in those systems ... or, in which various kinds of properties inexplicably emerge out of systems exhibiting complex sorts of behavior. Instances of all of the foregoing scenarios have been demonstrated on numerous occasions.

Nonetheless, demonstrating the reality of the foregoing sorts of phenomena does not prove or force one to conclude that any given process for which one does not have a ready explanation concerning how such events are possible must be the result of some chaotic, complex, spontaneous, self-organizing, or emergent dynamic that automatically generates what cannot be otherwise explained. For example, unless one can show scientifically that a particular set of inorganic and organic interactions is capable of spontaneously organizing itself in a way that leads to life as an emergent property when certain thresholds of self-criticality have been reached in the context of complex systems behavior -- where initial conditions are of considerable importance -- then, all of the foregoing terminology constitutes little more than a bunch of buzz words that purport to explain things but, in reality, do nothing of the sort.

To claim that life is due to a sequence of phenomena that are built on layer after layer of spontaneously emerging properties arising out of systems that have become – and are continuing to become -- increasingly complex as a result of the accumulation of, and ensuing interaction of, the foregoing sorts of emergent properties might be a meaningful way of engaging a great deal of data, but it is entirely too vague to be of any scientific value.

Furthermore, claiming that since we seem to have no other explanation for how life arose, then, life "must have" arisen through such an inexplicable -- but determinately emergent -- set of processes might be an interesting conjecture. Nevertheless, unless one can

| Explorations |

explicate the inexplicable in demonstrable, provable ways, then, there is no science present ... just conjecture.

Many scientists believe that the structural character of the universe gives expression to, and is the result of, a set of natural laws capable of being discovered through a reiterative process that rigorously pursues observation, experiment, and critical analysis in an attempt to produce a coherent, consistent, accurately reflective portrait of some facet of reality. Consequently, scientists tend to believe that the universe and all it encompasses – including life – must be the result of some set of natural forces and principles that have the capacity to generate, among other things, the phenomena we experience.

In other words, life is considered to be an inevitable product of the interaction of chemical and physical laws. Given the right set of chemical ingredients, forms of energy, kinds of forces, environmental conditions, and sufficient time, then, according to the foregoing way of thinking about things, the emergence of life will occur.

However, an on-going problem for scientists is that they have had a heck of a time trying to figure out what the right set of chemical ingredients, sources of energy, forces, environmental conditions, and so on are. Indeed, to date, scientists have not been successful – not even remotely so -- in their attempts to show that life is, in fact, an inevitable outcome that is rooted in the interaction of a determinate set of naturally occurring physical/material events.

Many scientists believe there are three general steps that lead to the dance of life. First, one throws into the evolutionary pot an array of carbon-containing molecules, together with an assortment of other kinds of inorganic molecules that can spice things up. These molecules might have arisen on Earth, and/or they might have come to Earth via asteroids and comets, or they might even somehow have found their way to Earth from somewhere in the cosmic void.

Secondly, scientists presume that the structural character of one's pot is sufficiently complex that it permits a variety of processes to take place that are capable of: Bringing together, concentrating, and assembling the molecules initially present in such an evolutionary pot. This complexity is believed to extend to the structural properties of the interior of the pot that needs (if the theory is to have a chance of being correct) to consist of the right sort of surfaces, textures, and minerals, to be able to help catalyze and compartmentalize an array of molecular reactions that, supposedly, lead to the emergence of complex molecules such as: Proteins, nucleic acids, lipids, and carbohydrates.

Thirdly, the dynamic of interacting molecules within the right kind of evolutionary pot eventually establishes networks of metabolic pathways that are able to sustain themselves, compete for resources, and self-replicate. Such systems are believed to give expression to a set of characteristics that have varying degrees of capacity for survival and, as a result, forces such as natural selection and genetic drift begin to push and pull populations of organisms in different directions as a function of the interaction between the capabilities of those sorts of organisms and the degree to which environmental conditions lend support to, or are antagonistic to, those capacities.

Aside from the many problems that are entailed by the foregoing tripartite narrative (and there will be more discussion concerning such problems shortly), people often get bogged down with trying to determine when, exactly, life emerged during the aforementioned three-step process. Some people identify the beginning of life with the appearance of the first systems that were capable, in some sense, of self-replication via RNA and/or DNA.

Other individuals believe the beginning of life is synonymous with a capacity to establish metabolic pathways. Still other individuals refer to the capacity to form semipermeable membranes as marking the emergence of life. And, finally, there are those who believe that appropriate combinations involving all of the foregoing capabilities are necessary for life to exist.

I believe the foregoing kinds of considerations are rather premature. Before one even addresses the issue of 'what is life?' one must account for how the order necessary for underwriting the emergence of capacities -- such as: Self-replication, metabolism, and semipermeable membrane formation -- arose out of a assortment of interacting carbon-containing molecules and a variety of other inorganic molecules. The primary issue is not a matter of figuring out how to differentiate life and non-life, but, rather, the primary issue is a matter of trying to determine how functional order arises out of circumstances comprised of elements and forces that do not, on their own, exhibit such functionality or order.

To begin with, there are 80-90 years of collected data indicating that various kinds of molecules occurring in living organisms are capable of being fashioned in the laboratory under the right kind of experimental conditions. However, there is little, or no, evidence indicating that the chemical interactions occurring on early Earth went about their business in the manner in which laboratory experiments suggested might have been the case.

Are the laboratory experiments being alluded to in the foregoing paragraph rather suggestive? Of course, they are ... but being suggestive is not proof of anything.

By their very nature, experiments require the organizational capacities of one, or more, experimenters in order for those experiments to be able to take place. Experimenters bring materials together in a specific manner (e.g., amounts, sequence, length of time, and conditions) and ensure that those materials are subjected to a certain set of events within an environment that is highly regulated.

When things are done in the foregoing manner, various consequences follow. But, what happens when materials and forces are left to their own devices, sans experimenter ... will the same kinds of consequences that are observed in the laboratory also occur?

Maybe! However, the issue is whether, or not, those sorts of consequences will inevitably occur independently of the ordered conditions of a laboratory experiment.

Experiments can provide a proof of concept – that is, experiments can demonstrate that certain kinds of consequences are possible and follow from certain kinds of conditions. Nevertheless, there is no guarantee that the natural world will necessarily give expression to the conditions and circumstances that are necessary for 'interesting' kinds of consequences to emerge.

For example, let's consider a classic experiment conducted back in the early 1950s, under the guidance of Harold Urey – a Nobel Prize winning chemists -- by Stanley Miller, a second-year graduate student. Among other things, the tabletop simulation of early Earth conditions had a 5-inch, 300-milliliter glass flask that was two-thirds full of water that supposedly represented the ocean.

Depending on circumstances, ocean water comes in a variety of forms. The saline content of that water can vary, as can its temperature, pH value, and mineral content ... all of which can impact the rates and character of whatever sorts of reactions might take place in that kind of a medium.

Moreover, on early Earth, surface waters would have been bathed relatively continuously in a certain, unknown amount of ultraviolet light. As a result, whatever reactions might have taken place in the liquid medium also might have been quickly degraded as a result of the presence of that ultraviolet light ... and the impact of ultraviolet light on organic molecules is only part of the broader problem of photolysis in which the presence of light has the capacity to degrade the reactants and products of various reactions.

In addition, ocean water would have been subject to tidal forces, currents, and storms of varying intensities. How tides, ocean currents, and storms might have affected chemical reactions is a further set of considerations that need to be factored into one's analysis of the possible significance – or lack thereof – of the Miller/Urey experiment.

The bottom line is that what might take place in a flask filled with water that is hooked up to other experimental equipment is not necessarily indicative of what might take place on early Earth. No matter what geological period one is considering, ocean water is a much more variable and complex medium than is 'ordinary' water.

The aforementioned 300-milliliter flask of water was hooked up to a 10 inch, 5-liter flask filled with a number of gases that are fairly reactive – namely, hydrogen (H_2), methane (CH_4), and ammonia (NH_3). In addition, the latter flask contained two metal electrodes that were intended to serve as the experimental counterpart to lightning strikes.

Opinions concerning the composition of the atmosphere on early Earth have gone through a number of fairly significant changes since the Miller/Urey experiment. For example, seven, or so, years, after the Miller/Urey experiment had been completed, the evidence from additional geological and geochemical experiments/analysis tended to indicate that the atmosphere of early Earth consisted, to a large extent, of carbon dioxide and nitrogen.

Unlike hydrogen, methane, and ammonia – which are reactive gases – carbon dioxide and nitrogen are less reactive than the gases used in the Miller/Urey experiment. What is more important, however, is that the updated version of the atmosphere of early Earth was quite different from the composition of the atmosphere envisioned by Miller/Urey.

Consequently, what might happen in a flask containing a set of reactive gases does not necessarily have much relevance with respect to what might have happened in the actual early Earth atmosphere. The latter atmospheric environment might have contained different gases that were less reactive than the Miller/Urey experimental set-up.

Furthermore, other than involving electricity, I'm not quite clear about how the electricity delivered through two metal electrodes is much like what happens when lightening strikes. The sparks in the Miller/Urey experiment involved 2-4 watts of energy, whereas lightening strikes deliver the equivalent of approximately 8000 watts.

Moreover, the experimental sparks were fairly regular and in the same area. Lightening strikes, on the other hand, are sporadically intermittent and tend not to regularly visit the same, confined area again and again.

Unless, of course, one wishes to include the interfacing of the Catatumbo River with Lake Maracaibo in Venezuela where lightening strikes occur up to 280 times per hour, ten hours a day, and between 140 and 160 nights of the year. And, if one did wish to factor such possibilities into the matter, one would introduce an array of problems for the reactants and products of chemical reactions that would arise in any context involving that kind of a constant barrage of powerful, electrical discharges.

One of the problems being alluded to in the foregoing paragraph is that whatever chemical reactions might have been helped along with one lightening discharge might very well have been disrupted or destroyed with subsequent lightening strikes. No one has performed experiments simulating the Catatumbo River/Lake Maracaibo conditions, so, it is hard to determine what might, or might not, have taken place under those sorts of conditions.

The two flasks in the Miller/Urey experiment were linked up with one another via glass tubing. At one point along the tubing, a condenser section was set up, and the flask containing the water was heated on a continuous basis by a relatively low intensity source of energy that was intended to simulate the condition of evaporation that was believed to be present on early Earth.

Once the Miller/Urey experiment started, the experiment was permitted to run over several days. After a few days, the formerly clear flask water began to become yellowish in color, and, as well, the area of the electrodes was exhibiting some blackish residue.

Miller subjected the residue and the water to chemical analysis. His primary tool in this aspect of the experiment was paper chromatography -- a process that helps to differentiate chemical molecules from one another – and Miller discovered the presence of glycine ($C_2H_5NO_2$), the least complex member of the amino acids that make up the proteins of life.

Miller re-ran the experiment. This time he let it proceed for a week, and, as well, he turned up the heat in the flask containing the water so that the latter slowly boiled.

At the end of seven-day experimental period, Miller again used the process of paper chromatography to separate out whatever molecules might be present in the water. He discovered the presence of a wide array of organic molecules, including quite a few amino acids.

The foregoing is all very interesting. However, the Miller/Urey experiment also raises a lot of questions above and beyond the problems already noted in earlier comments.

For instance, the experimental apparatus was sealed and involved a continuous circulation of chemical components that were regularly exposed to: Relatively low-intensity, electric sparks; conditions of condensation; and being passed through boiling water. Why should one suppose that conditions on early Earth also consisted (in part or whole) in a similar sort of environment that involved: Materials being sealed off from the rest of the world; continuous circulation of the same components; regular doses of low-intensity electric sparks;

regular and consistent conditions of condensation, as well as boiling water ... all for a period of no more than a week?

To the foregoing question, one can add several other issues. For example, whatever chemical residues accumulated – under questionable conditions -- over a period of a week, likely would be subjected also to the continuous, degrading actions of a wide variety of hydrological, ultraviolet, photolytic, and other environmental forces (e.g., acidity, alkalinity, etc.).

What would survive from an interacting set of synthesizing and degrading forces is anybody's guess. One cannot necessarily assume that, over time, the forces of synthesis would necessarily overpower the simultaneously occurring forces that served to undermine and degrade whatever the forces of synthesis might have brought forth.

On May 15, 1953, Miller's two-page article – '*A Production of Amino Acids Under Possible Primitive Earth Conditions*' – was published in *Science*. While the foregoing title was technically correct, what might possibly have been the case on early Earth is not necessarily how things actually were back then, and, therefore, the title of Miller's article is also potentially misleading if what he considered to be 'possible' didn't accurately reflect actual, early Earth conditions.

Since the 1953 paper was released, a great many other experiments have been conducted that were able to demonstrate how, under certain conditions, different molecules that played important roles in the biology of life could be produced experimentally. For example, in 1960, by heating a concentrated solution of hydrogen cyanide (HCN), John Oró was able to synthesize considerable amounts of adenine – one of the five nucleobases from which nucleotides are formed as well as being a central component in adenosine triphosphate (a major source of energy for many biological reactions).

The Oró experiment is very suggestive in relation to the origin of life issue. That is, the experiment is suggestive provided there were concentrated solutions of hydrogen cyanide on early earth, and those solutions were heated in just the right way, for just the right amount of time, and were not subsequently subjected to any of the forces (e.g., water, light, acidity, alkalinity, and temperature) of molecular degradation that have been present on Earth from a very early time.

| Explorations |

Later on in the 1960s, Leslie Orgel demonstrated that if one froze water rich in organic molecules, then, as water crystals grew in the freezing water, this had the effect of concentrating the organic molecules that remained in solution within the portions of water that had not, yet, frozen. Therefore, Orgel prepared dilute solutions of hydrogen cyanide and slowly lowered the temperature of the solution to -20 degrees Centigrade.

Orgel's experiment led to the production of small amounts of highly, concentrated HCN. Moreover, over a period of weeks and months, the HCN molecules were observed to establish linkages involving up to four HCN molecules.

Oró's experiment (outlined earlier) required concentrated solutions of HCN to be <u>heated</u> in order for adenine to be synthesized. How did the concentrated brine of HCN produced by freezing dilute solutions of HCN in Orgel's experiment come to be sufficiently heated for the right amount of time (and the process of thawing, for example, might not entail sufficient heat) to yield small amounts of adenine?

Well, one way of responding to the foregoing question is to hypothesize that heating might not have been required. Ten, or so, years later -- in the mid-1970s -- Stanley Miller and several colleagues repeated the Orgel experiment.

When the initial portion of this replicated experiment was completed, the researchers stored the flasks in a freezer, waited more than twenty years, and, then, proceeded to analyze the contents of those flasks. They found a fair amount of adenine had been produced while in a frozen condition.

Low temperatures tend to slow down the rate of reactions with respect to the synthesis of various molecules. However, given a long enough period of time, cold, freezing conditions will not necessarily inhibit the formation of more complex molecules from taking place.

However, what If Orgel's experimental solution contained other kinds of organic molecules as well as HCN, how would this have affected his results? If those solutions were: Acidic, alkaline, exhibited a high saline content, and/or contained various assortments of minerals suspended in solution, how would any of these added factors affect Orgel's experiment?

| Explorations |

How likely is it that one might find water-based solutions on early Earth that contained dilute amounts of <u>only</u> HCN? Such solutions might be possible, but how likely were they?

Any answer that one gives to the foregoing questions will be fairly arbitrary. This is because we don't actually know what the conditions for any <u>particular</u> part of early Earth actually were even if we might know what some of the <u>general</u> conditions were that prevailed at that time.

Over the years, a wide variety of prebiotic experiments sought to fill in the gaps with respect to how a variety of molecules of importance to the origin of life might have arisen under "possible" conditions with respect to primitive Earth. However, as was the case with the Orgel, Oró and Miller experiments, just how likely any of those possible conditions might have been is not known with any high degree of certitude.

Furthermore, even if -- for the purposes of argument -- one were to accept the idea that all of the "possible" conditions described in a whole set of different experiments might have reflected actual conditions in different areas of early Earth, there was still another, major hurdle to get over. How can one be sure that all of the different sets of conditions (e.g., temperatures, pH conditions, energy sources, chemical materials, atmospheric conditions, degrees of concentration, and so on) that were needed -- according to an array of experiments -- to produce different kinds of molecules important to life would necessarily have taken place in close proximity to one another?

After all, one might grant – and this would require a person to overlook quite a few problems and questions -- that the conditions established in various experimental set-ups could have reflected actual conditions in different parts of early Earth. Nevertheless, how did all of the molecules synthesized under an array of variable, experimental conditions come together in one small area – say, the size of a cell -- in order to be able to form functional, metabolic pathways?

No scientist (or group of scientists) has been able to do a <u>single</u>, self-contained experiment that simultaneously: (1) Simulated all of the conditions said to be necessary for producing the array of molecules essential to life as we know it, and, then, (2) observed the products of those differential conditions proceed to self-organize into functional, integrated, metabolic pathways that were capable of underwriting the existence and complexity of the simplest of living organisms. Therefore, even if one grants the possibility that individual components important to the existence of life were, somehow, synthesized on early Earth – and this is, by no means, a foregone, scientifically proven conclusion – nevertheless, there is no explanation for how all of those components came to be functionally organized in one place, no bigger than a cell.

Furthermore, one cannot take the mass of data concerning the prebiotic conditions of early Earth that have accumulated over decades of so-called research and try to claim – with a straight face – that it all gives expression to the best scientific theory we have concerning the origin of life issue. The fact that a bunch of scientists – some of whom won Nobel Prizes – spend time in a laboratory, formulate hypotheses, conduct experiments, draw conclusions, and come up with this or that equation, does not mean that what they have done constitutes science or is scientifically viable.

Many scientists have developed theories concerning the origins of life. Many religious people have developed theories concerning the origins of life.

Many scientists criticize the latter individuals because the religiously inclined have no viable, provable account of how the dynamics of life came into being even though such people use terms like 'creation science' and 'intelligent design' in order to give the appearance of having put forth a scientific theory of some kind. What is appropriate for the goose is also appropriate for the gander.

Therefore, since scientists have not been able to put forth any viable, provable account of how the dynamics of life came into being through purely physical/chemical means, then, despite the fact that scientists use terms like the 'science of evolution' and the 'scientific method', scientists are really no further ahead in the origin of life explanation lottery than religious people are. There is no 'best available scientific account of the origin of life' because there is no science in this area that is capable of demonstrating itself to be reliable.

Just because people refer to themselves as scientists and spew forth a lot of hypotheses, speculations, conjectures, opinions, and experimental results, this doesn't automatically render what they say and do in this respect to be of any scientific value. Nor does their position as scientists automatically award them scientific bragging rights with respect to people who are religiously inclined and have immersed themselves in activities called creation science and intelligent design.

If one doesn't know the truth of things, then, irrespective of what phrases might be used involving the word "science" or "scientific", one is ignorant. If one doesn't know the truth of something, then it becomes an exercise in foolishness to try to claim that one unproven, allegedly scientific theory/account is better, more scientific than some other unproven, allegedly scientific theory/account.

All attempts to scientifically account for the origin of life – whether through creation science or "mainstream" science – are equally inept and riddled with an array of problems. There is no "best scientific account" concerning the origin of life ... there is just ignorance all the way around.

Educators – the sort of people Dobzhansky was addressing in his previously discussed, *American Biology Teacher* article ('*Nothing in Biology Makes Sense Except in the Light of Evolution*') -- who want to teach a theory concerning the origin of life or which – purportedly – deals with the nature of speciation as being scientific -- when such theories entail little more than ignorance at virtually every crucial juncture -- seem to be under a misunderstanding when it comes to the process of education. Ignorance is ignorance, and it shouldn't be packaged as being anything other than ignorance.

There is no such thing as scientific ignorance. There is just ignorance.

What we don't know when it comes to a scientific account of the origin of life is close to 100%. The "best scientific account" that we have concerning the origin of life is that we have no idea how, or if, the origin of life can be demonstrably explained in terms of known scientific laws and principles.

Proponents of evolutionary biology have gone to court on many occasions defending the idea that students are, in effect, being educationally abused when those students are forced to take courses in the public school system that are imbued with the biases and misconceptions of the proponents of creation science and intelligent design. However, the fact of the matter is that students are no less educationally abused when they are forced to take courses in the public school system that are imbued with the biases and misconceptions of the proponents of evolutionary biology.

Biases and misconceptions are just that. Propagating bias and misconceptions as being anything other than what they are is not an exercise in learning how to do science, or learning how to become scientific.

If educators want to teach science in science classes, then assist students to develop the sort of critical understanding that allows them to be able to differentiate the wheat from the chaff with respect to the search for truth concerning the origin of life issue. Educators need to assist students to learn, on the one hand, about the lacunae, problems, unknowns, missteps, and unanswered questions that saturate the whole field of origin of life research, as well as many facets of the field of evolutionary biology, and, on the other hand, educators need to assist students to learn that at the present time there is no scientific theory concerning the origin of life that is even remotely viable.

To try to do anything else in a classroom (whether elementary, high school, college, or university) would constitute an exercise in educational abuse. Unfortunately, the judges who issue decisions concerning cases involving the proponents of evolutionary biology versus the proponents of creation science or intelligent design biology don't seem to even understand the nature of the issues about which they are making legal judgments ... judgments that will affect the lives of millions of students.

| Explorations |

Over the last 40 years, or so, a new approach -- with respect to trying to provide a scientific account concerning the origin of life issue -- has gained a certain amount of traction in at least some scientific circles. This new approach is referred to as the 'hydrothermal hypothesis.'

By way of background, one of the sticking points for a lot of origin of life theories up until the 1970s circulated around the issue of water. It was an inconvenient truth that the presence of water tended to resist and/or undermine certain, essential, chemical reactions (that are important to life) from proceeding vary far, if at all ... water is Janus-like in its capacity to both help facilitate as well as help undermine a variety of chemical reactions.

Another possibility, however, began to bubble to the surface of consciousness beginning in the late 1970s. Jack Corliss, an oceanographer, took the submersible, research vessel Alvin to the bottom of the ocean, and in the process, he discovered incredible networks or ecosystems of life that were flourishing in conditions of tremendous pressure, no sun light, and the very high temperatures that exist in various undersea volcanic vents.

When water is subjected to high pressures (say, a kilobar – a thousand atmospheres -- or more), together with sufficiently high temperatures (say, 175 degrees Celsius, or more), then, the dielectric constant of water goes down. In many ways water becomes like an organic solvent under these conditions.

As a result, water tends to behave very differently under the foregoing sorts of conditions than it does at much less extreme temperatures and pressures. Perhaps, therefore, the physical and chemical differences that manifest themselves in water under conditions of high pressure and high temperature might be able to permit certain kinds of chemical reactions to proceed that might not be able to take place when placed in water at the sort of temperatures and pressures that exist in many places on the surface of the Earth or in the top several hundred feet of the ocean.

For example, consider pyruvate (CH_3COCOO^-) -- a source of energy that, among other things, helps to subsidize many reactions taking place within one, or another, metabolic pathway. When glucose, a six-

| Explorations |

carbon atom, is split, first into two pyruvate molecules due to the presence of the right kind of catalytic enzyme, and, then, subsequently, the pyruvate molecules are split into still smaller molecules – again, due to the presence of the right kind of enzyme -- energy is released along the way, and this energy is used to help advance various reactions that will not occur spontaneously ... that is, on their own.

In addition, if one combines pyruvate, carbon dioxide, and the right kind of enzymatic catalyst, one can generate a molecule known as oxaloacetate [$HO_2CC(O)CH_2CO_2H$]. This latter molecule has further uses within certain metabolic pathways of living organisms.

However, when pyruvate is left to its own devices in water – that is, without the presence of the right sort of catalytic enzymes – it tends to break down into smaller molecules. These latter molecules contain only one or two carbon atoms, and a result cannot be combined with carbon dioxide to produce the four-carbon molecule, oxaloacetate ... at least not at normal room temperatures and pressures, and not without the presence of an appropriate kind of catalyst that can speed up the reaction rates of such chemical components, and not in the presence of water.

What would happen if one were to combine water, pyruvate, as well as carbon dioxide and subject those ingredients to various conditions of high temperature (say, 150 to 300 degrees Celsius) and high pressure (say, 500 to several thousand atmospheres)? Would one obtain molecules of oxaloacetate or anything else of interest to the origin of life issue?

Harold Morowitz and Robert Hazen -- along with the assistance of Hat Yoder and George Cody -- undertook the foregoing experiment ... or, at least, a facsimile thereof. They placed water and pyruvate (both liquids) into a gold tube -- the size of a long grain of rice – and introduced carbon dioxide gas into the tube via the way of a chemical known as oxalic acid dihydrate ($H_2C_2O_4 \cdot 2H_2O$) that decomposes into carbon and water at temperatures above 100 degrees Celsius.

The open end of the gold tube into which the various chemical reactants had been introduced was sealed up using a complex process involving a carbon-arc welder, a graphite rod and liquid nitrogen -- at a temperature of -196 degrees Celsius that was used to keep the other end of the gold tube sufficiently cool so that this would help prevent the pyruvate – which tends to be fairly volatile under certain conditions -- from boiling away when the carbon-arc welding process went about its sealing business at the other end of the tube.

The small, rice-sized, gold tubes (there were three of them) were, then, placed within a complex arrangement consisting of: a platinum holder, nickel metal cylinder (served as the electric furnace), ceramic filler rods, ceramic end caps, thermocouple wires, all packed within a white aluminum powder. The foregoing arrangement was, then, attached to a steel plug that is capable of retaining pressure while, simultaneously, providing a means of insulating an assortment of wires through which an electric current flows that controls the amount of temperature/heat being applied to the gold tubes.

Finally, all of the above is sealed within a metal container. This container is capable of withstanding a pressurized gas (argon) being pumped into the contraption and once pumped in will subject the gold tubes to the same sort of pressure.

The pressure selected for the experiment was two kilobars or 2000 atmospheres. The temperature was set at 250 degrees Celsius and was controlled by a computer.

The whole, experimental set-up was permitted to run for several hours. Supposedly, the conditions established through the experiment were intended to simulate the conditions that might be found several miles down in the ocean along one, or another, volcanic vent.

Following the aforementioned two-hour experimental period, a combination of gas chromatography and a mass spectrometer was used to analyze the contents of the gold tubes (after they were opened). Those contents didn't reveal the presence of oxaloacetate – as the researchers thought might be the case -- but the contents did contain thousands of other molecules of various descriptions.

Among the molecules that were synthesized were alcohols and sugars. In addition they discovered complex molecules that contained dozens of carbon atoms ... some of which formed the sort of branching structures and rings that are similar to various kinds of branching and ring structures that are found in living organisms.

The researchers drew certain conclusions from their experiment. More specifically, among other things, they felt they had demonstrated

– in a proof of concept sort of manner – that hydrothermal conditions of great pressure and high temperature were capable of generating a vast array of molecules that might have played various roles along the way toward the prebiotic origins of life.

There are a number of problems that permeate the foregoing experiment. For example, where does one discover hydrothermal conditions – except, perhaps, in a laboratory – such that a set of circumstances lasts for only several hours and takes place under very carefully controlled, sealed conditions of temperature and pressure in which a chemically inert gold tube presses in on the primary chemical reactants without permitting any outside agents (of a possible reactive nature) into the reaction chamber?

What would have happened if the experiment had gone on for a thousand or a million or a billion years rather than for two hours? We don't know, and, yet, the former set of possibilities is far more likely than a two-hour experiment, so, really, what does the experiment outlined above actually teach us?

After all, if you pressure-cook certain foods for several hours at an elevated temperature, you might get a tasty meal. If you cook the same dish for several thousand, million, or billion years, the meal might not be so tasty … or suggestive with respect to the origin of life issue.

Even assuming there were real-world hydrothermal conditions that provided a niche within which certain chemical ingredients could be completely sealed for, say, a two-hour period, what happens to those contents once the container is breached and its contents are released into the ocean waters that are circulating through a given volcanic vent? We don't know because – for a variety of reasons (not the least of which is an inability to maintain control over a wealth of variables in such a situation) -- no one has performed that kind of an experiment.

What happens if the innermost, sealed container in actual, non-laboratory based conditions does not consist of a soft, relatively inert material such as gold? Will we get the same results?

Or, approaching issues from a slightly different direction, let's take the experiment at face value. One sets up an experiment, and one gets some interesting and unexpected results.

| Explorations |

What does any of this 'unexpectedness' do for the origin of life issue? How will all of the unexpected molecules and molecular fragments fit into an attempt to explain how life might have arisen from such a concoction?

Could life have arisen from some arbitrary set of ingredients subjected to some arbitrary set of conditions? Maybe, but, to the best of my knowledge, Morowitz, Hazen, Yoder, and Cody, didn't discover life in their gold tubes, and, therefore, one is left to ponder and critically reflect on the possible significance, if any, of what they discovered.

The researchers were expecting one thing – some molecules of oxaloacetate – and got a whole lot of something else. They seemed to believe that what they actually got was some sort of emergent set of properties, and, perhaps, conducting other kinds of similar experiments -- at different temperatures or pressures, and with different ingredients -- might lead to an array of additional sets of emergent properties ... that is, entities that were not anticipated prior to running such experiments but that showed up, nonetheless, and entailed some interesting possibilities.

When one performs an experiment and that experiment does not yield the results one expected, one hasn't stumbled upon emergent properties. Rather, one has come across evidence pointing to one's ignorance concerning the nature of the forces and principles that are likely to be operative with respect to the dynamics of a given set of conditions that have been set in motion by one's experiment.

Claiming that those sorts of allegedly emergent phenomena might, somehow, lay the basis for constructing a provable account of, or explanation for, the origin of life seems rather strained ... to say the least. The only emergent dimension of such an experiment is that one comes to learn some things that one didn't know before.

If one piles emergent properties upon emergent properties upon emergent properties (and so on indefinitely) one doesn't necessarily end up with life. One might end up, however, with some new facts ... facts that might, or might not, have something of relevance to disclose with respect to the origin of life issue.

| Explorations |

John Holland is one of the individuals who helped bring the field of emergent modeling into prominence. He used computer algorithms – that is, a programmed system or network of operational rules -- to simulate various phenomena.

He believes emergent properties can be shown to be a function of the kinds of selection rules one uses to model the phenomenon out of which such properties emerge. Moreover, he believes that the degree of complexity inherent in some, given emergent phenomenon might be closely related to the number of lines of programming code that are needed to faithfully simulate or reflect the properties of such a phenomenon.

In his 1998 book: *Emergence: From Chaos to Order*, Holland indicates that the idea of emergence is so complex that formulating a concise definition for the phenomenon is unlikely to take place. Furthermore, he admits that he has no concise definition to offer in conjunction with the notion of emergent behavior.

Nevertheless, Holland's perspective in relation to the problem of trying to concisely define the phenomenon of emergence could be quite prescient. After all, there really might be a realm of emergent phenomena that do not necessarily share a set of overlapping, operational selection rules, and, therefore, such phenomena tend to resist being reduced down in a way that could be encompassed by any kind of concise definition that would be capable of capturing the variability and complexity of those sorts of phenomena.

On the other hand, Holland's opinion about whether, or not, the complexity of emergent phenomena renders them resistant to concise definition might be steeped in a certain amount of confusion about what emergent phenomena actually are … or are not. In other words, can one – or should one -- automatically assume there are an array of special dynamics that give expression to something called "emergent phenomena," or is the idea of "emergent properties" just a catch-all term that tends to camouflage the presence of considerable ignorance with respect to how various things work in the universe.

For example, as previously noted, Harold Morowitz and Robert Hazen held a tentative hypothesis that if one subjected water, pyruvate, and CO_2 to sufficiently high pressures and temperatures one might be able to produce molecules of oxaloacetate despite the

| Explorations |

absence of an enzyme to help facilitate the process. However, their experiment produced something quite different than the molecules of oxaloacetate that had been anticipated as possible outcomes if one ran the experiment at issue -- namely, the experiment yielded an array of thousands of unanticipated molecules.

What were the dynamics underlying the differences between what was expected and what actually occurred? Were there some sort of special, emergent dynamics that were taking place or did the researchers just not understand how things work under certain conditions?

What was actually happening in the sealed rice-sized gold tubes containing water, pyruvate, and carbon dioxide that were being heated to 250 degrees Centigrade, as well as being subjected to 2000 atmospheres of pressure? The fact of the matter is we don't know.

Was the heat primarily responsible for the synthesis of unexpected molecules? Was the pressure primarily responsible for the production of the unanticipated? Was the cooling down period that preceded opening the gold tubes primarily responsible for yielding outcomes that had not been predicted? Was the combination of heat, pressure, time, and cooling down primarily responsible for what took place, and why weren't the researchers able to predict such an outcome? We don't necessarily know how pressure, temperature, and certain ingredients interact with one another across various ranges of values.

Do molecules that are inert under "normal" conditions remain so under more extreme conditions? Are their various thresholds of pressure and temperature that if surpassed will give expression to certain kinds of phenomena that, currently, we do not understand? What underlies such thresholds and why do they occur at some junctures and not others? What are the limits, if any, that might exist in relation to the interaction of pressure, temperature, and various substances across a range of values? What impact does the amount of time that transpires during the experiment have on how pressure, temperature, and molecules combine together to generate products?

I'm not sure that I see any emergent phenomena that are taking place in the Morowitz-Hazen experiment. I do see an awful lot of unanswered questions and considerable ignorance concerning the

| Explorations |

238

physics and chemistry of what is transpiring inside the gold tubes during the experiment ... questions and ignorance that all tend to revolve around not knowing why what was observed to happen in the experimental outcome was able to take place.

To refer to the unexpected and unanticipated as giving expression to the dynamics of emergent phenomena doesn't really explain anything at all. In fact, such a way of talking might constitute little more than a certain kind of magical thinking in which causal attribution is assigned to a hypothetical entity – namely, emergence – whose actual, specific dynamics cannot be verified ... and that might not even be an actual phenomenon (just a way of descriptively referring – if rather vaguely -- to phenomena whose internal dynamics lie beyond the horizons of our understanding).

Furthermore, the capacity to develop a computer algorithm – as Holland and others have done -- to simulate a phenomenon doesn't necessarily – in and of itself – prove that the phenomenon being modeled or simulated is a function of the sort of operational or selection rules that are contained in the algorithm. Such simulations/models only demonstrate that, to varying degrees of accuracy, a computer can mimic certain behavioral properties by means of a given algorithm that has been set in motion by a working computer that has the capacities needed to run the algorithm successfully.

A psychopath can mimic the emotional behavior of 'normal' people. However, the psychopath did not necessarily generate his or her own behavior in the same way that normal people generate their emotional behavior.

A painter can simulate, with considerable accuracy and attention to detail, some of the visual properties of a scene of nature or the external characteristics of a person. However, the manner in which a painter arrives at her or his terminal juncture (i.e., the existence of a finished picture) is not the way in which nature arrives at its terminal juncture (i.e., the existence of the natural phenomena or person being painted).

A computer simulation might be able to model some of the behavioral properties of certain real-world phenomena. This does not necessarily mean the processes (computer algorithms and real world phenomena) underlying the respective surface behaviors are the same.

The possibility that one might not be able to predict what a computer algorithm will generate if given enough time is not an expression of emergence. It is a statement of ignorance concerning how the dynamics set in motion by that computer algorithm will unfold over time.

For human beings, trying to follow the dynamics of the foregoing processes is too complicated. There are too many variables for a person to be able to keep track of simultaneously so that an individual can understand what is happening from second to second in real time.

For a computer, the issue of understanding an algorithm is irrelevant. All the computer does is to run the program for a specified time (both the parameter of running and stopping are specified by something other than the computer), and things end up wherever they end up. However, if one were to ask the computer to predict the outcome of the algorithm prior to the program being run, the computer would be in no better position (without running the program) than a human being is as far as giving a reliable prediction is concerned because ignorance has central prominence in both cases.

So-called emergent properties are as 'mysterious' to a computer as they are to human beings. In both cases, neither the computer nor the human being is capable of predicting how, respectively, a given algorithm or comparable real-world dynamic will unfold over time.

There is no emergent phenomenon going on in either case. There is just ignorance about the character of the outcome and how such an outcome arises from the dynamics that are inherent in a computer program or a real world context.

When someone says that life is a quintessentially emergent phenomenon, what is that person trying to say? Generally speaking, individuals say this sort of thing when they don't understand how life is possible but wish to be able to continue to believe that various physical laws (both known and unknown) are capable of coming together and giving rise to life in ways that his or her current understanding does not grasp.

| Explorations |

In other words, such people tend to believe that somewhere, somehow, the right combination of forces and elements came together within the right sort of circumstances and conditions to be able to give rise to some kind of living protocell. Thus, life is an emergent property of the interacting combination of the right set of unknown: Forces, elements, circumstances and conditions.

Every time someone – either with a computer on in a lab – is able to run an experiment leading to unexpected or unanticipated results that appear to be somewhat suggestive in relation to origin of life issues, then, those kinds of results are considered by some individuals to constitute evidential support for the possibility that life also arose through a similar process of unexpected and unanticipated outcomes.

For some individuals, emergent properties and emergent behavior seem to become the answer to every unknown issue involving the origin of life. However, such 'answers' never explain or account for anything in specific detail, and, consequently, just how certain kinds of underlying dynamics are capable of generating life is always left unaddressed, and the resulting gap in understanding is papered over by using the term: 'emergent behavior'.

Emergence is not a scientific term. It is a philosophical one, and it entails many of the same kinds of ambiguities and arbitrary assumptions that characterize any number of philosophical positions.

Furthermore, dressing up the idea of emergence in scientific clothing doesn't make the concept any more rigorous. For example, one can talk all one likes about how: Far from equilibrium conditions are capable of creating conditions involving the flow of energy that dissipate that flow in unexpected and unanticipated ways and, in the process, gives rise to certain kinds of ordered structures of energy flow that are quite different from what takes place near equilibrium conditions ... and, if one likes, one can quantify the whole description with lots of spiffy equations and mathematical expressions.

Nonetheless, however scientifically valuable such accounts might be in conjunction with describing or modeling an array of phenomena, there is no, or little, transfer value when it comes to explaining the origin of life. In other words, there is no scientist (or group of scientists) who has (have) come up with a far from equilibrium scenario that reliably and demonstrably accounts for precisely how the dissipative structures that constitute different life forms (or the dissipative structures inherent in various kinds of metabolic pathways) arises in various kinds of far from equilibrium conditions.

| Explorations |

242

Before moving on, the reader [(?) ..., readers (?) -- see Introduction] should understand that there are two broad kinds of hydrothermal vents. They are referred to as black smokers and white smokers, and each kind of vent system gives expression to different sets of chemical and physical conditions.

Black smokers arise in connection with volcanic activity in the depths of the ocean. The 'black smoke' is not actually smoke but consists of a acidic mixture of metal sulfides and seawater heated to temperatures of around 400 degrees Centigrade under tremendous pressure from the ocean depths in which black smokers exist (one of the deepest, if not the deepest, black smoker discovered to date resides in the Cayman Trough, a little more than 3 miles below the ocean surface).

The material surrounding the channel-way that rises up through the black smoker chimney system is made from various kinds of sulfur minerals. This material has precipitated out from the heated, metal sulfide solution that is churning up through the black smoker chimney.

Black smokers increase in height as a result of the continuing precipitation of the aforementioned sulfur minerals. The growth rates of the chimneys built up from the precipitants vary with conditions, but those structures can reach heights of several hundred feet before beginning to fall apart after 20,000 years, or so.

White smokers, unlike black smokers, are not a function of volcanic activity. Instead, the interaction of seawater with mantle-derived rocks releases energy in the form of heat along with a variety of gases, including: Hydrogen, hydrogen sulfide, carbon dioxide (which, given the right conditions, can lead to the formation of methane), and nitrogen (which, given the right conditions, can lead to the generation ammonia).

The foregoing heated solution is not nearly as hot as the seawater mixture that churns up through black smokers, but the solution in white smokers does contain a great many electrons in the form of reduced reactants. White smokers are alkaline in character.

Moreover, while white smokers sometimes form chimney-like structures similar to black smokers, white smokers more often form complex, interconnecting structures made of materials precipitating out of the 'white smoke' rising from and through such structures. The white color of the "smoke" that emanates from white smokers comes from the calcium, silicon, and barium compounds contained in the hydrothermal mixture associated with such structures.

The arrangement of bubble chambers and compartmentalized units in white smokers are roughly the size of living cells. They form extended, interconnected, microscopic, networks of porous materials.

The existence of each kind of smoker has inspired various researchers to conjecture that life might have arisen in one or the other form of hydrothermal vent system. The minerals, gases, pH conditions, surface structures, and compositional materials that are associated with the respective smokers are considered by various researchers to be ideal "breeding" grounds for an array of chemical reactions that might lead to life.

The amazing, but different, ecosystems that are found living in harmony with each of the respective smokers have suggested to some individuals that, perhaps, life arose as a function of the physical and chemical conditions present in one, or the other, kind of smoker. The task then becomes a matter of showing how life could have arisen in the underlying physical and chemical conditions associated with one of those two kinds of smokers ... or, perhaps, both.

While acknowledging the differences between the two aforementioned sorts of smokers, much of what is said in this section of the present chapter, is directed toward the general kinds of problems that are likely to be encountered by both modes of smokers. For example, irrespective of whatever the particular physical and chemical conditions of a given smoker might be, if one hopes to develop a plausible theory concerning the origin of life, one must account for how various modes of order arise in those different kinds of conditions that are capable of establishing an array of interacting, metabolic pathways that will perform the functions that are able to initiate and sustain living organisms.

In short, the physics and chemistry of each smoker are different. Nevertheless, the ultimate problem facing both of the smokers is the same – namely, how does one induce a set of basic physical and chemical reactions to form, first, more complex biomolecules and, then in turn, to assemble such biomolecules into functional, self-sustaining

| Explorations |

metabolic pathways before they disassemble under the onslaught of a variety of forces involving: temperature, water, pressure, pH values, unfavorable thermodynamic conditions, changing geological conditions, and competing chemical reactions.

| Explorations |

Stanley Miller – whose classic 1950s experiment was discussed earlier – believed that life must have formed somewhere within the area between a few centimeters and several hundred meters, or so, relative to the surface of oceans/lakes. This area is known as the Photic Zone, and it represents the depth to which light – considered by many evolutionary biologists to play a primary role in the origin of life – will penetrate in a given body of water.

Miller and others were critical of the hydrothermal vent hypothesis that maintained life might have formed near the bottom of the ocean along volcanic vents. Among other reasons, Miller and many other similar-minded researchers felt that the heat from such vents would have destroyed more molecular precursors to life (e.g., amino acids and ribose sugars) than they would have created.

Various experiments have been conducted in an attempt to shore up some of the perceived weaknesses (such as the Miller criticism noted in the preceding paragraph) that are associated with the hydrothermal vent hypothesis. For instance, in the period spanning 1999 and 2000, Jay Brandes designed a number of experiments to try and address a few of the theoretical problems with which the hydrothermal vent hypothesis was faced.

One of the experiments Brandes performed involved the amino acid leucine [$HO_2CCH(NH_2)CH_2CH(CH_3)$]. This is an important biomolecule (that is, a molecule known to play various roles in living organisms).

When leucine is subjected to temperatures of, say, several hundred degrees Centigrade, under conditions of elevated pressure, leucine tends to decompose fairly quickly (in a few minutes). However, when leucine is exposed to the foregoing sorts of conditions in the presence of an iron-sulfur mineral known as pyrrhotite, the amino acid is able to survive for a number of days.

Pyrrhotite is significant because it is a fairly common component in oceanic volcanic vents. Moreover, while the means through which pyrrhotite is able to help prevent the break down of leucine seems to be somewhat elusive, the implication of the Brandes experiment is as follows: One cannot automatically assume that the biomolecules which might arise in hydrothermal vents will necessarily and automatically

| Explorations |

decompose when exposed to conditions of high temperature and pressure since there are various kinds of minerals existing in those vents – such as pyrrhotite -- that might be able to help stabilize those biomolecules and extend their molecular lives.

Findings from other experiments also have suggested that if amino acids can establish strong bonds with various kinds of minerals, they might have a better chance of remaining intact for a longer period of time than in the absence of such mineral bonds. The implication of this research is that, perhaps, there were conditions in hydrothermal vents that facilitated boding between various kinds of minerals and different amino acids, and, in the process, helped preserve the molecular identity of those amino acids in extreme conditions.

Whatever truths are entailed by the foregoing sorts of experiments and research, they sound somewhat strained when it comes to trying to account for the origin of life. Simply because one can demonstrate that the life of a molecule might be extended for a short period of time under certain circumstances, this does not necessarily have any relevance to what might have actually happened on early Earth or what needed to happen on early Earth if the origin of life is to be explained purely in terms of the laws of physics and chemistry.

The fact there is evidence to show that something could have happened does not mean that this is what actually did happen. A lot of prebiotic experiments and research seems to resonate with the words that the Marlon Brandon character, Terry Malloy, voiced in the movie: *On the Waterfront* – namely, "I coulda' been a contender."

A lot of things could have been, but are not. It remains to be seen whether various prebiotic pretenders turn out to be bums or real contenders. However, for the most part a lot of those researchers just seem to be caught up in their own fantasies of what "coulda' been" or should have been or might have been if things worked the way their ideas claimed was possible.

Does extending the life of a molecule from a few minutes to a few days really appreciably change anything as far as accounting for the origin of life is concerned? Do we know whether, or not, <u>all</u> the biomolecules of life <u>regularly</u> established bonds with various minerals and that these sorts of arrangements lasted sufficiently long to enable the biomolecules to enter into reactions with other biomolecules while still subjected to the extreme conditions of hydrothermal vents? Do we know whether, or not, the existence of the biomolecule-mineral bonds would have interfered with the ability of the attached biomolecules to interact with other biomolecules?

Unless all of the foregoing questions – plus many others -- can be answered in definitive terms, one is not necessarily dealing with something of scientific value as far as the origin of life issue is concerned. The aforementioned experiments and research do not constitute evidence in favor of a scientific account for the origin of life because we really don't know what, if any, relevance those findings have with respect to the actual conditions in any given hydrothermal vent on early Earth.

For example, hydrothermal vents tend to exist in very unstable, geological conditions. How long do vents last in such unstable conditions?

During the first year, or so, of this century, the submersible vehicle Atlantis was involved in the discovery of an alkaline vent system located on an underwater mountain known as the Atlantis massive, roughly 9 miles from the Mid-Atlantic ridge. Some of the vents found there were nearly 200 feet tall.

One of the white-smoker, alkaline vents found on the Atlantis massive was dubbed the 'Lost City'. It has been estimated to have been venting for 40,000 years – twice the length of time usually associated with the life-span of black-smoker, acidic hydrothermal vents that had been discovered many years before.

20,000 to 40,000 years is not a very long period of time for nature to work with and through which to catalyze the basic molecules of life and, then, assemble them into some network of metabolic pathways. Even if one were to arbitrarily add on several hundred thousand years to the life span of white smoker vent systems (and there is little, or no, evidential basis for extending the life-span of various kinds of smokers in this way), one still needs to assume a great deal to suppose that, somehow, the first prototypes of life emerged in such vent systems.

One might be willing to concede that some minerals could extend the lifetime of certain biomolecules under fairly extreme conditions of

| Explorations |

temperature and pressure. Nevertheless, we really don't know if any given hydrothermal vent would be around long enough for the foregoing sort of possibility involving mineral-biomolecule bonds to be able to make any difference as far as the origin of life is concerned.

Research also has been done which demonstrates that a variety of relatively common minerals – such as the sulfides of copper, iron, nickel, zinc or cobalt (as well as the oxides of some of the foregoing minerals) – have the capacity to promote (catalyze) the addition of carbon atoms to other molecules under certain conditions ... one of which involves elevated temperatures. Thus, mineral-rich hydrothermal vent systems might be excellent sources for the building of more complex biomolecules as carbon atoms are added to, among other possibilities, hydrogen molecules.

If one considers the fact that there are, and have been, tens of thousands of deep ocean ridges in the oceans of the world that are peppered with various kinds of hydrothermal vents, and, then, if one throws in millions of years of time through which the mineral-rich hydrothermal vents will be permitted to do their work of preservation and catalysis, then, someone might – and there are those who have – come to the conclusion that an abundance of biomolecules of varying degrees of complexity must have been formed in and around hydrothermal vents. Seemingly, one is off and running – perhaps taking a lead – in the explanatory races with respect to the origin of life issue as one imagines all manner of metabolic pathways that might emerge as different combinations of minerals worked their catalytic magic in the hydrothermal vents ... or, so, the theory goes.

Even if one were to grant each and every possibility outlined in the last few pages – and, for a variety of reasons, I am not inclined to do this because, among other things, far too many unproven assumptions are necessary to make the hydrothermal scenario work -- none of the granted possibilities, either alone, or in combination with one another, accounts for how functional order arises out of the morass of biomolecules that might have been generated through hydrothermal vents.

The assumption is made that given so much biomolecular material with which to work, then, surely, functional, metabolic pathways must have arisen again and again. The problem is that there is absolutely no proof such an assumption is rooted in reality.

To be sure, some of the prebiotic experimental and research data are highly suggestive. There are interesting speculations. There are promising conjectures. There are intriguing possibilities ... but there is absolutely no scientific proof that the hydrothermal vent hypothesis is true.

One can imagine whatever one likes, but that is all one ends up with: imagination. It is an exercise in magical thinking in which someone supposes that because he or she believes something must be true, then, this is the way reality must be.

As far as the hydrothermal vent hypothesis is concerned, in order to have any chance of demonstrating a truly scientific explanation for the origin of life, one must show that hydrothermal vents will produce functional proteins, lipids, nucleic acids, and carbohydrates. This has not been done.

Moreover, in order to have any hope of demonstrating a truly scientific explanation for the origin of life, one must show that hydrothermal vents will produce workable metabolic pathways capable of performing not just a few, minor biological functions but everything that is necessary for such pathways to be able to continuously sustain themselves over a period of time. This has not been done.

Furthermore, in order for there to be some possibility of demonstrating a truly scientific explanation for the origin of life, one must show that the metabolic pathways that do arise (assuming they do) will form integrated networks that are able to replicate and pass on such capabilities in a manner that permits additional, independent, integrated, biologically functioning networks of metabolic pathways to become established. This has not been done.

Maybe the day will come when one, or more, individuals will be able to successfully meet all of the foregoing three challenges. However, today is not that day.

The hydrothermal vent hypothesis is not a scientific hypothesis. Rather, it is a conjecture in search of scientific proof.

| Explorations |

One could assemble a library of scientific facts concerning the hydrothermal vent conjecture ... and, indeed, there are many large library-like collections containing that kind of technical material. However, unless one can show how a given library of facts can prove the truth of the hydrothermal vent conjecture, one doesn't have a scientific theory.

Instead, one has a conjecture to which various scientific facts have been attached. This situation is somewhat akin to the way certain prebiotic research has indicated that a biomolecule sometimes can become bonded to a mineral that might help to prolong the life of the former biomolecule through an unknown mechanism and, therefore, with no real understanding of whether, or not, those facts are actually capable of sustaining the lifetime of the conjecture for any length of time.

Claiming that a library of scientific facts is <u>consistent</u> with the hydrothermal vent hypothesis does not make that conjecture either true or scientific. In order to be able to assess the relevance of such claims, one needs to critically examine the nature of the 'consistency' that is being claimed in order to understand in what way, if any, an allegedly scientific fact is capable of establishing a viable, demonstrable, concrete bridge between the hydrothermal vent conjecture and a sustainable account of the origin of life.

As intimated a page, or so, back, there are no scientific facts that are said to be consistent with the hydrothermal vent conjecture/hypothesis that are capable of establishing a viable, demonstrable, concrete bridge between that conjecture/hypothesis and a sustainable account of the origin of life. Consequently, whatever scientific facts are claimed to be consistent with the hydrothermal vent hypothesis or conjecture are of an entirely inessential kind because they cannot prove what needs to be proved as far as the origin of life issue is concerned.

If one needs to travel from Boston to Seattle, and one finds oneself in Atlanta, then, being in Atlanta might be considered by some to be entirely consistent with the character of the stated journey. Nonetheless, one's presence in Atlanta also tends to raise a lot of questions about, whether, or not, one will ever make it to Seattle or whether one even knows where one is going or what one is doing.

The same sorts of questions tend to arise in conjunction with the idea of consistency when considering the hydrothermal vent hypothesis. If one needs to reach the destination of having a viable account for the origin of life, and one is wandering around a library of scientific facts trying to figure out if, or how, any of those facts will enable one to travel from the hydrothermal vent hypothesis to the truth, one's status is sort of like the situation described in the previous paragraph.

In other words, one started out on one's journey in Boston (the hydrothermal vent hypothesis). Now, however, one finds oneself in Atlanta (the library of scientific facts) on the way, possibly, to Seattle (the truth), and, unfortunately, claims of consistency don't possess a whole lot of value under such circumstances because they don't necessarily get one any closer to one's destination ... however interesting and intriguing the possibilities in Atlanta might appear to be.

| Explorations |

A key metabolic pathway in living organisms is the citric acid cycle. This is also known as the TCA (Tricarboxylic Acid) cycle, as well as the Krebs cycle.

This pathway consists of a handful of relatively small compounds made up of just three molecules: carbon, hydrogen, and oxygen. The molecules are: (1) oxaloacetate, (2) citrate, (3) isocitrate, (4) α-ketoglutarate, (5) succinyl-CoA, (6) succinate, (7) fumarate, and (8) malate. In addition, two-carbon atoms from pyruvate are inserted into the beginning of the cycle in conjunction with acetyl CoA.

During the course of the TCA cycle a variety of molecules are produced that are important building blocks for the synthesis of other biomolecules ... including amino acids, sugars, and lipids, as well as molecules that serve as a source of energy in the form of ATP (in bacterial cells and plant mitochondria) and GTP (in animal mitochondria). However, each step of the cycle requires the presence of a different enzyme that catalyzes a specific reaction by helping to rearrange the bonds and relationships among the carbon, hydrogen and oxygen molecules involved in the cycle with the help of coenzymes or cofactors (NAD – nicotinamide adenine dinucleotide – and FAD – flavin adenine dinucleotide) that accept or donate electrons at certain points in the cycle.

In the mid-1960s, some microorganisms were discovered that ran the foregoing metabolic pathway in reverse. Not surprisingly, this newly discovered process was referred to as a reverse citric acid cycle.

What was surprising, however, is that a certain point in the cycle, citric acid split up into a molecule of oxaloacetate and acetate, and, in the process, opened up the possibility for an additional metabolic cycle to be established provided that a few modifications were made in relation to the acetate molecule. Consequently, the reverse citric acid cycle seemed to constitute a metabolic pathway that had a potential capacity for self-replication.

Some people entertained the idea that the reverse citric acid cycle might have been closely related to the first metabolic pathways contained in primitive protocells. Among other things, this possibility had the virtue of giving expression to a self-replicating process that –

| Explorations |

253

at least in principle – doubled its potential with each completion of the cycle.

Of course, there was still the problem of having to account for, among other things, the origins of the 9 enzymes and several coenzymes that made the cycle possible. However, if one returns to the topic of the sulfide and oxide minerals that were explored earlier in this section, then perhaps, those minerals -- along with other components that either circulated in the hydrothermal vents and/or were part of the structure of those vents – might have been able to help facilitate (i.e., catalyze) different steps in the cycle and, therefore, helped sustain the cycle until the right sort of enzymatic proteins came into existence that would be able to introduce added efficiency and speed to various reactions taking place within the reverse citric acid cycle.

The idea of sulfide minerals serving as interim catalytic-like agents in protocells is rendered somewhat more plausible by the fact that at the core of a variety of modern enzymes are groupings of sulfur, iron, or nickel molecules. Perhaps, modern enzymes somehow arose from the simple beginnings of sulfur, iron or nickel sulfide minerals when aspects of the latter became incorporated into amino acid complexes that resulted in a protein with enzymatic properties.

Unfortunately, all of the foregoing possibilities are really little more than speculation. For instance, no one has shown that an array of sulfide minerals (and/or oxide minerals) has the potential to be arranged in just the right sort of sequential way and with just the right amount of sufficient catalytic activity to make a reverse citric acid cycle work at all ... let alone within a plausible time frame for such a system to be able to survive and replicate amidst conditions involving extreme temperatures and pressure as well as existing in an environment that is not necessarily all that stable from a geological point of view.

Moreover, no one has shown how sulfide minerals with catalytic properties were able to transition to proteins with catalytic properties. In other words, how does a person go, on the one hand, from: (1) A metabolic-like system regulated by a sequence of conveniently placed sulfide minerals within a compartmentalize niche of some given hydrothermal vent, and, on the other hand, to: (2) A nucleic acid based system of coding that gives rise to a metabolic pathway that is regulated by enzymes that contain cores involving iron, nickel, or sulfur molecules?

George Cody, Robert Hazen, and Hat Yoder of the Carnegie Institute group conducted a number of experiments in the latter part of the 1990s that were intended to study the behavior of citric acid in conditions of high temperature and pressure. These conditions were intended to simulate what might have happened in the vicinity of various hydrothermal vents on early Earth.

Cody analyzed the results of those experiments. He determined there were two kinds of reaction cycles that tended to take place under the conditions specified by the experimental design, and he labeled them alpha and beta pathways.

The alpha pathway begins with citric acid breaking down into acetate and oxaloacetate molecules and, therefore, mimics what also can be observed to occur in the reverse citric acid cycle. However, under the experimental conditions, the foregoing oxaloacetate further degrades into pyruvate plus carbon dioxide, and, then, the pyruvate molecules decompose into acetate.

Irrespective of whatever combination of reactants and minerals were used in the experiments, the researchers could not get pyruvate to generate oxaloacetate. Consequently, the alpha pathway could not even get the reverse citric acid cycle started, let alone find a way to move on to the other steps of the reverse citric acid pathway.

The beta pathway discovered by Cody seemed more promising because it was rooted in a carbon dioxide produced series of successive reactions that yielded molecules with five, four, and three carbon atoms respectively. However, with one exception (aconitate) these carbon-containing molecules were different kinds of five-, four-, and three-carbon molecules than the ones that characterized the reverse citric acid cycle.

Cody also uncovered some evidence indicating that the beta-pathway that sometimes occurred during the experiments he was analyzing had the ability to be reversible in the presence of nickel sulfide. This suggested that the beta-pathway might be able to form a closed metabolic loop.

| Explorations |

However, there was an absence of certain other kinds of evidence in the foregoing experiments. More specifically, there was no data that showed that the beta-pathway gave expression to a metabolic potential that might be able to generate the sort of biomolecules that are synthesized in either the citric acid cycle or the reverse acid cycle ... biomolecules that play important roles as building blocks with respect to the synthesis of additional biomolecules – such as amino acids, sugars, and lipids -- which are intimately involved with the process of life as we know it.

Furthermore, Cody's analysis did not appear to demonstrate that the beta-pathway associated with the experiments his group ran was capable of producing ATP or GTP ... a key source of energy in biological systems. In fact, given that the molecules that showed up in the beta-pathway were mostly different from the molecules found in the reverse citric acid cycle, the very molecules that made up the beta-pathway might constitute an obstacle with respect to the formation of either ATP or GTP.

For example, the molecule, succinyl-CoA, plays an essential role within the citric acid cycle by helping to bring about the synthesis of ATP and GTP. Succinyl-CoA accomplishes this through holding on to the energy generated during the oxidation of the α-ketoglutarate molecule by means of a thioester bond. When the latter bond is hydrolyzed, the path has been cleared for the synthesis of ATP and GTP.

It is uncertain whether, or not, any of the molecules in the beta-pathway analyzed by Cody might be capable, under suitable circumstances, of preserving energy in the same way that succinyl-CoA does. If none of the molecules in the beta-pathway is capable of achieving this step, then a very important element is missing from the beta-pathway even if -- as Cody feels might be the case -- that pathway was capable of forming a closed metabolic loop.

A few more problems can be added to the foregoing considerations. One set of such problems is similar to an aforementioned issue.

For example, let's assume one begins with something like the beta-pathway that possesses nickel sulfide to serve as a catalyst of sorts. Given such a starting point, one must be able to account for how a nucleic acid base pairing system -- that encodes for proteins with enzymatic capacities that might have some nickel atoms at their core -- arises from the aforementioned, non-nucleic acid base pairing starting point.

There are still more problems or questions that need to be explored in conjunction with the beta-pathway possibility. For example, what about the other metabolic pathways that will be necessary in order to be able to take functional advantage (i.e., to help a given protocell to survive) of the molecules that are produced via the beta-pathway?

How did these other metabolic pathways come into existence? How did they become integrated with the biomolecules that are supposedly being synthesized through the beta-pathway?

A metabolic pathway that operates in the way that the reverse citric acid cycle does is not sufficient unto itself as an explanation for the origin of life. It needs to be augmented by, and integrated with, a variety of other metabolic pathways, which, in turn, are involved with still other metabolic pathways ... and this principle of additional, integrated, complementary metabolic pathways applies to the beta-pathway scenario as well.

Moreover, all of these complementary metabolic pathways need to be set in a context that consists of an appropriate sequence of the right kind of sulfide and oxide minerals (or other, alternative, catalytic agents) that are capable of making such metabolic pathways functional. Even if one were to grant that the beta-pathway formed closed metabolic loops, this is not enough ... in other words, that loop must be demonstrated to be both functional (i.e., capable of producing useful biomolecules), as well as connected to other metabolic pathways that can make use of what is being synthesized through the beta-pathway.

None of the foregoing issues were part of the Cody analysis of the beta-pathway. Therefore, if the beta-pathway is to be considered a viable candidate with respect to explaining the origin of life, then a lot more works needs to be done.

Moreover, as it stands -- and quite apart from the problems arising in conjunction with the need to account for additional metabolic pathways to complement the beta-pathway – the beta-pathway idea is missing some important ingredients. Among other things, and as indicated earlier, one doesn't even know whether the beta-pathway has any biologically relevant functionality with respect to the molecules that are produced through it when citric acid is subjected to conditions of extreme temperature and pressure.

It is not enough to show that a given pathway might form a closed loop. One also has to be able to demonstrate that the pathway has a potential functional value for helping to account for the origin of life.

Apart from – but also related to – the beta-pathway, there are a number of other issues that need to be addressed. For example, assuming that the reverse citric acid cycle (or something very much like it) might have been one of the first metabolic pathways to become established in the times of early Earth, how was the transition made from the reverse citric acid cycle to the 'normal' citric acid cycle?

Any number of possibilities might be advanced to address such a problem. However, there is no definitive evidence to show that any particular one of those possibilities is the right one (i.e., that it accurately reflects what happened).

An even more important issue has to do with the emergence of the DNA code? No one knows how this came about, and there aren't even any reasonable conjectural candidates for consideration.

The hydrothermal vent hypothesis maintains that metabolic pathways might have arisen in conjunction with various sulfide and oxide minerals that populated those vents. Aside from the previously noted problem of having to come up with a credible scenario for how an array of such minerals came to be arranged in just the right way and with just the right sort of catalytic activity to be able to give rise to functional, metabolic pathways, one must also be able to provide a credible account for how such prototypes transitioned into a coded set of nucleic acid base pairs that was able to incorporate the metabolic information contained in the sulfide mineral based metabolic pathways despite the fact that the system of coded nucleic base pairs seem to have nothing to do with arrays of sulfide and oxide minerals that have a structure and composition that is quite dissimilar from nucleic acid base pairs.

If one cannot explain how the transition from sulfide mineral-based metabolic pathways to nucleic acid-based metabolic pathways was accomplished, then one is left with several problems. The first problem is the huge hole that exists in any origin of life account that might be associated with such an inability to bridge the aforementioned transition issue.

The second problem is as follows: One will have to consider the possibility that the DNA/RNA coding system arose entirely independently of whatever primitive protocells might have formed that are based on the sorts of sulfide/oxide mineral metabolic pathways that often are envisioned to have arisen in conjunction with the hydrothermal vent hypothesis. Among other things, such a possibility suggests that all of the prebiotic research connected with trying to show how biological systems might have been given their start through various kinds of inorganic and organic chemistry that made use of networks of sulfide and oxide mineral pathways of catalysis in the context of hydrothermal vents is relatively worthless because none of that research really explains how the nucleic acid base pairings came to contain the sort of information that made the former sort of functionally integrated metabolic pathways possible.

In short, the degree of difficulty with respect to the problem of accounting for the origin of life via physics and chemistry has just doubled. One not only has to explain how functional sulfide mineral-based metabolic pathways arose, but, one also has to explain how quite different nucleic acid base pair systems arose that were able to independently solve the same set of problems involving metabolism that had been at least partially solved by the sulfide mineral approach to forming functional metabolic pathways that were facilitated by the presence of catalytic agents.

As a side note, and before moving on to other issues, all of the difficulties that saturate sulfide/oxide mineral–based accounts concerning the rise of metabolic pathways also befuddle various theories (e.g., Graham Cairns-Smith) which claim that certain kinds of mineral-laden clays could have served as a catalytic medium that might have brought about metabolic pathways through which important biomolecules might have been synthesized. If one analyzed the previous discussion concerning the role that sulfide minerals might have played in the hydrothermal vent hypothesis approach to the origin of life issue, and one substituted the word "clay" whenever terms such as "sulfide minerals" or "oxide minerals" appeared, all of the problems that have been pointed out with respect to the latter terms (e.g., sulfide minerals) would carry over to the clay-based theories.

Whatever strengths and properties might be associated with the idea of clay serving as a template, of sorts, for the origin of life, those strengths and properties are not enough to overcome the problems permeating that idea ... problems that already have been raised in conjunction with the sulfide/oxide mineral-based theories. Not the least of such problems is the relative dearth of evidence that is capable of demonstrating precisely how clay-based theories were able to generate the sort of functional metabolic pathways that are needed to provide a viable means of accounting for the origin of life.

| Explorations |

If life is not to be a one-and-done proposition, there must be a way of storing information that contains instructions for generating an integrated set of structural and dynamic properties that not only are needed for survival but which also can be transferred in an manner that permits similar, but independent units of instructional storage to arise. Some individuals – such as Sidney Fox – have tried to account for the foregoing sort of informational storage process through the notion of protenoids (protein-like entities).

Protenoids consist of a sequence of amino acids that are synthesized through various chemical and physical conditions ... conditions that, given enough time, will lead to the formation of chains of peptides (i.e., protenoids) that are theorized to have the sort of properties that -- when arranged in appropriate sequences -- can synthesize nucleotides. In turn, these nucleotides serve as the storage units for an array of operational instructions that are not only necessary for a protocell to be functional in a biological sense but, as well, are necessary for the transmission of that information in a way that can assist other protocells to arise, function, and enable the same sort of information to be passed along down a line of molecular, if not cellular, descent.

Potentially, amino acids are capable of linking up with one another in an enormous array of possibilities that extend far, far, far beyond even a realm of arrangements that entails hundreds of trillions of combinations. The vast number of such combinatorial possibilities seems to pose a rather significant problem for anyone who might want to provide a rational, credible account for how a set of, say, 20 amino acid combinations from amongst an array of such enormous possibilities came together in just the right way to be able to synthesize the right kind of nucleotides that, in turn, would come to form a sequence of base pairs that were capable of leading to the synthesis of the same set of amino combinations from which similar sequences of nucleotides could be synthesized again and again.

There is exactly zero proof indicating that any of the evolutionary scenarios concerning the origin of life is capable of explaining in a convincing manner how the foregoing mass of combinatorial possibilities was able to give rise to the sort of functional network of metabolic pathways that are necessary to account for even the simplest forms of life. Of course, one could assume that everything somehow happened in a just-so way, but assuming one's conclusion in such a fashion tends to be a sign of the presence of magical thinking rather than the presence of a rigorous, critically reflective, methodical process of science.

Hope, however, springs eternal ... even in the minds of people who consider themselves – or are considered by others – to be scientists. So, let's consider a few more ideas.

In 1982 Thomas Cech and Sidney Altman uncovered the existence of ribozymes. Ribozymes consist of RNA molecules that not only are able to store information but, as well, are able to catalyze certain kinds of biochemical reactions.

The discovery of ribozymes offered a possible way to eliminate a dilemma with which origin of life theories had been confronted prior to 1982. More specifically, although everyone conceded that both proteins and DNA/RNA were necessary for life, no one could figure out a plausible account for which of the two ingredients come first.

Did the origin of life process start with DNA/RNA and subsequently lead to the synthesis of proteins? Or, alternatively, did the origin of life process begin with proteins (as Fox and a few others maintained) and this, in turn, led to the synthesis of DNA/RNA?

Ribozymes appeared to resolve the foregoing problem rather nicely. A biomolecule had been found that, seemingly, might be able to take on the roles of both proteins and DNA.

While, in principle, ribozymes appeared to have explanatory potential with respect to addressing the aforementioned chicken-and-egg priority issue in relation to the origin of life, there also were some outstanding questions swirling about that notion. For example, even though ribozymes were capable of catalyzing some reactions, did ribozymes have the capacity to catalytically facilitate all manner of reactions?

If the answer to the foregoing questions is no, then, there are determinate limits to the catalytic properties of ribozymes. Depending on the nature of such limits, ribozymes might not constitute as big a treasure trove with respect to be able to provide a credible evolutionary account for the origin of life as some theorists might have hoped.

Ribosomes (not to be confused with ribozymes) consist of a complex integration of proteins and strands of RNA. In combination, the foregoing two components of ribosomes assist cells to bring about the assembly of proteins.

Initially, scientists believed that the proteins in ribosomes were primarily responsible for the sort of catalytic activity that facilitated the linking up of amino acids with one another during the formation of various proteins. Eventually, however, research determined that ribosomal RNA, not proteins, played the lead role in the assembly of proteins.

There was a further tantalizing piece involving the origin of life puzzle that complemented the discoveries involving the role of RNA in ribozymes and ribosomes. RNA nucleotides (or closely related molecular structures) are found in some coenzymes that play important roles in, among other reactions, the citric acid and reverse citric acid cycles that were discussed earlier in this chapter.

Finally, research also has uncovered the existence of what are sometimes referred to as 'riboswitches'. These are segments of RNA found in messenger RNA that are capable of regulating some aspects of gene expression by turning certain genes on and off through the way in which their conformational shapes change when binding to various kinds of molecules.

Many people today are familiar with the term "junk DNA". This phrase was introduced in 1972 by Susumu Ohno, a Japanese geneticist, as a way of referring to the fact that only about 2% of the human genome consists of genes that actually code for proteins, whereas the other 98% of the genome consists of, apparently, useless, nucleotide residues.

The traditional picture of protein synthesis was that a given gene codes for, and is transcribed into, messenger RNA. Messenger RNA helps bring about the assembly of the protein that was specified by the gene that led to the appearance of messenger RNA.

In 2001, a more complex picture began to emerge. Among other things, researchers discovered that something called "microRNA"

| Explorations |

(sometimes consisting of as few as 22, or so, nucleotide sequences) was capable of binding to various segments of messenger RNA, and, as a result, the microRNA was able to modulate the activity (or expression) of the messenger RNA molecules.

In addition, researchers discovered that what had been considered to be useless or junk DNA was coding for the tiny sequences of RNA known as microRNA. These small, coded segments of RNA were performing a vast array of regulatory functions within cells.

For example, consider the protein myosin that plays a major role in orchestrating the activity of heart muscles. Researchers uncovered the fact that microRNA sequences were tucked away in one of the introns associated with the production of myosin.

An intron is a nucleotide sequence that is removed by RNA splicing during the translation of messenger RNA into – in this case -- a myosin protein. The intron that is removed during RNA splicing was considered to be useless or junk RNA that for 'reasons' lost in the distant past had, nonetheless, been retained and still was able to code for the transcription of such sequences ... and, as a result, the segment of the DNA sequences coding for the useless messenger RNA was considered to be a junk form of base pairings as well.

Yet, lo and behold, the intron was not useless. It contained information that helped regulate the activity of myosin in a variety of circumstances.

Among other things researchers found that such microRNA sequences helped heart muscles to respond in various ways to the presence of, among other things, thyroid hormones. In addition, researchers discovered that as the nature of the microRNA changed, then so too did the manner in which heart activity was regulated also change.

An obvious question that emerges in conjunction with the foregoing findings is the following one. How did all of the regulatory information become embedded within the DNA genetic sequences so that it could be removed from the messenger RNA sequences in the form of introns and, then, subsequently be released to perform regulatory functions in conjunction with whatever protein had been assembled and according to whatever set of conditions happen to prevail at the time the protein was assembled and began to go about its functional business?

Both the hydrothermal vent hypothesis and the prebiotic soup conjecture concerning the origin of life have no plausible, credible, evidence-based way of responding to, or accounting for, the emergence of regulatory order in living systems. Consequently, since order plays such an essential, defining role in making life what it is, neither the hydrothermal vent hypothesis nor the prebiotic soup conjecture really give expression to a viable scientific, evolutionary theory for the origin of life.

Furthermore, neither of those perspectives constitutes the best available scientific theories of the origin of life. This is because neither of those perspectives gives expression to a scientific theory in any meaningful sense of the word.

They each consist of little more than speculations, assumptions, and pieces of isolated, disconnected, and highly questionable data. Such data might have been derived through scientific means, but this is not sufficient to qualify the ideas that make use of such data as being scientific in nature.

As has been shown throughout this chapter, those pieces of data cannot withstand any sort of rigorous critical analysis. After the dust of such a process of considered, critical reflection clears, neither the hydrothermal vent hypothesis nor the prebiotic soup conjecture has been able to plausibly and credibly demonstrate how the pieces of data that have been gathered together over more than 60 years of extensive research would be capable of permitting one to bridge the huge gap that separates, on the one hand, the hydrothermal vent hypothesis or the prebiotic soup conjecture from, on the other hand, a coherent, detailed, consistent, evidence-based account concerning the origin of life.

The inability of science (on so many levels) to generate a successful theory concerning the origin of life issue does not leave one with the best available scientific account for the origin of life. The failure of science in this respect leaves one with no scientific theory at all.

The presence of scientists does not necessarily render a theory scientific. The presence of experimental research conducted by scientists does not necessarily transform the pieces of data that come from such research into a scientific theory. The writing and publishing of an array of articles, books, and essays that are steeped in scientific jargon, terminology, and technical calculations does not necessarily mean that the subject matter of those books, articles, and so on constitutes a scientific theory.

Something is scientific when one can demonstrate -- through the use of reason and empirical data -- that the claims being made in the name of science are capable of being defended in a way which demonstrates that the reasoned, evidence-based system of understanding underlying those claims is able to accurately reflect, to varying degrees of specificity and predictability, those facets of reality to which the claims allude. Evolutionary theories concerning the origin of life have not been able to satisfy – even in minor ways -- the foregoing challenge, and, therefore, those theories are not scientific ... they are just theories, hypotheses, and conjectures, and they do not deserve being assigned the label of "scientific".

Notwithstanding the foregoing considerations, ribozymes, ribosomes, riboswitches, and microRNA represent independently derived forms of support for the idea that, perhaps, RNA should be at the heart of any origin of life scenario that sought to explain how certain capacities – that is, storing information, transmitting it, and handling whatever catalytic activities might be necessary to facilitate such storage and transmission activities -- were possible.

As appealing as all of the foregoing facts concerning RNA sound (and a set of theories known as the 'RNA world hypothesis' were constructed and updated through such facts), nevertheless, there are a variety of problems inhabiting and threatening the RNA world hypothesis. To begin with, having a potential means to store and transmit information involving operational instructions for setting up metabolic pathways that can be catalyzed in appropriate ways is one thing.

However, the origin of such operational instructions is quite another matter. The existence of ribozymes, ribosomes, riboswitches, microRNA, or any other RNA-based capacity does not explain how the set of operational instructions that coordinate and regulate the activity of ribozymes, ribosomes, riboswitches, microRNA, or other RNA-based capacities came into existence. Ribozymes, ribosomes, riboswitches, and microRNA only have biological value when they are capable of operating at a time and in a way and in a place and for a duration that is capable of producing what is needed for cells to be functionally viable.

Therefore, without an appropriate script and directorial oversight, ribozymes, ribosomes, riboswitches, and microRNA are somewhat limited in their capacities to explain origin of life issues. They are sort of like a group of actors who, individually, might possess certain acting talents but, nonetheless, if those actors are left to their own devices to give expression to an array of arbitrary actions, then those actors will not necessarily be able to produce a qualitatively coherent, sensible, and functional film (i.e., explanatory account).

Furthermore, despite decades of trying to find a plausible way of generating RNA molecules from simple precursors under various kinds of simulated early Earth scenarios, no scientist or group of scientists has been able to successfully synthesize RNA. In addition, no one has come up with a plausible mechanism (either in the context of some variation on the hydrothermal vent hypothesis or in relation to some version of the primordial soup scenario) for inducing RNA molecules to link up with one another under early-Earth-like conditions.

To varying degrees, scientists understand how ribozymes, ribosomes, riboswitches, and microRNA work in functional cells. However, scientists have little, or no, understanding about how those RNA-related components came to be organized in a way that, along with other factors, gave rise to functional cells.

| Explorations |

[In passing, I find it interesting that Stanislaus Burzynski -- the person who discovered Antineoplastons and their possible role in the etiology of cancer (something that was explored in the first chapter) -- had stumbled upon the discovery of a group of small peptides that seemed to have a regulatory function with respect to preventing various kinds of cancer from being able to gain a foothold in individuals. One wonders if there might be a variety of microRNA segments that code for such peptide sequences.

Perhaps cancer is caused by a variety of factors (carcinogens) that inhibit the expression of those sequences of microRNA that are responsible for the presence of Antineoplastons in healthy individuals. By using antineoplastons as a treatment for cancer patients, Dr. Burzynski might have been introducing countermeasures for an acute or a chronic problem involving the expression of those segments of microRNA that, normally speaking, regulate the generation and activity of Antineoplastons in healthy individuals.]

| Explorations |

| Explorations |

Extinction

The vast majority of organisms that have appeared on, or in, the Earth at one time or another have become extinct. Various species are going extinct on a regular basis, and this tendency gives expression to a background rate against which existing life forms play out various possibilities with respect to forces of natural selection that determines whether, or not, such life forms will become part of that background rate.

The average lifespan for species, in general, is approximately 5 million years. However, the lifespan for any given species might be as little as a hundred thousand years, or as long as 15 million years.

The 'normal' background rate of extinction seems to run around 10 to 20%. In other words, out of every 100 species, 10 to 20 of the members of the larger set of species will become extinct over a million year period ... which works out to be roughly .00001-.00002% of existing species per year.

Occasionally, a type of extinction occurs that deviates substantially from the aforementioned background rate. These are events involving mass casualties resulting in the disappearance of numerous species within – geologically speaking -- a relatively short period of time.

Extinction events might be caused by an array of conditions. Among such possibilities are: Massive volcanic eruptions, relatively rapid changes in climate, large meteor impacts, the release of considerable quantities of methane from hydrates (methane that becomes entangled within a crystalline form of water and, in the process, forms a structure that is similar to ice), and so on –

An array of evidence collected over many years indicates that as many as 17 relatively minor, kinds of mass extinctions have taken place since life first appeared on Earth. For example, there were many large mammal species that became extinct by the end of the last ice age, 10,000 years ago.

On the other hand, there have been, at least, five 'events' involving mass extinctions that are considerably larger than the minor forms of extinction being alluded to in the last paragraph. These major instances of mass extinction usually encompass at least 40% -- if not more -- of the life forms existing at a given time.

| Explorations |

The mass extinction events for which evidence exists are as follows. The first 'event' happened in the late Ordovician period some 440 million years ago; (2) a second 'event' occurred in the late Devonian period roughly 370 million years ago; (3) a third 'event' took place near the end of the Permian period approximately 250 million years ago; (4) a fourth 'event' occurred near the end of the Triassic period around 200 million years ago; and, finally, (5) the so-called KT 'event' occurred near the end of the Cretaceous period some 65 million years ago (the 'K' refers to the Greek word for chalk – kreta – which is commonly found in rock strata that tend to mark the boundaries of the Cretaceous period, and 'T' refers to the Tertiary period that followed the Cretaceous period). A mass extinction 'event' might consist of just one dynamic (such as large scale volcanic eruptions), or that kind of event might involve several kinds of dynamics that interact with one another.

There might well have been additional events entailing mass extinction. However, clear-cut evidence for such possibilities is missing due to problems involving a lack of fossils, along with various difficulties associated with being able to establish precise dates for such events.

Nonetheless, there is evidence that at least one other mass extinction event apparently took place in Precambrian times, some 560 to 550 million years ago. Initially discovered in the Ediacara Hills of Australia -- but subsequently found among the fossils in many other locations throughout the world -- there were a variety of animals (including the first fossils that could be seen with the naked eye) that existed in Precambrian times. However, during the latter portion of the Precambrian period, those animals disappeared from the fossil record.

The mass extinction event that occurred during the latter stages of the Ordovician period seemed to involve mostly marine fauna of one kind or another. The available evidence concerning that event suggests it might have been due to relatively rapid changes in climate as tropical-like temperatures were replaced by much cooler conditions.

The second mass extinction event for which there is a fairly substantial amount of evidence took place late in the Devonian period. Instead of consisting of one event, this mass extinction event seemed to be the result of a series of extinction events that occurred approximately 360 million years, or so, ago.

Armored fish, aquatically skilled cephalopods, and other organisms became extinct as a result of whatever events were going on during those days. Opinions on the nature of the cause of the extinctions vary, but one of the possibilities mentioned is that Earth might have been hit by a fairly sizeable asteroid or comet late in the Devonian period.

The largest of the foregoing five events took place near the end of the Permian period, 250 million years ago. It might have wiped out 90%, or more, of all life forms that were in existence at the time.

Many species involving both flora and fauna were involved in the foregoing mass extinction event. Furthermore, the species that were affected inhabited both land (e.g., insects, reptiles, plants, and amphibians) as well as water environments (e.g., most of the marine groups that had been dominant during the Paleozoic era disappeared or were severely decimated during this event).

The fourth mass extinction event occurred fairly late during the Triassic period. This event seemed to affect mostly aquatic life forms, but many water-based families of species became extinct at approximately the same time.

As arrays of species were disappearing during the late Triassic mass extinction event, there were other species that arose in, and around, the time of the Triassic mass-extinction event. For instance, quite a few modern groups – such as mammals, turtles, and crocodiles – began to appear at this time.

The KT 'event', which took place approximately 65 million years ago, eliminated an incredible array of species ... including the life form (dinosaurs) that had dominated the Earth for roughly 135 million years. The reign of dinosaurs had begun during the Triassic period and extended until the end of the Cretaceous period when the Earth was hit by a sizable asteroid in Chicxulub, Mexico on the Yucatan peninsula.

However, there were many species of life other than dinosaurs that disappeared as a result of the KT event. A great deal of research indicates that as many as three-quarters of all plant and animal species extant at the time of the event soon disappeared.

| Explorations |

The impact of the aforementioned asteroid created conditions that were somewhat similar to those that various scientists have claimed might arise in conjunction with a 'nuclear winter' scenario. Among other things, under such circumstances, the atmosphere would have became filled with so much debris due to the impact of an asteroid, as well as ensuing fires, and so on, that the light of the sun likely would have become blocked out for a substantial period of time (perhaps, years), and this could have eliminated a variety of species in several ways.

For instance, not only would some species die out due to the relatively rapid drop in temperature that would occur in the aftermath of the asteroid strike, but, in addition, plankton and plants would have become unable to perform photosynthesis since light from the sun likely would have had difficulty penetrating a debris-filled atmosphere. The extinction of plants and plankton would lead, in turn, to the demise of whatever species relied on such plants and plankton as a food source, and, this, subsequently, would lead to the disappearance of whatever forms of life fed on the consumers of plants and planktons ... etc., etc., etc.

Let's briefly review the time frame for the five mass extinctions for which evidence exists. The first in a series of five mass extinction events took place 440 years ago. Following another 70 million year period, a second mass extinction occurred. 120 million years later, life forms underwent a third mass extinction that eliminated up to, at least, 90% of all species. 50 million years further down the temporal road, a fourth mass extinction occurred. Finally, a fifth mass extinction took place approximately 135 million years later in which three-fourths of all forms of plant and animal life disappeared.

In other words, within a period of 185 million years, life on Earth was substantially extinguished in vast numbers including one instance of mass extinction that eliminated at least 40% of life forms existing on Earth at that time, as well as second mass extinction event that was calculated to have wiped out between 90-95% of all life forms, along with a third mass extinction event that extinguished three-fourths of all life forms existing at the time. Moreover, during that 185 million year period, there were 6 additional substantial, but much more limited, extinction episodes.

| Explorations |

Normally speaking, when many people speak about evolution, what they have to say is couched in terms of what might transpire over many hundreds of million of years. Nonetheless, a variety of extinction events – both major and minor -- tend to induce one to critically reflect on what might have been going on within an extraordinary period of 185 million years ... a period of time in which life was reduced down to 10% of its former number of species, and, then, over the next 120 million years, life forms were again reduced by three-fourths of their numbers ... plus whatever mass extinctions occurred as a result of the event that occurred near the end of the Triassic period ... along with a number of other minor – but still substantial – instances of mass extinction.

How did life recover sufficiently from being nearly extinct some 250 million years ago to becoming sufficiently robust that it was able to withstand another major extinction event 50 million years later? How did new life forms rise like Phoenix from the ashes during that 50 million year period?

Alternatively, how did that which happened with respect to life, between 65 million years ago and the present time, occur? In other words, how does one go from a point in which three-fourths of life has been wiped out to the present state of biodiversity?

Following each mass extinction event, a variety of new flora and fauna appeared on the scene – such as when mammals, crocodiles, and turtles emerged in, and around, the time of the mass extinction of the late Triassic period, or in relation to the rapid radiation of animals with shells that occurred following the mass-extinction event associated with the Precambrian period.

The foregoing data tend to indicate that, theoretically speaking, one no longer has the usual luxury of having hundreds of millions of years to work with in order to try to account for how various evolutionary events might have taken place. Instead, one is dealing with time frames of 50 and 65 million years respectively.

Of course, 50-60 million years is still a very long time. Nonetheless, the time within which the recovery of life must take place and, in the process, give expression generate many new forms of life is considerably truncated from time frames consisting of hundreds of millions of years.

| Explorations |

Furthermore, one cannot necessarily pinpoint the place, time, or circumstances when a given species first shows up. The fossils found in geological strata, together with various methods of dating, might be able to provide a general framework for the appearance of a given species, but the precise time, place, circumstances, and means through which a species became a thing unto itself appears to be relatively hidden (and this is part of the branching problem discussed in a previous section of this chapter).

In addition, the problems surrounding the emergence of new life forms following mass-extinction events can be intensified somewhat relative to the aforementioned time frames of 50-65 million years. Consider the following.

The Cambrian explosion -- or radiation – that predates all five of the mass extinction events -- began approximately 540 million years ago and lasted for roughly 20 million years. During that relatively brief period of time, the general body-plan for many of the major phyla of modern metazoans, or members of the Animal Kingdom, came into existence, and, as well, there was considerable diversification of other kinds of organisms such as phytoplankton.

In addition, the fossil record indicates that certain kinds of complex organisms arose during the Cambrian explosion that appeared to be unlike any phyla existing today. Obviously, these sorts of organisms subsequently became part of the background extinction rate.

Many evolutionary biologists -- since, and including, Darwin -- tend to agree that during the Cambrian explosion the phyla for all modern animals seemed to simultaneously emerge in the fossil record within a relatively short period of geological time. The problem that arose from such an acknowledgement had to do with the need to explain how so much diversity emerged – relatively speaking -- so quickly.

Since the time of Darwin, some researchers (including Darwin himself) suspected that the incomplete nature of the fossil record might contain a great of information concerning the nature of the explosion ... that is, if such fossils had been discovered rather than missing. In other words, the perspective advocated by a variety of individuals inclined toward the theory of evolution suggested that if

| Explorations |

the fossil record were to become more complete, not only would the evidence needed to explain the explosion have been readily available, but, as well, such data would have been able to demonstrate that the evolutionary branching process entailed by the Cambrian explosion was relatively uniform and gradual.

The foregoing contention might well be true. On the other hand, one could say something very similar in conjunction with almost any issue for which there is a relative death of evidence capable of supporting whatever one believes might be the truth concerning such an issue.

To be sure, the absence of evidence does not necessarily constitute evidence of absence. Nevertheless, an absence of evidence does not constitute any form of positive evidence either.

Stephen Jay Gould and Niles Eldredge developed an alternative approach to trying to account for evolutionary phenomena like the Cambrian explosion. The two paleontologists believed the fossil record contained very little evidence supporting Darwin's belief that evolution occurred through a process of gradualism -- that is, there seemed to be very little, overall, phenotypic change exhibited across the geological history occupied by the fossils for a given species.

This period of relatively limited, net, evolutionary change is known as a condition of stasis or a stage of equilibrium. However, from time to time, that condition of stasis or equilibrium is punctuated by periods of change in the fossil record.

These periods of change entail a process of speciation. New species arise within the context of small populations that have been separated geographically, ecologically, or in some other way from the ancestral population

This process of speciation is related to Ernst Mayr's founder effect notion. Small populations are moved from one adaptive peak (defining one species) to another, different kind of adaptive peak (defining a new species), by – somehow – moving through a valley in which such adaptive transitions tend to run up against forces of natural selection of one kind or another.

At some point, the newly minted species comes back into the picture via the presence of fossils. Consequently, if one just looks at the surface evidence (fossils), the emergence of the new species might appear to be strange and involve a seemingly inexplicable transition in the fossil record, when, in reality (or so the theory goes) the process of speciation has been perfectly 'normal' but took place off-stage (i.e., without fossil evidence).

Not all evolutionary biologists believe that the sort of speciation entailed by the theory of punctuated equilibrium is necessary in order for adaptive, evolutionary change to be able to occur. Such individuals believe that phenomena like genetic drift and/or an array of mutational events are capable of bringing about adaptive changes independently of the process of speciation outlined by Eldredge and Gould.

Moreover, the evolutionary biologists to whom I am alluding in the foregoing paragraph tend to claim that genetic constraints of one kind, or another, often prevent transitions in morphological character (i.e., evolution) from taking place. From the perspective of those theorists, genetic drift and/or mutational events are necessary before substantial phenotypic transitions (of an evolutionary nature) will be able to occur due to the manner through which genetic drift and/or mutations, of one kind or another, overcome previous genetic constraints.

Nevertheless, whether one believes that crucial evidence has disappeared in the mists of incomplete fossil records, or one advances a theory of punctuated equilibrium that revolves around the possibility of a certain kind of speciation process, or one maintains that adaptive change can arise through the phenomenon of genetic drift and/or a sequence of mutational events, there is an absence of any proof which shows that one plausibly can account for the apparently sudden emergence of life forms like the ones that seemed to occur during the Cambrian explosion.

All one has is a certain amount of data mixed in with an array of conjectures, assumptions, and hypotheses concerning those events. The dimension of proof is entirely absent.

Because technical terms and phrases -- along with a few equations – are often sprinkled among the conjectures, speculations, and assumptions, the aforementioned positions appear – at least to some individuals -- to be scientific in nature. Nonetheless, no real science is present.

As far as the theory of evolution is concerned, none of the essential dynamics have been proven. Nothing of a critical nature has been substantiated. Nothing of a fundamental nature has been confirmed. Nothing has been demonstrated as being likely to be true.

At best, whatever might have been proven, substantiated, confirmed or demonstrated tends to be entirely a function of surface phenomena. None of the deep, dynamic principles that are capable of bringing about the cause of so-called evolutionary change or bringing about the cause of the order that is manifested through the surface phenomena associated with what is alleged to be evolutionary change have been brought into the light of understanding.

Like the fossil evidence that might potentially exist but has not, yet, been discovered, so too, data consisting of direct, observational evidence involving the actual dynamics of punctuated equilibrium, genetic drift, and mutational events all occur off-stage, so to speak, and are unavailable to us except in indirect ways that rely more on the process of interpretation, assumption, and conjecture than they do on the presence of real concrete evidence.

Similar kinds of problems tend to permeate the periods of recovery that follow each of the periods of mass extinction. Within a fairly short period of time following such events – geologically speaking – there often appear to be Cambrian-like explosions of life forms that seem to come into view in relatively inexplicable ways.

How does one explain such phenomena? Ideas such as: an incomplete fossil record, or punctuated equilibrium, or genetic drift, or a set of mutational events – whether considered individually or collectively – are not scientific explanations for what occurred during the various explosion of life forms that followed mass extinction events, but, instead, those ideas are allusions to the possibility of explanations that, unfortunately, lack the presence of anything more concrete than various kinds of experimental data and research that are suggestive or interesting without being conclusive or compelling ... that is, there is an absence of any semblance of proof in conjunction with the aforementioned ideas.

| Explorations |

278

Those ideas – taken individually or collectively – might be correct. However, there is no proof this is the case.

How does an idea become scientific when there is no proof that such an idea actually accounts for what it purportedly explains? In the absence of proof certain ideas might provide one with a hermeneutical understanding that possesses a kind of meaningfulness that helps make sense of some facet of reality (as was discussed previously in conjunction with Dobzhansky), but what is meaningful and what is true are not necessarily coextensive.

The time-frame issue becomes even more acute when one comes to the matter of human evolution. Instead of talking in terms of 50-65 million years as in the case of some of the mass extinction events, or speaking in terms of the 20 million years associated with the Cambrian explosion, the time frame for human evolution supposedly occurs over a period of 2-3 million years.

Some evolutionary biologists wish to extend the foregoing 2-3 million year period by an additional 3-4 million years -- and more will be said about this in the next section of the current chapter. However, whether one is speaking in terms of a time frame lasting 2-3 million years, or one is talking in terms of period of time lasting 6-7 million years, one still is dealing with a theory that claims that an incredible array of complex phenomena took place with a relatively short period of time – indeed, apparently, such events took place within a frame of time that is significantly shorter than any other time frame in evolutionary history as far as the emergence of significant new capabilities is concerned.

More specifically, during a period of time covering anywhere from two to seven million years (which is still 13 to 18 million years less than the time frame for the Cambrian explosion and 32 to 47 million years less than the time frame for the recovery of life following the late Permian and KT extinction events respectively), evolutionary biologists claim that very complex capacities involving: Language, creativity/inventiveness, reason/logic, insight, problem-solving, various kinds of genius (e.g., artistic, musical, mathematical, or mechanical), memory, imagination, reflexive consciousness, spirituality, hermeneutical activity, morality, and the like came into existence. There are libraries filled with conjectures concerning all of the foregoing phenomena, but what is missing from those documents is: Compelling evidence that the individuals producing such documents know – in specific, demonstrable terms -- how any of the foregoing capabilities came about; or, compelling evidence that the authors of those documents know how the origin of life came about; or, compelling evidence indicating that such individuals know how new forms of life arose following mass extinction events.

Of course, someone might counter with the possibility that the rudiments of intelligence, reason, logic, language, creativity, memory, morality, imagination, insight, reflexive consciousness, and so on might have begun to take root in various earlier species, and, if this is the case, then trying to shrink the time frame in the manner that is being suggested in the previous paragraph is quite misleading. This, certainly, is a possibility.

However, the underlying problems don't really disappear in conjunction with such a counter proposal. Instead, the character of the problems that must be explained merely shifts a little.

Firstly -- and <u>assuming</u> that the foregoing possibility is correct -- one must be able to account for how any of the rudimentary capacities for logic, language, and so on were initially able to arise prior to the appearance of hominid-like creatures. To offer a date, or related evidence, for <u>when</u> those kinds of capabilities might have first begun to emerge is not enough.

One must be able to provide a detailed, concrete account of what the nature of the dynamics was that led to the emergence of even the most rudimentary, primitive forms of those abilities. No such evolutionary account exists.

Secondly, one must be able to account – in specific, concrete terms -- for the dynamic history of transitions or transformations that led from the rudimentary editions of the aforementioned capabilities to their modern, human counterparts. No such evolutionary account exists.

Finally, whether one considers the time-frame for the emergence of advanced cognitive/mental abilities to be between two and three million years, or one broadens that time frame somewhat and contends that the emergence of those sorts of cognitive/mental

| Explorations |

capabilities started between six and seven million years ago, one is not really specifying precisely when, or how, any of it took place. In other words, the mental capabilities at issue didn't necessarily take two to three million years or six to seven million years to evolve ... those time frames merely mark the period of time within which – we know not where, what or how – something happened.

Contending that advanced cognitive/mental capacities emerged during a two-to-three million year period or maintaining that they emerged during a six-to-seven million year period is not necessarily the same as, or equivalent to, the claim that it took two to three million years or six to seven million years for those capabilities to evolve. Since we don't know how – or precisely when – such capabilities emerged, we really have no idea how long it took for any of those abilities to appear on the scene.

To be sure, the idea that some sort of significant set of gradual steps was necessary to produce a complex phenomenon seems to be somewhat easier to wrap understanding around with respect to how something might have happened than is the notion that events might have taken place in some non-gradual manner. However, as pointed out earlier, irrespective of whether things took place relatively gradually or relatively quickly, establishing a time frame of whatever length of time doesn't actually tell us when or how something happened – only that whatever happened, happened somewhere within that period.

For instance, the late Permian mass extinction event was followed by a 10 million year fossil gap in the oceans of the Earth. This gap extended into the early Triassic period.

The rich, multi-mile-long reefs consisting of large walls made from, among things, the remnants of coral life – systems of reefs that were prominent during the Permian period -- had all disappeared. Moreover, up until the present time, paleontologists have been unable to discover any evidence within the geological strata covering ten million years relative to that period of history -- involving both the extinction event of the later Permian period and the early part of the ensuing Triassic period -- which suggests the presence of any kind of reef structures during that time frame.

| Explorations |

Apparently – at least according to the fossil record -- all that survived in the world's oceans following the late Permian mass extinction event were five species of shelly organisms consisting of: Four bivalve creatures (Unionites, Claraia, Promyalina, and Eumorphotis), along with one kind of brachiopod (Lingula). On land, one reptilian form (Lystrosaurus) appeared to dominate life (constituting as much as 95% of all life forms).

Nothing else – as far as visible life forms are concerned -- appears to be present for the next 10 million years. Then, slowly, evolutionary events seem to begin to pick up speed as life moves into the middle part of the Triassic period.

The foregoing data appears to indicate that evolution went on a holiday for 10 million years. What happened?

There is always the possibility that paleontologists simply haven't yet been able to discover the evidence that is out there somewhere waiting to be found and, if discovered, would provide the proof that evolutionary changes constituted an on-going, robust set of phenomena in the oceans of the world following the late-Permian mass extinction. This is a possibility but it is not a scientific one.

Such a possibility becomes scientific when one has the necessary evidence to back up that kind of a claim. Until the time when the necessary sort of evidence is forthcoming, the aforementioned possibility is merely a non-scientific conjecture or speculation.

In passing, the reader might wish to note that paleontologists have found all manner of fossils (non-marine deposits) elsewhere in the geological strata corresponding to the early Triassic period. However, these plentiful findings are limited to just a couple of species: Clararia and Lystrosaurus.

If the 10 million year gap is genuine – that is, it constitutes reliable evidence indicating that evolution was at a standstill – one is presented with several puzzles. What prevented evolution from taking place, and what got it going again?

Given – i.e., assuming -- that the post-extinction environment had been so toxic and obstacle-riddled that life – let alone evolutionary change – was not possible, then, how did five species of shelly creatures, plus a reptile, manage to survive and, given that they

| Explorations |

survived, why didn't they evolve? Moreover, if evolution was not possible in the post-apocalyptic period following the late-Permian mass extinction, then what was it that had to change in order for life to once again begin to evolve? And, finally, once conditions conducive to the dynamics of population biology began to appear, what was it that actually happened so that things – evolutionarily speaking – could once again begin to move in more diversified directions?

If 90-95% of life forms on Earth had become extinct due to the late-Permian event, whatever remained is likely to have been scattered in the form of relatively small populations. Small populations tend to limit the variation that is available to the gene pool of such species, and this raises several problems.

To begin with, how does a population of limited variability find a way to survive for 10 million years despite – presumably -- changing conditions? This is not to say that such a question cannot be answered, but, currently, we lack sufficient evidence -- concerning both the precise ecological conditions of the early Triassic period, as well as the capabilities of the few species that were living in those conditions -- that would be needed to address that kind of a question with any degree of compelling credibility.

Secondly, given the likelihood of such limited genetic variability, how did the capabilities arise that permitted the relatively few species of life existing in the early Triassic to begin to evolve in relation to variable conditions of natural selection? Moreover, why did it take 10 million years for such variable capabilities to emerge?

What kind of a system of genetic drift and/or series of mutations would enter into stasis for 10 million years, and, then, suddenly (relatively speaking) begin to become active again? Did allegedly random events of either variety (i.e., genetic drift and/or mutations) suddenly stop occurring for that period of time, and, if so, why did this happen?

Seemingly, evolutionary theory is a lot like Archimedes's notion when he is alleged to have claimed words to the effect of: "Give me a place to stand, and I will move the Earth." It is all about leveraging the assumption that there is a place where one can stand and through which one can accomplish what one claims is possible.

Similarly evolutionary theory is largely a function of looking for a place to stand (the evidence) from which one can uncover (move) the weighty conjecture concerning the nature of so-called evolutionary change. However, finding the requisite standing place in relation to evolutionary theory is, in many respects, as elusive as realizing Archimedes thought experiment might prove to be.

Many people – including quite a few scientists -- will argue that theology and religion are not scientific in nature because those systems of thought can't prove their assertions or because theology and religion have no reliable, intersubjective means through which to uncover the kind of empirical data that is needed to be able to advance a compelling and demonstrable case for any of their claims concerning the nature of reality. Fair enough.

However, the epistemological status of evolutionary theory appears to be very much like that of religion and theology. The former system of thought can't prove any of its assertions concerning the underlying cause of the sort of changes that occur in life forms over time that are said to be evolutionary in nature, and, furthermore, evolutionary theory doesn't seem to be rooted in any reliable, intersubjective means through which to uncover the kind of empirical data that is needed to be able to advance a compelling and demonstrable case for any of its claims concerning the nature of reality.

Everyone agrees that things – including life – change. Nevertheless, no one has any proof capable of being agreed upon by the vast majority of individuals that the reason(s) why things change is (are) because the nature of reality is 'X'.

Yet, the hermeneutical musings of scientists – which are devoid of proof when it comes to evolution -- are said to be scientific in nature, while the hermeneutical musings of theologians and people of religion are said to be non-scientific in nature. This seems to be a distinction without a difference.

Some people who are inclined toward an evolutionary perspective concerning the nature of reality (including life) might wish to argue that one must become a scientist in order to truly understand the extent to which the theory of evolution is capable of proving itself.

| Explorations |

Similar arguments have been -- and continue to be -- advanced by theologians and proponents of this or that religion.

In other words, the sort of argument that sometimes emerges from the evolutionary and religious perspectives is that a person can only understand the nature of the truths that are given expression through a particular belief system by becoming the right sort of technical expert within the context of that framework. When one acquires such expertise, one will be able to see the truth of things.

This is an exercise in framing. One's understanding is being shaped, organized, and manipulated to accept a certain point of view as being true quite apart from whether, or not, there is any way to independently show that what is being said concerning the nature of reality is true in the way such perspectives claim is the case.

Scientists tend to insist that theologians and people of religion play the game of evidence and proof according to strict rules. There are no presumptive freebies permitted in such a game.

Every claim must be backed up with proof. And, this is as it should be.

Amazingly, however, people who advocate an evolutionary point of view apparently do not believe they are required to play the aforementioned game by the same set of strict rules of proof and demonstration. People who are inclined toward an evolutionary perspective tend to refer to their claims as being scientific without ever having to prove the scientific character of those claims.

Such individuals consider what they believe to be scientific even though what they believe constitutes a system of thought that is largely incapable of demonstrating the truth of any of its essential claims concerning the nature of reality or how reality supposedly works. The proponents of evolution continuously grant themselves all manner of presumptive freebies in relation to underlying assumptions – such as randomness – but insist that this is an entirely different matter than when theologians and people of religion try to assume their way through this or that claim.

In evolutionary theory, every branch -- as well as the trunk and the underlying root system -- of the tree of life is held together via assumptions. One cannot conceptually move from a prebiotic root system to the trunk of the evolutionary tree of life without making a huge number of assumptions, nor can a person theoretically move from that trunk to a given branch, nor can an individual hermeneutically move from one evolutionary branch to another branch without assuming that changes – considered to be largely random in nature (either via a series of just-so mutations or the vagaries of genetic drift) – come about in such a way that the dynamics of those changes cannot actually be observed but must be assumed to have occurred in the way they were claimed to have occurred.

| Explorations |

The Evolution of Human Beings

As recently as the late 1990s – less than 20 years ago – the mainstream evolutionary account concerning the emergence of human beings ran somewhat along the following lines. At some point prior to 4.4 million years ago, the initial member of the life forms that are referred to as hominins branched off from various kinds of primates, and, then, approximately a little over two million years later, the genus, Homo, arrived on the scene.

Hominins refers to a group of species and genera that are considered to be more closely related to human beings than they are to chimpanzees and bonobos (sometimes referred to as pygmy chimpanzees). The basis of this relationship of closeness involves, among other features, varying degrees of: Exhibiting an upright posture; being bipedal, and having a larger brain relative to chimpanzees and bonobos.

In addition, the hip/pelvis region of hominins was much shorter and more bowl-shaped than that of apes ... a feature that helped stabilize bipedal movement as well as assisted hominins to stand in an upright position. There were also various characteristics involving leg length and the type of bones in the feet that tended to differentiate (to a degree) various members the hominins from chimpanzees and bonobos.

The hominins encompass a variety of genera with which Homo sapiens, along with a number of other human-like species (very broadly construed), have been grouped for purposes of comparison, and those genera include: Homo, Australopithecus, Paranthropus, Ardipithecus, and Kenyanthropus. Currently, the Homo genus classification consists of at least eight species: Homo habilis; Homo rudolfensis; African Homo erectus (also known as Homo ergaster); Homo erectus (from Asia); Homo neanderthalensis; Homo floresiensis; Homo heidelbergensis, and Homo sapiens.

Between, on the one hand, the advent of the first hominin more than 4.4 million years ago and, on the other hand, the rise of the genus Homo several million years later, there were additional hominin species that appeared on the scene -- including at least six species of Australopithecus, two species of Paranthropus, and several editions of

Ardipithicus. What any of these life forms have to do with one another is uncertain and the subject of a great deal of debate.

The, now famous, "Lucy" (discovered in Ethiopia in 1974) is a member of the species Australopithecus afarensis. Her species stumbled onto the evolutionary scene roughly 3.2 million years ago and survived for about 900,000 years before becoming extinct.

A hundred thousand, or so, years later – somewhere around the three million year mark -- the Paranthropus group of hominins begins to show up. One or another species from this group managed to survive for a little less than several million years before disappearing.

Several hundred thousand years later, roughly around the two million year mark, the earliest versions of the Homo genus begin to arise. Of the eight editions of the Homo genus that we know about, only one species – Homo sapiens – still survives.

According to the late 1990's, mainstream version of events, hominins did not begin to leave the African continent until about 1 million years ago. These hominins migrated into various areas of the world and began to give rise to a variety of species in the Homo genus.

For example, according to the 1990s version of human evolution, Homo neanderthalensis became established in Eurasia and appeared to flourish for several hundred thousand years. Eventually, that species became extinct when – from the perspective of the predominant view of the late 1990s – that species was completely supplanted some 28,000 to 30,000 years ago (possibly through combat, competition, or both) by the smarter, tool-making, symbol-manipulating Homo sapiens.

A variety of evidence uncovered during the last 20 years has changed the foregoing picture substantially. For example, fossil research from Dmanisi, in the Republic of Georgia, suggests that hominins might have left Africa (around 1.78 million years ago) nearly three-quarters of a million years earlier than the roughly one million years ago that was believed to have been the case in the late 1990s, and, in addition, that migration might have been accomplished completely independently of the Homo genus that, previously, had been thought to have begun the African exodus.

Moreover, additional research conducted on the Indonesian island of Flores could push the aforementioned exit of hominins back even further than the evidence discovered in Dmanisi, Georgia. Moreover, the small brain and body of the species Homo floresiensis found on Flores suggest that this organism might have descended from an earlier species of Australopithecus or something similar to the Australopithecus.

In addition, the Flores data indicates there were versions of the genus Homo that had survived at least another 13,000-15,000 years beyond the period 28,000 to 30,000 years ago when Homo sapiens supposedly replaced Homo neanderthalensis. In other words, dating-data indicate that there are hominin fossils from the island of Flores that place Homo floresiensis in that locality as late as 17,000 years ago ... 13,000 to 15,000 years after Homo neanderthalensis allegedly became extinct.

Another pocket of data, based on fossils found in the Djurab Desert, indicates that hominins might have first arisen in the vicinity of Chad rather than in East Africa. In addition, the Djurab evidence suggests that the first hominins might have appeared some two million years earlier than previously thought ... pushing back the origins of hominins to approximately seven million years ago.

Furthermore, relatively newly discovered evidence in Malapa, South Africa by Lee Berger – a paleoanthropologist at the University of Witwatersrand in Johannesburg, South Africa -- is changing perceptions about where the Homo genus actually might have begun. Such research raises the possibility that the Homo genus could have first emerged in the south of Africa rather than in eastern Africa as earlier believed.

As well, views about the species Homo neanderthalensis and its relationship with Homo sapiens also have undergone a substantial transformation over the last 20 years of research. For example, evidence has been discovered indicating that Neanderthals seemed to have had some ability to make tools, and the members of this species also appeared to exhibit a capacity for some degree of symbol-based traditions that were reflected in the systems of jewelry, feathers, and paint that adorned their bodies.

Moreover, whereas in the late 1990s experts believed Homo neanderthalensis and Homo sapiens did not interbreed, nevertheless, more recent analysis of DNA samples indicates otherwise. Collectively speaking, anywhere from 3 to 20% of Homo neanderthalensis genes might have been passed on to various populations within the genus of Homo sapiens ... including some genes that might have helped confer a certain amount of enhanced immunity.

Current evidence also indicates – at least to some individuals – that the history of hominins does not necessarily tell a story in which one species or genus replaces another in some sort of linear fashion. Rather, the evidence suggests that a number of different hominin groups might have overlapped somewhat and, in the process, interacted with one another to an unknown degree, and if this is the case, then, sorting out which – if any – particular group begat another becomes a much more difficult task.

For example, the earlier picture of human evolution maintained that Australopithecus – which began to show up in fossil remains found in southern Africa during the 1920s – was supplanted, eventually, by the taller, larger-brained species Homo erectus that showed up in Asia (Java and China) and that eventually – supposedly -- evolved into Homo neanderthalensis, followed by Homo sapiens. Thus, at a certain juncture in mainstream evolutionary thinking, Australopithecus, Homo erectus, and Homo neanderthalensis were all considered to be part of the direct lineage leading to Homo sapiens.

The discovery of fossils by Louis and Mary Leakey in Olduvai Gorge in Tanzania, East Africa initiated a process of re-thinking the evolution of hominins. Part of this re-conceptualizing of hominin history was rooted in an ability to date the geological strata in which fossils were found through independent means (e.g., magnetic and volcanic data) that permitted researchers to establish roughly accurate starting and ending points concerning the rise and fall of various hominin species.

Moreover, an array of newly discovered evidence indicated that hominins did not necessarily form a sequence of organisms – with one kind of hominin life form succeeding from a previous species of hominin -- but, instead, different kinds of hominin sometimes overlapped with one another. For instance, data indicated that two different genera -- Homo habilis and Paranthropus boisei – contemporaneously inhabited the same region of East Africa for thousands of years.

Whether, or not, the two foregoing genera were directly ancestral to Homo sapiens is uncertain. Whether, or not, the two aforementioned genera engaged in some degree of interbreeding similar to what occurred with Homo neanderthalensis and Homo sapiens is also unclear.

Since the findings of Mary and Louis Leakey began to move thinking about the evolutionary history of hominins in different directions, a variety of evidence has arisen indicating that as many as – possibly -- six species of the Homo genus were extant at various times during the last one hundred thousand years. To what extent any of those species interacted or interbred with one another is unknown, and, as a result, we are faced with the possibility that there might have been a multiplicity of lineages underlying the Homo genus.

Consequently, the question of who was related to whom -- if at all -- and in what way -- if at all -- makes reconstructing the history of hominins much more difficult. Evolutionary connections – or possible connections – no longer seem to be as straightforward and linear as once appeared to be the case.

Some of the foregoing issues might be better addressed as new hominin fossils are uncovered. However, relatively speaking, hominin fossils have been difficult to unearth (and, this is also the case in conjunction with chimpanzees and various other African apes ... all of whom have a relatively impoverished fossil record).

Nevertheless, many paleontologists find comfort in the fact that only about 3% of the land area that is encompassed by Africa has been scoured for, among other things, hominin fossils. Many researchers believe a much larger sample of land mass will have to be explored before anyone can claim that the fossils which have been found can be said to constitute a fairly representative sample of evidence as far as the evolutionary history of hominins is concerned.

When one throws in the findings from the islands of Flores and Java in Indonesia, along with the fossils discovered in Zhoukoudian, China, together with the newly discovered treasure trove of fossils associated with Malapa, South Africa, one realizes that there could be a great many more pieces of the puzzle involving human evolution in particular, as well as hominin evolution in general, that are out there somewhere, waiting to be found. However, whether, or not, such pieces of the puzzle will be found or actually are out there waiting to be found is, at this time, unknown.

In the meantime, there are a number of questions that should be raised. For example, the species Homo floresiensis that was found on the island of Flores in Indonesia and survived until approximately 17,000 years ago was small-brained and, possibly, linked to some Lucy-like exemplar from one, or another, of the various Australopithecus genera found in East Africa, and, therefore, one might ask: What did either Homo floresiensis or some progenitor form of Australopithecus have to do with Homo sapiens?

How did Homo floresiensis get to the island of Flores? Where did they come from? Who were their direct ancestors?

Even if one were to uncover fossil evidence that provided a much more robust evidential lineage that linked some form of Australopithecus to the rise of Homo floresiensis, what implications – if any -- would this have for the origins of Homo sapiens? For example, how was the transition made from the small brain of Homo floresiensis to the much larger brain of Homo sapiens, and why should one be forced to suppose that Homo floresiensis and Homo sapiens have any common connection whatsoever?

We do not know where Homo floresiensis came from. Although the possibility exists that this species might have had some evolutionary connection (still unproven) with a small-brained ape-man or ape woman, Australopithecus, found in East Africa, the origin of Homo floresiensis is an on-going mystery.

The reasons why Homo floresiensis is classified as a hominin are, in general, fairly clear. It possesses a variety of anatomical characteristics (such as being bipedal and having a capacity to stand upright, as well as a few other features) that seem to place it in closer evolutionary proximity to different hominins (including Homo sapiens) than to either chimpanzees or bonobos.

| Explorations |

However, why consider Homo floresiensis to be part of the human family? Even if this species is linked to a form of Australopithecus in East Africa that suggests hominins might have exited Africa more than two million years ago, what, if anything, does this have to do with the evolution of Homo sapiens?

One could raise similar questions in conjunction with the seven million year old fossils found in the Djurab Desert in Chad. Those fossils might be hominin in nature, but what is there about that discovery that demonstrates they are direct, or even indirect, relations of Homo sapiens?

The discoveries in the Djurab Desert might be able to push back the history of <u>hominins</u> several million years. However, why automatically assume that those fossils also push back <u>human</u> evolution several million years as well?

Unless one can demonstrate determinate evolutionary links between the Djurab fossils and Homo sapiens, one really has no basis for claiming that the former fossils require researchers to extend the evolutionary history of Homo sapiens by several million years. The general category of hominins is one thing, and the particular category of Homo sapiens might be quite another thing.

Something is considered a hominin because of how that life form relates more closely – across an array of anatomical characteristics – to human beings than such organisms relate to chimpanzees and bonobos. To say that something is hominin does not necessarily render it human in some sense despite the presence of whatever anatomical similarities it might share with human beings.

For instance, Homo neanderthalensis and Homo sapiens interbred. Nonetheless, ancestral origins of both Homo neanderthalensis and Homo sapiens are something of a mystery.

Both of those species might have arisen from Homo erectus (aka Homo ergaster) that first appeared – as far as current fossil evidence indicates – between 1.9 and 1.6 million years ago. On the other hand, the newly uncovered fossils from Malapa, South Africa might, or might not, indicate there was some alternative ancestral path to either Homo neanderthalensis, or Homo sapiens, or both.

However, what, if anything, do the foregoing possibilities have to do with hominins in general? Did Homo erectus descend from some form of Australopithecus or Paranthropus or Ardipithecus? Did the Malapa, South African life forms descend from Australopithecus or Paranthropus or Ardipithecus, and, if not, from what did they descend?

Currently, we don't know the answer to any of the foregoing questions. Consequently, it seems premature to conflate the history of hominins with the possible history of Homo erectus, and/or Homo neanderthalensis, and/or Homo sapiens.

Approximately 2.9 to 2.4 million years ago – roughly around the time when the Lucy line of Australopithecus became extinct – two new life forms (both quite different from Lucy's Australopithecus family) showed up in the fossil record. One of those life forms belonged to the Homo genus, while the other life form belonged to the genus Paranthropus.

The genus Paranthropus is a member of the hominin group. However, it does not appear to be part of the ancestral tree of Homo sapiens ... again underlining the fact that not all members of the hominin group are necessarily human in some essential or fundamental sense of the term -- despite the presence of characteristics that incline researchers to consider them to be closer, in a certain sense, to human beings than to chimpanzees and bonobos.

The other member of the hominin group that appeared on the scene about the same time as the Paranthropus genus is considered to be the very first exemplar of the Homo genus. The general body form of that life form possessed certain features that, to a limited degree, are somewhat reminiscent of Homo sapiens.

In addition, this alleged ancestor of Homo sapiens also had a much larger brain than anything that preceded it and was capable of making various kinds of very simple tools. Nonetheless, the brain-size of this species was much smaller than that of Homo sapiens or even the species Homo erectus that appeared roughly a million years later after the aforementioned founding member of the Homo genus appeared on the scene.

Between 1.9 and 1.6 million years ago, Homo erectus (aka Homo ergaster) arose. The body features of this species were virtually indistinguishable from Homo sapiens, and, as indicated in the last paragraph, the brain-size of Homo erectus was larger than the life form that arose approximately a million years earlier and that is thought to have gotten the Homo genus its start.

Did the first exemplar of the Homo genus descend from some edition of the Australopithecus genus that became extinct around that time? We don't know.

Did Homo erectus descend from the foregoing, groundbreaking form of Homo genus? We don't know?

Did either Homo neanderthalensis or Homo sapiens descend from Homo erectus? We don't know.

Home erectus is believed to have migrated out of Africa and, eventually, populated various parts of Asia and Europe. Did Homo neanderthalensis interbreed with Homo erectus – much as Homo sapiens interbred with Homo neanderthalensis – but, nonetheless, was a separate species that had arisen in some way independent of Homo erectus -- as also might have been the case in relation to Homo neanderthalensis and Homo sapiens?

How did the larger brain-size (relative to, say, Australopithecus) of the first member of the Homo genus arise? How did the still larger brain-size of Homo erectus emerge during the million years that separated those first two members of the Homo genus?

We don't know the answer to either of the foregoing questions. Consequently, the genus Australopithecus might not have anything to do with the origins of the Homo genus, even though Australopithecus is considered to be a member of the hominin group.

In addition, there is little, or no, evidence indicating that the genus Paranthropus has anything to do with the origins of the Homo genus, and, yet, Paranthropus is considered to be a member of the hominin group. Moreover, the genus Ardipithecus seems even less likely (due to its even more ancient pedigree) to have anything to do with the origins of the Homo genus (although it might have some evolutionary connection to Australopithecus), and, yet, Ardipithecus is considered to be a part of the hominin group ... although, to be sure, this issue is not without its share of controversy.

For example, in 2009 a 4.4 million year old, fairly intact skeleton was discovered in the Afar region of Ethiopia by a group of researchers led by Tim White. The remains were designated as the species ramidus in the genus Ardipithecus and were given the nickname, Ardi.

Ardi was a mixed mosaic of physical characteristics. More specifically, Ardipithecus ramidus exhibited anatomical features that were conducive to both traveling through the trees (e.g., long, curved fingers; a divergent big toe; relatively flat feet), as well as features that would have aided bipedal movement (e.g., the backward flexibility of minor toes, along with a certain degree of stiffness in the foot).

In short, Ardi suggested that the presence of anatomical features that might have facilitated climbing and arboreal locomotion didn't necessarily preclude the possibility of the simultaneous presence of other anatomical features that might have been conducive to some degree of upright posture and bipedal movement. A life form could be considered to be hominin even though there were some ape-like anatomical features that were present.

Again however, while the foregoing considerations indicate there might be compelling reasons for extending the definition of what constitutes a hominin, nonetheless, such an extended way of characterizing hominins might have little, or nothing, to do with determining the origin(s) of human beings. This is especially the case if evidence cannot be found – and none has been discovered to date due to a relative lack of fossil evidence -- which demonstrates that Ardipithecus ramidus is some sort of direct (if distant) antecessor to human beings.

Does Ardipithecus ramidus have anything to do with the rise of Australopithecus anamensis, which, in turn, might have possible progenitor links with Australopithecus afarensis (Lucy)? We don't know, but even if it did, the jump from Australopithecus afarensis to the Homo genus is a fairly big one (and the difference in brain size forms only one part of the explanatory chasm existing between the two genera).

As pointed out earlier in this section, some researchers believe that Homo floresiensis might have had some sort of connection with Australopithecus afarensis (Lucy). Nonetheless, even if one were to assume such an unspecified connection, there is little, or no, evidence

| Explorations |

297

to indicate that Homo floresiensis had any direct connection with the rise of Homo sapiens.

Three years after Ardi was discovered, another set of fossil remains was unearthed ... also in the Afar region of Ethiopia. The remains were found in 2012 at a site called Burtele – approximately 48 kilometers from where Ardi was discovered -- and consisted of eight small bones that belonged to a foot and, perhaps not surprisingly, was referred to as the Burtele species.

The Burtele foot has been dated as being contemporaneous with Lucy, but that foot is also quite different and more anatomically archaic than anything found in Australopithecus afarensis. While the big toe of the Burtele foot appears to indicate that the species to which the foot belongs is a hominin of some kind, nonetheless, there are other features of the Burtele foot that are more reminiscent of Ardi than Lucy ... that is, there are features associated with the Burtele foot that seem to be consistent with some degree of arboreal locomotion as well as with a degree of bipedal motion.

Did the species to which the Burtele foot belongs arise from Ardipithecus ramidus? We don't know, but even if there is a connection, of some kind, between Ardipithecus ramidus and the Burtele foot species, we don't know what, if anything, any of this has to do with the origin (s) of Homo sapiens.

The foregoing issues are rendered even more complex when one takes the idea of homoplasy into consideration. Homoplasy refers to situations in which different species acquire similar characteristics independently of one another.

More specifically, two species, separated by several million years, might each be associated with a certain amount of evidence indicating that they both possessed some degree of capacity with respect to being bipedal. Nonetheless, one cannot automatically conclude that the two species are evolutionarily linked together because both species might have acquired the capacity to be bipedal independently of each other.

Notwithstanding the foregoing considerations, the last common ancestor between hominins and chimpanzees is estimated to have existed between six and ten million years ago. Moreover, that last "common ancestor" is likely to be situated in the context of a population rather than as a function of a single individual.

A population would permit an array of the "right" combination of hominid genes to align themselves in a subset of that last common ancestor population. This subset of the common ancestor population could branch off subsequently from the rest of the larger population.

Even if one assumes that all of the foregoing is true, none of those "givens" establishes what the nature of that last common ancestor population might have looked like, or, even more importantly, how the genes necessary for hominin-like characteristics arose in that population and came to be aligned in some sub-set of that common ancestor population. Furthermore, even if one were able to establish what the nature of the last common ancestor population might have looked like – at least in general terms – this only gets us as far as the rather amorphous collective referred to as hominins.

The origins of: Homo sapiens, Homo erectus (Asian not African), Homo floresiensis, Homo neanderthalensis, and Homo Heidelbergensis continue to be shrouded in mystery. The relationships of various members of the Homo genus with one another also are largely shrouded in mystery.

Among some researchers, there is speculation that Homo heidelbergensis might be the predecessor of either Homo neanderthalensis, or Homo sapiens, or both. In turn, Homo heidelbergensis – again, rather speculatively – has been linked with some, unknown antecessor of the Homo genus, and the foregoing unknown antecessor of Homo heidelbergensis is conjectured to have arisen from some unknown member of Homo ergaster (African) or Homo erectus (Asian).

The foregoing family tree might turn out be correct. At the moment, however, the possible family tree is constructed from little more than assumptions, speculations, and conjectures.

Researchers maintain that the members of the hominin group are all more closely related to human beings than those members are related to chimpanzees and bonobos. However, beyond this, we really don't know, or understand, very much.

| Explorations |

All humans are members of the hominin group. Nonetheless, not all members of the hominin group are necessarily human in any essential way.

Contrary to what some researchers are suggesting, the origin of Homo sapiens might not date back from six to ten million years. Furthermore, those life forms that are hominin and which do date back from six to ten million years might have little, or nothing, to do with the origins of Homo sapiens.

To claim, as some evolutionary biologists do, that human evolution covers a period of, at least, from six to ten million years seems to be -- potentially at least – somewhat misleading. Such a claim assumes that being human – rather than being hominin-like – began from six to ten million years ago, and, yet, there is no proof that this is the case.

There is no concrete, detailed explanation for how different members of the hominin group acquired the similarities that make them more similar to human beings than it makes them similar to chimpanzees and bonobos. Furthermore, there is no concrete, detailed explanation for how or when different members of the hominin group branched off from one another ... if they actually did branch off from one another.

Homo floresiensis has a brain size that is much smaller than most other members of the Homo genus. However, that species has enough of the right sort of other physical characteristics that permit it to be classified as a member of the Homo genus.

The brain size of Homo floresiensis suggests that it might have evolved from some form of Australopithecus. Nonetheless, two different genera are being linked here, and, therefore, one has to provide an account of how Homo floresiensis acquired all of the properties that make it a member of the Homo genus rather than some kind of Australopithecus.

Moreover, to say that floresiensis belongs to the Homo genus doesn't necessarily make that species human in some sense. In fact, one is confronted with the question of what exactly does it mean to be human.

| Explorations |

In terms of gross, physical properties, there are a number of features that differentiate human beings from other members of the hominin group. Among those properties one finds the following characteristics: short toes; arched feet; strong knee joints; enlarged femur head; short, broad pelvis, long, flexible waist; barrel-shaped rib cage; low shoulders; twisted humerus; strong wrist; long, opposable thumb; forwardly placed opening for spinal cord; chin; small canine teeth; and a large brain.

According to the theory of human evolution, the foregoing characteristics did not arise all at once like Athena allegedly arose fully formed from the head of Zeus. Those features were supposedly acquired at different points in evolutionary history.

For instance, seven million years ago, small canine teeth and the forwardly placed opening for the spinal cord arrived on the scene. Roughly 3 million years later (at the 4.1 million year mark), strong knee joints were acquired. Around 3.7 million years ago, short toes and arched feet came into being. Approximately 3.2 million years ago, the long thumb and short, broad pelvis showed up. Two million years ago, the twisted humerus and low shoulders appeared on the scene. A hundred thousand years later – 1.9 million years ago – long legs, enlarged femur heads, and a long, flexible waist arrived. 1.6 million years ago, the barrel-shaped rib cage arose. Several hundred thousand years later, strong wrists were acquired. Approximately one million years ago, a large brain emerged, and 800,000 years later, the modern chin evolved into place.

How any of the foregoing features came into being is unknown. How all of the aforementioned features collectively found their way into Homo sapiens is unknown.

| Explorations |

The story of human evolution – along with the story of evolution in general -- might be somewhat like the phi phenomenon in psychology. In this perceptual illusion a sequence of flashing lights is perceived as forming one continuous motion. In point of fact, the illusion consists of a series of separate events that are interpreted to give expression to continuity.

In the phi phenomenon a given flashing light is not what causes a subsequent bulb to flash. Moreover, the sequence of flashing lights is not set in motion by, or caused by, the first light that goes off during the sequence.

Each instance of a light flashing is a separate event that occurs within the context of a timed sequence in which only one light at a time is flashing. Nonetheless, the sequence and timing of a series of such separate events appears to create the illusion of continuous motion.

This is the same sort of phenomenon that is at the heart of motion pictures. When a sequence of static images of a certain kind is flipped at, or run with, sufficient speed, an observer experiences a sense of continuous motion or action, when, in reality no such action is present in any single image ... there is only a series of static images.

Similarly, in evolution, one encounters an illusion that is created by a sequence of images (the moment to moment dynamics of a population) that supposedly appear to give rise to subsequent species. However, with the exception of potentially limited cases such as Darwin's finches (touched upon in an earlier section of this chapter), there is nothing that evolutionary theory can point to in the way of hard evidence (as opposed to conjectures) that is able to demonstrate how the trunk and branches of the tree of life were all produced through the process of speciation ... and not just some of those branches involving cases similar to Darwin's finches that emerge in the context of the principles of population biology.

Assumptions are made – e.g., random mutations, and/or genetic drift, and/or punctuated equilibrium, and/or speciation – that, allegedly, connect a given species with subsequent ones. Nevertheless, the point when the transition is made from one species to another via natural processes is rather ill defined and seems more like an illusion

| Explorations |

created by a series of discrete events than it has been demonstrated to constitute a process of continuity.

Evolutionary arguments – including the ones involving human evolution -- seem to be somewhat like a film maker trying to claim that static images or individual frames are actually connected to one another in some sort of <u>causal</u> manner, and, therefore, those images or frames are not really static and independent from one another but are linked in some mysterious fashion as a dynamic function of the images themselves. Of course, the static images of the filming process are connected together because that process permits one image after another to be collected, stored, and run but the connection among those frames, relative to one another (rather than as a function of the filming process), is sequential not causal.

Moreover, in a film, there are people – such as the editor, director, and producer – who help shape the sequence in which individual frames are spliced together in order to give the impression that a certain set of actions has taken place. However, in evolution, whatever takes place through processes of genetic drift, mutation, punctuated equilibrium, and speciation are considered to be entirely independent of what occurred before, or what happened after, those sorts of 'evolutionary' events.

Natural selection plays the role of editor, director and producer. Nevertheless, natural selection is not interested in generating one kind of action sequence rather than some other kind of action sequence.

More specifically, natural selection doesn't worry about whether, or not, a given set of physical, chemical, geological, hydrological, and atmospheric factors will interact in such a way at a given point in time and space that those factors are capable of enabling a given life form or metabolic pathway or biomolecule to be able to survive rather than becoming extinct. In short, the forces of natural selection are described as operating quite independently of whether they are conducive to the creation, continuation, or extinction of some given precursor to life or some given form of life.

Consequently, events that are allegedly of an evolutionary nature might actually be static images that are entirely independent from one another. Yet, advocates of evolution seem to want to insist there is a connection among those static images that is caused by genetic drift, mutations, punctuated equilibrium, and/or speciation and, therefore, evolution constitutes a process of continuity rather than discontinuity with respect to the transition of one species to another ... but this might be an illusion of perceptual understanding rather than the actual nature of reality.

One can grasp how a filming and editing process can result in a sequence of film that gives expression to a continuous story that makes sense. Nonetheless, one has more difficulty grasping how the process of natural selection can result in a sequence of living events that gives expression to a continuous story that makes functional sense.

In the filming/editing process the presence of human intention on the part of the editor/director/producer, together with the intelligence of the observer, is responsible for the sense of order that is contained in the sequence of images. In natural selection there is no intention or intelligence that is present, and, consequently, one has a bit more difficulty trying to figure out how the interaction between, on the one hand, the forces of natural selection and, on the other hand, the random, independent events of genetic drift and/or mutation are responsible for the sense of order that emerges again and again across species – from the beginning of life until the present time.

To be sure, one is able to understand how the forces of natural selection that are present at a given point in time and space might act on a chemical/physical system and, in the process, permit that system to continue on because there is a set of compatibilities between the properties of that system and the characteristics of the forces of natural selection that are engaging those properties. Nevertheless, one has a harder time understanding how random, independent events are capable of continuously providing just the right sort of features to feed into the dynamics of the forces of natural selection so that life is able to arise and, then, radiate out in a diverse array of functional forms for some 3-4 billion years.

At heart, evolutionary theory appears to be something of an illusion. Not only do the dynamics of speciation seem, as previously outlined, to be engulfed in a phi-like phenomenon, but, as well, the manner in which allegedly random events generate the functional order that makes any given species – including humans -- capable of adapting to prevailing conditions of natural selection also seem illusory in nature as well.

| Explorations |

Some Evolutionary Roots of Psychology

Not too long ago I watched a TED talk (TED is an acronym for 'Technology, Entertainment, and Design') by Alison Gopnik. Dr. Gopnik has done some very interesting research in conjunction with learning and development -- research that makes her an important part of the trend in psychological sciences over the last 10-15 years that has altered the way in which many people (both professional and lay people) think about some of what goes on in the mind of young children (say, 1-4 years of age).

In a variety of ways, infants and young children are much more sophisticated explorers of their universe than many people give them credit for. Indeed, in some ways, young children might be better and more open explorers than adults are.

Unfortunately, all too many adults are socialized out of realizing some of their inherent potential for learning and development via the very process of schooling that many people assume is how human beings maximize their capacities for learning about the world. There are many ways in which schooling interferes with and undermines the process of learning as children are induced – through techniques of undue influence -- to accept an educational institution's view of some given issue ... such as the theory of evolution.

With the foregoing considerations in mind, several points seem worth mentioning in conjunction with Dr. Gopnik's TED presentation. To begin with, she seeks to place her work in an evolutionary context that, in and of itself, is unremarkable since many researchers in psychology do the same sort of thing these days.

Nevertheless, at certain points during her talk, Dr. Gopnik refers to neurochemistry, neurotransmitters, and so on, as if the mere use of that sort of terminology fully explains what is going on in the brain or how the brain and mind are connected, when, in point of fact -- as is also the case in relation to evolutionary theory -- no one has shown in a rigorously empirical manner how either neurochemistry or neurotransmitters came into existence or how they are able to generate: consciousness, thinking, reasoning, logic, memory, creativity, understanding, and so on.

| Explorations |

To be sure, various aspects of neurochemistry are correlated with mental functioning. However, correlation is not causation, and until the precise causal steps are nailed down, then, reducing mind to brain constitutes a bit of myth making, not science.

A second point concerning Dr. Gopnik's presentation involves the work of Thomas Bayes. Bayes was an eighteenth-century mathematician who invented a form of statistical thinking that is capable of leading to improved descriptions of a system based on a computational technique that incorporates new data into one's calculations ... calculations that are able to improve, to a certain extent, upon some initial probability model with which one began in relation to the system or situation being explored by an individual.

Dr. Gopnik suggests that young children are capable of running Bayesian-like computations in order to work out which hypothesis concerning an aspect of reality is more likely to be true based on their experiential interaction with such an aspect of reality ... something that even adults might have difficulty working out -- at least this would be the case if adults were required to use and apply the mathematical properties of Bayes' theorem to arrive at an answer.

However, one might respectfully suggest that although on the surface there might be certain parallels between Bayesian probability methods and the manner in which children try to work their way through various possible solutions to a problem, it does not follow that children are engaged in some sort of Bayesian computation ... anymore than an outfielder in baseball necessarily uses calculus to track down a fly ball. Yes, there is a process of reasoning and logical analysis taking place in the mind of the child, but this does not necessarily mean that Bayesian mathematical methods are being employed ... although one is entitled to say there is, at the very least, an analogical relationship between what children are capable of doing and Bayesian statistical techniques.

In fact, one might speculate that Bayes original idea was a specific, concrete, creative application of the sort of mental capacity to which Dr. Gopnik refers in her presentation as being present in children. In other words, it is our inherent capacity to learn from experience and, in the process, update our understanding of such experience that might have served as the inspiration for Thomas Bayes theorem and that reflected some of what had been taking place in his mind when he went from an initial understanding of something, and, then transitioned to an improved version of that idea through the incorporation of new experiences by means of a mathematical model.

In short, Bayes might have worked out a formal, mathematical model that captured, in a limited way, certain facets of the aforementioned more general capacity to be able to learn from experience by incorporating what we learn into our previous understanding. As such, Bayes theorem is an analog for a cognitive process that takes place in human beings – including children – but those cognitive processes transcend Bayes theorem even though that theorem does reflect certain aspects of what occurs during the process of seeking to understand some given phenomenon or dimension of experience.

Even if one were inclined to accept Dr. Gopnik's idea that children operate in accordance with Bayesian probability functions, one is still faced with a considerable conundrum. How did human beings acquire the capacity to think in that manner? What were the specific, evolutionary steps that made that sort of capacity possible?

The idea of evolution appears to be used by Dr. Gopnik as sort of a convenient, but very vague, background, rhetorical prop through which to frame her audience's understanding with respect to how things might have come to be the way they are. Supposedly -- or, so the evolutionary story goes -- we got to our present level of cognitive ability through evolution, and, yet, no one -- including Dr. Gopnik -- ever provides a detailed account of how those kinds of capacities actually came into being.

Everything is run through the presumptive lenses of evolutionary interpolation and extrapolation. In the process of framing things in the foregoing manner, understanding becomes steeped in mythological-like elements.

I do not say the foregoing as someone who seeks to advance either a Creationist position or some sort 'intelligent design' notion. Instead, I say what I do as a hardnosed empirical skeptic who, like Cuba Gooding in the movie: 'Jerry Maguire' is saying: "Show me the money."

| Explorations |

If one cannot produce the blow-by-blow empirical account of how things came to be the way they are (and the pages of this chapter suggest that the proponents of evolution cannot accomplish this in any credible fashion), then one is not talking about science. Rather, one is dabbling in philosophy while seeking to leverage the halo-like effect of the term: "science'.

Evolutionary theory might guide much of modern thinking in a variety of areas – especially in relation to psychology. Unfortunately, a great deal of that thinking is rooted in the sort of speculative philosophy and assumptions that cannot be proven and, consequently, is not rooted in real science ... even as evolutionary theory seeks to clothe itself in scientific jargon in order to give the impression of being scientific without having to meet the standards of actual substantive rigor.

Many people, of course, might respond to the foregoing by saying words to the effect: 'Well, of course, everyone admits there are many lacunae in evolutionary research, but it is the best available scientific theory to account for a wide array of phenomena ... indeed, if one rejects evolutionary theory, then with what do you propose to replace it?"

The foregoing is like a prosecutor saying: "Well there is very little actual, concrete evidence indicating that the person we have in custody is responsible for the crime with which he is being charged - although there is considerable circumstantial evidence and, as well, there are many expert witnesses who are willing to testify, according to their biases, that the right individual is in custody) -- but, gee, since there is no other viable suspect, why don't we just go along with the idea that the guy we have in custody is guilty ... after all, do you have anyone who would serve as a better suspect?"

A person doesn't have to offer up an alternative theory that explains things better than evolution does. One only has to understand that the available evidence does not support or justify holding on to the suspect of evolution simply because that suspect is the only entity our state of ignorance and limited imagination can conjure up to account for the action in question.

Unlike my evolutionist friends, I am not afraid to say that I do not know what the truth of the matter is. Notwithstanding such an acknowledgement, nevertheless, when one looks carefully at various accounts concerning the origins of life, or even the origins of novel, biological capabilities, existing evolutionary accounts leave one deeply dissatisfied. There is almost no intellectual rigor (despite the presence of scientific sounding jargon) present in those arguments, and I see no reason why I, or anyone, should adopt a theory that is so steeped in a cloud of unknowing and, yet, simultaneously, assume that evolutionary theory constitutes good science ... because this is just not the case.

Talking with many individuals who are advocates of the theory of evolution is like interacting with a bunch of K-street, Washington lobbyists who yammer away trying to induce people to support their grandiose, but rather empirically shaky and self-serving ideas. Being convinced of the truth of something is not necessarily the same thing as being correct concerning that to which one is so passionately attached.

Unfortunately, if one should express some sort of resistance to the marketing campaign of the evolutionists (as I am doing now), then look out, for the proverbial stuff is likely to hit the fan. Labels and epithets often soon follow -- such as: 'That person is anti-science'; or, 'that individual is a 'luddite''; or, 'such people are standing in the way of intellectual progress', or 'that person is hopelessly irrational' -- when all one is doing is pointing out (concretely and not theoretically) that there is a wealth of empirical and conceptual problems that beset the theory of evolution across an array of issues -- starting with the 'origin of life' matter, and extending into such topics as: the origins of consciousness, reason, logic, memory, creativity, morality, cognitive development, and so on.

| Explorations |

Evolution's Black Box

In engineering and science, a black box is at the epicenter of an unknown set of processes. One can talk about what arises out of those processes as an output, and one can talk about what some of the inputs might have been that are fed into that box and, to varying degrees, might have helped shape what transpires within that box, but the actual character of the dynamics of the black box that makes such outputs possible is a mystery.

At the heart of evolutionary theory are a series of black boxes. For example, consider the DNA code.

In 1953 James Watson and Francis Crick worked out the general, double helical structure of the DNA molecule. Within the context of that helix, they knew guanine and cytosine paired off with one another to form some rungs in the helix, and, as well, they knew that adenosine and thymine linked up together to form other rungs in the double helix.

In their April 25 letter to *Nature* magazine -- which introduced their discovery to the world -- they also intimated that the aforementioned pairing arrangements might serve as the basis for a copying system in which either of the strands making up the helix could serve as a template for the generation of the other, complementary strand. What the two researchers didn't know at that time was just what any given sequence of bases actually meant, and, in fact, it would take another ten years before an answer, of sorts, could be offered in relation to the meaning of the DNA code.

The term "of sorts" is used in the foregoing paragraph because the answer that took ten years to work out concerned discovering what the sequences meant. That answer, however, had no clue how such a system of coding came into being.

There are two questions swirling about the DNA code. One question concerns the nature of the code, while the other question has to do with how that code came into existence, and scientists largely have been preoccupied with – and only have answered -- the first question.

Let's take a look at the first question noted above. What is the code?

| Explorations |

There are four different bases in DNA. There are 20 amino acids.

How are the two kinds of molecules related? What is the "meaning" of any given base with respect to the generation of amino acids?

A one-to-one correspondence between a base and an amino acid doesn't work. There are too many amino acids, and, therefore, one base pair could call for any one of five, or more, amino acids, and, as a result considerable confusion would enter into the process of translating a given base into the particular amino acid that was needed to help form this or that protein.

If the DNA code consisted of a pair of bases, only 16 amino acids could be formed. In other words, if the code was a base doublet, then any one of four bases could appear in the first position, and, as well, any one of four bases could appear in the second position, for a total of 16 possibilities.

There would appear to be four possibilities too few to form the necessary 20 amino acids, and, as a result, a certain amount of confusion would be present. Such confused understaffing might tend to undermine the precision oriented nature of living organisms.

Eventually, several individuals (Sydney Brenner and Francis Crick) demonstrated that the DNA code – whatever it might turn out to be – had to consist of at least three bases. However, if any of the four bases could occupy any one of the three coding positions, then, this would lead to 64 possibilities (4 x 4 x 4), and this seemed to give more than three times as many possibilities as were needed to code for just 20 amino acids.

Quite a few suggestions were put forth during the next ten years in an attempt to identify the precise nature of the relationship between nucleic bases and amino acids. Eventually, researchers discovered that there appeared to be several levels of coding taking place.

On what might be considered the most outward level of coding, there was a degree of redundancy or degeneracy built into the DNA code. This meant that while some of the three-letter nucleic base words coded for just one amino acid, nonetheless, in another case six different three-letter nucleic base combinations coded for the same amino acid (e.g., leucine), and in still another instance, three, three-

| Explorations |

313

letter nucleic base combination coded for the same amino acid (e.g., isoleucine), or in a number of cases, sets of four three-letter nucleic base combinations coded for the same amino acid (e. g., valine, serine, proline, threonine, alanine, arginine, and glycine)

Moreover, there were three three-letter nucleic base combinations that didn't code for an amino acid. Instead, they represented stop signals.

The foregoing, several paragraphs outline the general structure of the code. In other words, they are part of the description that deals with what the code is.

What has not, yet, been explained is how the code came to be the way it is. For instance, how did a three-letter base combination come to mean "stop", and how did any given three-letter nucleic base combination come to 'mean' one, rather than another, amino acid?

Some researchers were not content with knowing how the code worked. They wanted to understand what processes led to the code assuming the form it did.

During their journey of discovery, they learned that different factors seemed to be associated with each of the three nucleic bases that made up any given three-letter nucleic combination. For instance, consider the first nucleic base letter of any triplet or codon ... some individuals felt it might code for much more than originally had been believed.

More specifically, in a cell, amino acids are synthesized in several different ways, and each of these ways begins with simple, molecular precursors. Research indicated that there seemed to be a relationship between the first nucleic acid base-letter that made up a given triplet (codon) and the identity of the precursor that began the process of synthesizing the amino acid being coded for by that DNA triplet sequence.

For instance, pyruvate – which, among other things, helps get the Krebs cycle started – is a precursor for the synthesis of certain amino acids. Researchers found that all of the amino acids that have pyruvate as a precursor are coded for by a three-letter nucleic acid codon that begins with the nucleic acid base 'T' or thymine.

| Explorations |

The foregoing relationship is very intriguing and interesting. Nonetheless, such a relationship doesn't really solve the underlying puzzle: How did the DNA code come to be the way it is?

In other words, how did the nucleic acid base thymine come to mean that the three-letter codon for which it was the first nucleic acid base-letter would code for one of the amino acids that uses the precursor pyruvate in its synthesis? Why didn't codons starting with thymine code for a precursor that initiated synthesis for a different kind of amino acid?

How did thymine come to "mean" or stand for pyruvate? What was the nature of the dynamic linking a nucleic acid base (consisting of a five carbon sugar, a phosphate group, plus a nitrogenous base) and pyruvate (CH_3COCOO^-)?

At what point in the evolutionary process was it determined that any given amino acids would be represented by this or that nucleic acid triplet and, in addition, determined that the composition of that triplet would begin with a nucleic acid base that specified the identity of the precursor that would initiate the synthesis of the amino acid being coded for by such a triplet? How did this sort of determination come about?

If the origins of life are rooted in black smokers, white smokers, and/or some Stanley Miller kind of scenario, and, as a result an interconnected set of metabolic pathways arose – in a manner that is not currently understood -- that were capable of initiating and sustaining life, then, how did the information contained in such a arrangement get transferred to a sequence of three letter codons? Moreover, how did that information get incorporated into the sequence of codons in a way that not only stipulated which triplet would stand for which amino acid but did so in a way that specified that the first letter of the codon would identify the precursor that was necessary for the synthesis of the amino acid being coded for in the triplet.

The foregoing, mysterious conspiring of events sounds even more preposterous than the idea that Francis Crick (the Noble Prize winning scientist who, along with James Watson, had established the basic helical character of DNA) came up with in an attempt to explain why the DNA code was the way it was. More specifically, Crick put forth an idea that he referred to as: "directed panspermia".

According to Crick, life on earth was the result of a seeding process in which a bacterial life form of extraterrestrial origin had been introduced into the planet Earth at some point in the distant past. Moreover, according to Crick, the seeding process was intentional and conducted by some sort of alien intelligence.

Crick's idea is more of an evasion than it is an explanation. Even if his idea were correct, it still doesn't explain how extraterrestrial bacteria or intelligent, alien life forms came into being.

Crick's conjecture notwithstanding, one is still left with two problems: (1) Accounting for how the DNA coding process acquired its system of linking nucleic acid base triplets with amino acids; (2) accounting for how the DNA coding process acquired its system for linking the first nucleic acid base letter in a given triplet to the identity of the precursor that would help initiate the synthesis of the amino acid being coded for by that triplet.

If the origins of life <u>are not</u> rooted in the prebiotic chemistry of black smokers, white smokers, and/or Stanley Miller-like scenarios, then how does one account for the millions of DNA sequences that would have to arise in order to be able to code for – mean, stand for, represent – different amino acid combinations in the form of peptides or proteins that played central roles in helping to make this or that metabolic pathway possible? In addition how did the DNA coding system acquire the ability to have the first nucleic acid base letter in any triplet code for -- mean, stand for, or represent -- the precursors that are needed to synthesize the amino acid being encoded?

No matter how one would like to proceed with respect to trying to account for the origin of life, one is faced with a deep mystery, puzzle, or problem. On the one hand, an individual can start with various scenarios involving prebiotic chemistry that -- in a way that is not currently understood – came together in a manner that eventually was able to transfer information about metabolic pathways to, or incorporated that information into, a DNA coding system. Or, on the other hand, a person can begin with some sort of scenario in which there is an accumulation of millions of nucleic acid base sequences over millions of years that somehow – in a way that is not currently understood -- came to give expression to a DNA coding system in which certain triplets came to represent specific amino acids, and, as well, those triplets came to give expression to a DNA coding system in which the first nucleic acid base letter in a triplet identified the precursor that was to be used to help initiate the synthesis of the amino acid being encoded by that triplet.

Neither of the foregoing two possibilities is any better equipped to explain or account for the origin of life than is Crick's notion of directed panspermia. None of the foregoing three possibilities constitutes a scientific explanation.

Just as certain research has pointed out the intriguing relationship (whose origins are a complete mystery) between the first nucleic acid base letter of a given triplet and the identity of the precursor that helps to initiate the synthesis of the amino acid being coded for by that triplet, similar research also has indicated that there appears to be a connection between the nature of the second nucleic acid base letter in a given triplet and the degree to which the amino acid being coded for through that triplet is soluble in water. More specifically, researchers have discovered that five out of six of the amino acids that are most insoluble (hydrophobic) in character have 'T', or thymine, as the second nucleic acid base letter for a given triplet, while all of most water soluble (hydrophilic) amino acids are coded for by DNA triplets that have 'A', adenine, as the second nucleic acid base letter in the triplet that is coding for such amino acids.

Once again, the puzzle of origins rears its ugly, inexplicable head. How did the nucleic acid base letter 'A' – adenine – come to code for, mean, or represent an amino acid that has the property of being highly hydrophilic when 'A' is the second nucleic acid base letter in a triplet coding for that amino acid? How did the nucleic acid base letter 'T' – thymine – come to code for, mean, or represent an amino acid that has the property of being highly hydrophobic when the second nucleic acid base letter in a triplet coding for that amino acid is 'T'?

In short, how did a nucleic acid base letter come to determine whether the amino acid being encoded would be hydrophilic or hydrophobic? How did the positioning of a nucleic acid base letter within a triplet come to mean, stand for, or represent the solubility of the amino acid being encoded?

| Explorations |

One also might ask why DNA triplets didn't code for lipids or carbohydrates, instead of coding for amino acids? The short answer, of course, is that this is just the way things are.

Nonetheless, the foregoing short answer doesn't really account for how and why DNA triplets got connected with amino acids rather than lipids or carbohydrates. This is especially the case given that the basic molecules that make up nucleic acids, amino acids, lipids, and carbohydrates are quite different from one another, and, consequently, there is no obvious reason why nucleic acids should be linked to amino acids rather than lipids or carbohydrates ... the arrangements that are in place with respect to the link between nucleic acid base triplets and amino acids seem to be rather arbitrary in character.

The third nucleic acid base letter in a DNA triplet is, to a great degree, fairly degenerate in character. Another way of referring to this state of affairs is to say that the third nucleic acid base letter often tends to be devoid of useful information ... that is it is information free.

For example, consider the amino acid, glycine. A triplet coding for glycine is GGG (guanine times three).

However, the final nucleic acid base letter 'G' in the triple guanine codon could be 'A' – adenine – or 'C' – cytosine – or 'T' – thymine, and each of those triplets would still code for glycine. The identity of the nucleic acid base letter holding down the third position in the DNA triplet doesn't seem to matter.

Yet, the third nucleic acid base letter in a DNA triplet does matter in certain instances. For example, the amino acids tryptophan and methionine are encoded, respectively, by TGG and ATG, but if the final 'G' in either of these triplets is changed to 'T' – thymine – or 'A' – adenine – or 'C' – cytosine – one will not be coding for the same amino acid but, rather, a different amino acid is being encoded or a 'stop' signal is being indicated.

One finds similar triplet specificity when it comes to stop codes. TAA, TAG, and TGA are all stop codons, and, yet, if the character of the nucleic acid base letter occupying the third position in the triplet is altered to some other nucleic acid base letter, one will get an amino acid and not a stop signal.

| Explorations |

There are eleven triplets among the 64 possible DNA combinations of the four nucleic acid bases that are a little less concerned with the identity of the third nucleic acid base letter than, say tryptophan or methionine are, but, nonetheless, those eleven triplets will not permit just any nucleic acid base letter into the third position of the triplet. For example, phenylalanine will permit either 'T' – thymine – or 'C' – cytosine – in the third position of the DNA triplet and either triplet will code for phenylalanine, but if the third position of the triplet is occupied by 'A' – adenine -- or 'G' – guanine – one will get the amino acid, leucine, not phenylalanine.

How did TTT and TTC come to stand for phenylalanine but not leucine? How did TAA, TAG, and TGA come to 'mean' stop rather than some amino acid? How did TGG and ATG come to represent tryptophan and methionine respectively?

How did the third position in a nucleic acid base triplet come to be significant in some instances but not others? How did the third position in a nucleic acid base triplet become semi-important in some cases (for example, phenylalanine, tryptophan, histidine, glutamine, and asparagines – to name a few) but not in other cases (e.g., leucine and glycine)?

Some researchers have proposed that the primordial code was a function of doublets (two nucleic acid base letters), and, at an unknown point during the process of evolution, there was some sort of codon capture dynamic that turned the doublet code into a triplet code. When such a switch-over occurred is not known, nor is it known how such a transition in coding took place, nor is it known how the initial doublet code came into being ... if any of this is the way things actually began.

Natural selection might account for why a given coding system was endorsed due the survival value that was entailed by such a system once it came into existence. Nonetheless, natural selection does not account for how either a doublet code or a triplet code came into existence or how the former (doublet) coding system transitioned later into a triplet coding system – if this is what took place rather than just being a conjecture.

DNA coding is one of many black boxes occupying the heart of evolutionary theory. No one knows how that coding system came into existence. No one knows how nucleic acid base letter triplets came to 'mean' amino acids rather than, say, lipids, or how nucleic acid base letter triplets came to mean one amino acid rather than another. No one knows how certain nucleic acid triplets came to mean 'stop' rather than stand for an amino acid of one kind or another. No one knows how some DNA triplets became very particular about the nucleic acid base letter occupying the third position in a codon while other triplets were less fussy (or not fussy at all) with the nucleic acid base letter that occupied the third position of a codon.

There are all manner of inputs that have been conjectured as – possibly – having helped shape the evolutionary process through which the system of DNA coding might have come to assume its central place among biological systems organisms on Earth. There are all manner of outputs that have been described as having arisen through the coding system of DNA.

Nonetheless, the origin(s) of the DNA coding system are steeped in mystery. Those origins entail a dynamic that is a total black box as far as evolutionary theory is concerned, and, as a result, at the present time there is no way to account for those dynamics in a scientific way.

| Explorations |

In 1883 Andreas F.W. Schimper conjectured that, originally, chloroplasts might have been part of a symbiotic relationship between nonphotosynthetic cells and certain kinds of photosynthetic bacteria. Chloroplasts are organelles that are found in the cytoplasm of both plants as well as algae, and those organelles contain molecules of chlorophyll pigments, along with various enzymatic proteins, that make photosynthesis possible as well as make possible the production of ATP – adenosine triphosphate -- one of the primary mediums of energy currencies in cellular life.

Schimper believed that over a period of time the symbiotic relationship between the nonphotosynthetic organism and certain bacteria transitioned into a permanent arrangement. As a result, two organisms began to function as one life form when various metabolic pathways of the two organisms were integrated while other metabolic pathways possessed by one or the other of the two organisms fell by the wayside.

Approximately forty years later, Schimper's idea was broadened to include mitochondria ... the double-membrane organelle found in the cytoplasm of eukaryotes (life forms that – unlike prokaryotes -- possess a true nucleus together with a number of cytoplasmic organelles such as the Golgi complex, lysosomes, and the endoplasmic reticulum). In other words, some biologists conjectured that mitochondria (which, among other things, are responsible for the production of energy-containing molecules in cells) originated in a symbiotic relationship between bacteria (purple bacteria to be specific) and some form of protoeukaryote (a primitive form of eukaryote) and, then, over time, the two life forms merged into one organism.

The underlying idea came to be known as endosymbiosis. This referred to a process in which some kind of protoeukaryotic life form would ingest bacteria (cyanobacteria – or some ancestor -- in the case of chloroplasts and purple bacteria – or some ancestor -- in the case of mitochondria) that established a symbiotic relationship (i.e., one from which both organisms derived benefit) and, eventually, that symbiotic relationship becomes transformed, somehow, into just one organism as the different kinds of bacteria became dedicated organelles -- i.e., chloroplasts or mitochondria – within a larger protoeukaryotic life form.

The idea of endosymbiosis was largely rejected and ignored for more than 70 years. However, during the 1960s, research revealed that chloroplasts and mitochondria are semiautonomous organelles that are capable of dividing on their own, synthesizing their own proteins, and they also contain DNA, mRNA (messenger RNA), tRNA (transfer RNA), as well as ribosomes (small particles consisting of rRNA – ribosomal RNA – and proteins that engage in protein synthesis).

With so many semiautonomous capabilities present in chloroplasts and mitochondria, the possibility of endosymbiosis no longer seemed to require such a large leap of imagination. Mitochondria and chloroplasts appeared to share many of the characteristics of various bacteria, and, so, if certain kinds of bacteria were ingested by a larger protoeukaryotic form of life, and this ingestion was followed by the establishment of some kind of symbiotic relationship, and, then, finally, the two life forms became integrated over a period of time, there seemed to be a plausible set of steps through which endosymbiosis might have taken place ... a theory that was more fully developed by Lynn Margulis.

The theory of endosymbiosis presumes that prior to the incorporation of certain kinds of bacteria into protoeukaryotic organisms, life forms were anaerobic – that is, such organisms relied on a form of respiration in which nutrients are converted into useful forms of energy and materials by moving electrons around through metabolic pathways that were centered on molecules other than oxygen. Organisms were required to operate in the foregoing manner because there was very little oxygen in the primitive atmosphere of early Earth.

At some point (between one and two billion years ago), certain forms of bacteria (known as cyanobacteria) acquired the ability to use pigments – such as chlorophyll – to capture energy from certain wavelengths of light and, then, transform that light energy into a form of chemical energy that was capable of subsidizing a variety of metabolic pathways through which an array of biomolecules were synthesized and subsequently used to sustain life processes. Prior to

| Explorations |

the advent of cyanobacteria, bacteria would have had to use some other molecule – such as molecular hydrogen or hydrogen sulfide -- as an electron donor (rather than chlorophyll) in the process of photosynthetic respiration.

The process of photosynthesis involving chlorophyll is a fairly complex process that aside from sunlight also uses water that is a very stable molecule and, therefore, resists giving up any of its electrons. In photosynthesis water is first broken open by orienting the water molecule in just the right way so that its electrons can be engaged one by one, and, in the process, oxygen is released.

Next, photosystem II – comprised of P680, the pair of chloroplast molecules that constitute one of several reaction centers – removes electrons from the aforementioned oxygen-generating process when that reaction center is activated by light of the right wave length (680 nanometers). The electrons that have been captured through photosystem II are, then, shunted down an electron transport system and along the way those electrons are used in the synthesis of ATP (a carrier of energy in the form of phosphoanhydride bonds) before being transferred to photosystem I – comprised of P700, the pair of chloroplast molecules that constitute the second of two reaction centers that are activated by light of the right wavelength (700 nanometers).

This latter photosystem re-energizes the electrons involved in the process of electron transport before passing them on to NADPH (nicotinamide adenine dinucleotide phosphate), a coenzyme that accepts several electrons (and a proton) from photosystem I. NADPH subsequently becomes involved in a metabolic pathway that activates carbon dioxide and converts the latter molecule into sugar. The foregoing process is known as oxygenic photosynthesis.

Aside from all of the other useful results that arise out of this sort of photosynthesis (and which were outlined in the previous paragraph), one of the most eventful dimensions associated with it revolves around the oxygen that is released as a waste product. As oxygen was released into the atmosphere of the Earth 1-2 billion years ago, this gradually led to the disappearance -- for the most part -- of the materials (like hydrogen sulfide or dissolved iron) that certain anaerobic organisms used to survive. Consequently, these organisms found ecological niches that tended to be devoid of oxygen.

Nevertheless, somewhere along the evolutionary way, organisms capable of aerobic respiration arose, and, as a result, were able to oxidize glucose to carbon dioxide and water by using oxygen as an electron acceptor. In the process, a considerable portion of the energy released during those reactions was conserved in the form of ATP.

Once protoeukaryotic organisms arose that were capable of aerobic respiration, the stage was set for the appearance of eukaryotes that, in part – according to the theory of endosymbiosis -- involved the ingestion of purple bacteria or cyanobacteria that would become, respectively, mitochondria and chloroplasts. However, before bacteria could be ingested by a protoeukaryote, the latter organisms had to develop a capacity for endocytosis that constitutes a way of consuming extracellular materials – such as bacteria – through the infolding of a plasma membrane that is, then, pinched off as a membrane-bound vesicle containing whatever was taken in through this means.

There are at least 150 different kinds of eukaryotes that have within them diatoms (e.g., phytoplankton), photosynthetic organisms, and other small organisms living as endosymbionts within the larger organisms. The cell walls of the ingested life forms might have been stripped away and, as well, some of the cell structure of the ingested organisms might be whittled down in various ways, but what remains still continues to function ... at least for a time.

For example, various marine slugs have chloroplasts contained within some of the cells that line the digestive tract of such slugs. These chloroplasts come from the algae being eaten by those slugs, and they continue to operate their photosynthetic equipment for quite some time following ingestion.

However, these ingested chloroplasts do not divide or grow. And, within a few months, they stop functioning.

The process through which these chloroplasts are permitted to survive for a period of time rather than becoming completely disassembled during digestion is not known. Furthermore – and, perhaps, related to the foregoing point -- why this arrangement occurs in some marine slugs and mollusks but not in other kinds of mollusks is also unknown.

Given that such chloroplasts only survive for a time and cannot grow or divide suggests that certain integrating events have to occur in order to make the condition of endosymbiosis permanent. Consequently, the fact such symbiotic relationships between certain kinds of marine slugs and green algae can be established is likely only one of a number of steps that are necessary in order for a complete process of endosymbiosis to become a reality. What those steps are is not known.

There have been a variety of comparisons between, on the one hand, the rRNA sequences in chloroplasts and mitochondria, and, on the other hand, the rRNA sequences in various kinds of bacteria. The bacterial rRNA base sequences that match up most closely with chloroplasts are cyanobacteria, while the bacterial rRNA base sequences that seem most closely related to mitochondria are purple bacteria, and, therefore, those rRNA comparisons would seem to lend credence to the idea that, at some point, cyanobacteria – or a close relative -- were involved in the origin of chloroplasts, while purple bacteria served as the ancestral origin for mitochondria.

Nevertheless, while the existence of such rRNA comparisons is suggestive with respect to the idea of endosymbiosis serving as the basis for a possible evolutionary account concerning the origin of chloroplasts and mitochondria, those comparisons don't necessarily constitute proof for the idea of endosymbiosis. While rRNA comparisons do show a degree of similarity between two sequences, those similarities don't really reveal how the two things being compared came to share that similarity.

Evolutionary biologists, of course, believe that the rRNA sequence similarities in the things being compared indicates there was an evolutionary process that led from cyanobacteria to chloroplasts, just as there was an evolutionary process that led from purple bacteria to mitochondria. They just can't tell you what was involved in the nature of that evolutionary process.

Francis Crick might claim – if he were with us today – that an alien intelligence could have genetically engineered the bacteria, as well as the chloroplasts and mitochondria of eukaryotes, using similar

| Explorations |

325

methods, on the one hand, with respect to chloroplasts and cyanobacteria, and, on the other hand, in relation to mitochondria and purple bacteria because in each instance similar functional requirements were in effect.

Why should an alien intelligence have to re-invent the wheel? Similar designs are used in the respective cases because they serve similar functions.

Of course, back in the 1980s Francis Crick would have had no idea how any of the foregoing might have been accomplished by an alien intelligence. However, the existence of such ignorance would have placed him on even terms with his evolutionary colleagues.

Is the evolutionary account any better than Crick's notion of directed panspermia? Is it necessarily any simpler?

In order for the theory of endosymbiosis to be plausible, there are quite a few questions that have to be addressed in a satisfactory manner. For example, how did anaerobic organisms come into being? How did photosynthetic organisms involving molecular hydrogen or hydrogen sulfide as electron donors come into being? How did chlorophyll-based photosynthetic organisms arise? How did the transition from anaerobic respiration to aerobic respiration come about? How did eukaryotic life forms arise – with their true nucleus, and an array of organelles (e.g., Golgi complex, lysosomes, endoplasmic reticulum, endosomes -- both early and late) ... organelles that are not found in bacteria? How did the capacity for endocytosis come into existence? How did endosymbiosis become established ... that is, how did an ingested bacterium lose some of its functionality, while retaining other capabilities, and how did that former-bacterium become integrated into the cellular functioning of the larger organism?

There are no concrete, step-by-step, demonstrable answers to any of the foregoing questions. Every one of those questions is rooted in an evolutionary black box of unknown dynamics.

How did the DNA coding for each of the foregoing steps come into being? One might suppose that various genes were passed around through the process of conjugation (exchange of genetic material between two organisms) that led up to one, or another, of the

| Explorations |

foregoing steps, but where did the genes (and whatever capabilities they entail) come from?

At some point, the genetic buck has to stop. One has to be able to explain how any given biological capability became instantiated in genetic information.

Genetic <u>information</u> can't be passed around through the process of conjugation, insertion, and splicing until it has been raised to the status of information (having genetic meaning) from its previous condition of being genetic noise (being genetically meaningless). In addition, a scientific account must be given for the origins of the capabilities that are instantiated in the DNA sequences that are responsible for: anaerobic respiration, aerobic respiration, photosynthesis (involving chlorophyll, hydrogen sulfide, or whatever), cyanobacteria, protoeukaryotic life forms, endocytosis, endosymbiosis, and so on.

There are no scientific accounts that show the step-by-step process through which genetic noise becomes genetic information, or the step-by step process through which: anaerobic respiration, aerobic respiration, photosynthesis, cyanobacteria, protoeukaryotic life forms (including all the characteristics that distinguish them from bacteria and archaea), endocytosis, or endosymbiosis become encoded in DNA base sequences. Everything that permeates the foregoing issues is ensconced in conjecture, speculation, assumptions, and a great deal of ignorance.

For example, no one knows how the five basic dimensions of the process of photosynthesis came into being. No one knows how water was selected to be a source of electrons. No one knows how either photosystem I or photosystem II came into existence or why they came to revolve around wavelengths of 700 and 680 nanometers respectively. No one knows how all the steps involved in photosynthesis came to be organized and integrated into a functional metabolic pathway that could be fed into other functional metabolic pathways. No one knows how ATP came to play such a central role as a source of electrons, or how the production of ATP came to be incorporated into the process of photosynthesis.

| Explorations |

Where is all the science in the evolutionary theory of, in this case, photosynthesis? The science resides in some (but not all) of the inputs and in some (but not all) of the outputs.

Nonetheless, the dynamics of the evolutionary process itself remains locked in a black box surrounded by ignorance. There is no current scientific understanding that is capable of provably accounting for what took place, or is taking place, as a function of the dynamics contained within the black box referred to as evolution.

| Explorations |

Chapter 3: The Mentality of Neuroscience

Glial Mysteries

A traditional view of the brain's role in cognitive functioning is that the latter is due to the interaction of billions of neurons, as well as being a function of the dynamics transpiring within the trillions of synapses that constitute the interstitial, fluid-filled spaces that ebb and flow among neuronal shores. Surely, the sheer complexity generated by the activity of billions of neurons and trillions of synapses should be able to account for capabilities such as thinking, memory, language, imagination, creativity, genius, awareness, and so on.

One historical figure believed that the secrets of cognition could be induced to reveal themselves if the right sort of scientists were able to study just the right kind of brain ... a brain associated with the sort of mental brilliance, insight, understanding, and creativity that manifests itself only very rarely. The name of the foregoing 'cogninaut' is Dr. Thomas Hardy, and the brain he believed held the keys to unlock the mysteries of the mind belonged to Albert Einstein ... and, so, Dr. Harvey stole the brain of the recently deceased Einstein.

Dr. Harvey held at least several delusional beliefs in conjunction with the aforementioned "scientific" project. First, he believed – arbitrarily and, probably, quite falsely – that he had the right to abscond with the body part of a deceased human being, and, secondly, he believed – arbitrarily and, probably, quite falsely – that he had the right to decide with whom he would share portions of Einstein's brain.

Scientists – at least some of them -- often seem to think they have the right to tinker with the universe in any way they see fit ... another belief that is both arbitrary and, quite probably, false. Instead of looking for the source of Einstein's genius, Dr. Harvey should have been searching for the source of, if not cure for, delusional thinking ... 'physician heal thyself'.

For more than forty years, Dr. Harvey parceled out bits and pieces of the great man's brain. Apparently, those who were the recipients of such largesse failed to demonstrate the moral sense to neither ask for, nor accept, such a gift.

Surely, those who were granted access to remnants of Einstein's brain were aware that Einstein had not given Dr. Harvey permission to dispose of the brain of the Nobel Prize winner in any manner Dr. Harvey saw fit. Surely, those researchers knew that – somewhat like Herr Doktor Frankenstein – they were akin to people who might benefit from the grave-robbing inclinations of another human being.

On the other hand, perhaps they didn't know any of the foregoing. Maybe, they just presumed that Dr. Harvey had the requisite permission and authority to do what he did.

Or, perhaps, they were incurious about the whole situation and were simply anxious to get on with their careers and ambitions. Or, maybe they thought impolitic questions might get in the way of being able to be in touch with Einstein in a way that few others had ... a unique kind of one degree of separation.

Curiosity seems to have no limits except when it comes to determining the possible boundaries of moral propriety. For all too many scientists, knowledge of every kind is desirable except the sort of knowledge that might inform such dauntless explorers about whether what they are doing is right or wrong.

If people wish to argue that right and wrong are relative issues, then the burden of proof would seem to rest entirely with them. Moreover, if they are unable to prove that such a position is not an arbitrary perspective, then, some variation of the precautionary principle ought to govern the way forward.

In other words, one should be able to show that little, or no, harm will ensue with respect to oneself and/or in relation to others (including the environment) from one's intention to act. If one cannot do this, then, perhaps, one should refrain from proceeding on in circumstances fraught with such arbitrariness, uncertainty, and ignorance.

If Einstein had given his permission to Dr. Harvey and posterity to use his body as they deemed fit for the benefit of science and medicine, this certainly would lessen -- and, possibly, even extinguish -- culpability. However, to the best of my knowledge, such permission was not given, and history unfolded in one way rather than another.

Did any good come from Dr. Harvey's decision? Well, to answer that question, one would have to have a reliable means of deciding upon, calculating, and evaluating the criteria for what constitutes goodness.

Benefitting from something does not necessarily make that from which one benefits an expression of goodness ... though it might seem that way to the beneficiary. Presumably, all those who received brain snippets from Dr. Harvey benefitted in one way or another, but whether, or not, there was any demonstrable sort of good that emerged through the research done on Einstein's brain is a more complicated issue.

For example, whatever knowledge is acquired through scientific exploration must be weighed against the "collateral damage" that is done as a result of such a process of acquisition. What is acquired in the way of knowledge must also be weighed against the possible harm that might arise from the application of that knowledge.

Let's take a quick look at one example that is rooted in the case of Einstein's stolen brain. In 1985, an article by Dr. Marian Diamond and colleagues appeared in *Experimental Neurology*, a journal focusing on cutting-edge research in neuroscience. The title of the article was: "On the Brain of a Scientist: Albert Einstein."

The basic idea of the research underlying the journal piece revolved around the hypothesis that Einstein's genius was a function of the interplay of at least three regions of the brain believed to be responsible for (1) association, (2) abstraction, and (3) imagery. Consequently, she and her colleagues requested that Dr. Harvey send them tissue samples located in both the left and right hemispheres (to check if hemispherical dominance in the brain played any role), and, in addition, those samples should include sections from the prefrontal region (abstraction), the inferior parietal region (imagery), and the association cortex.

After receiving the requested samples, Dr. Diamond and her fellow researchers sliced the tissues into ultra-thin segments and dyed the latter to be able to highlight the presence of neurons in order to distinguish them from other facets of the brain tissues that were being studied. The samples from Einstein were then compared with similar tissue specimens (i.e., involving the same three regions of the brain in both hemispheres) from eleven, male, control subjects of variable ages between 47 and 80 (presumably deceased).

Somewhat surprisingly, perhaps, Dr. Diamond and her associates discovered absolutely no differences in any of the samples examined in relation to the character of the neurons found either in Einstein or in the eleven other control subjects. There appeared to be as many neurons in the sliced sections of the control subjects as there were in the samples from Einstein.

Apparently, genius was not a function of the interaction of the neurons in the association cortex, the prefrontal cortex, and the inferior parietal region, nor did hemispherical dominance appear to play any role with respect to genius. Indeed, if genius were a function of such dynamics, one would expect to find significant neuronal differences between the brain of Einstein and the brains of eleven individuals who had not been known to exhibit any signs of genius during their lives, but this was not the case.

The foregoing results notwithstanding, Dr. Martin and her colleagues did find one substantial difference between the brain tissue samples of Einstein and the tissue samples from the individuals serving as experimental controls. More specifically, the researchers discovered that in each of the brain regions studied, there were, on average, nearly twice as many non-neuronal, glial cells in the samples from Einstein as there were in any of the control subjects.

The largest differential in numbers of glial cells involved the inferior parietal cortex in the dominant, right hemisphere. This region (the inferior parietal cortex) of the brain is believed by many neuroscientists to be responsible for visual imagery, complex thought, and abstraction, and, therefore, the possibility emerged that, maybe, genius was a function of glial cells rather than neuronal activity.

There is at least one caveat to keep in mind with respect to the foregoing findings. More specifically, for reasons that are as inexplicable now as they were during the times of Camillo Golgi and Santiago Ramón y Cajal in the late 1800s and early 1900s, only a small number of neurons – possibly less than one in a hundred – are able to take on the stain of the dye used to highlight the presence and properties of a neuron.

Conceivably, therefore, the secret to genius might reside in the 99%, percent of the neurons that didn't show up during the staining process. One cannot compare what one cannot see.

Although the neurons that were visible in the aforementioned comparisons seemed to be roughly the same, there might have been substantial differences with respect to the neurons that didn't show up in the staining process. Moreover, given that it is the interaction of neurons that is considered by many neuroscientists to be the source of cognitive capabilities (including genius) – dynamics that are not captured by the static images that are expressed through staining – then, perhaps. the interaction of unknown millions of neurons (the ones for which staining doesn't work) might still hold the key to the difference between the brain of a genius and the cognitive functioning of individuals who are not geniuses.

Alternatively, maybe the interaction between the -- on average -- twice as many glial cells in the regions of Einstein's brain being studied (relative to the control individuals) together with the 99% of the neurons that couldn't be seen via the staining process might be able to account for the presence of genius. The problem is that we really don't know how neurons, on their own, or, glial cells, on their own, or, glial cells in conjunction with neuron cells, generate genius.

Possibly, genius is the result of one or more forces that lie beyond the horizons of glial and neuronal activity. Possibly, glial and neuronal cells play supporting roles for some other phenomenon that plays a more central role in the manifestation of genius.

The results published by Dr. Diamond and her colleagues in *Experimental Neurology* are interesting but quite inconclusive as far as being able to identify the nature of genius and how the latter arises out of brain activity. The significance of the, on average, twice as many glial cells in the three regions of Einstein's brain relative to the brains of the control subjects is suggestive but nothing more ... unless, and until, one can show what glial functioning has to do with the manifestation of genius, or abstraction, or imagery.

In the light of the inconclusive nature of the foregoing findings, one has difficulty understanding how someone might try to argue that the contents of the journal article concerning Einstein's brain justified the theft that helped make that article possible. In fact, even if much more determinate and significant data concerning the nature of genius had emerged from the research by Dr. Diamond and her colleagues, the calculus of justification still seems rather elusive and arbitrary.

| Explorations |

Notwithstanding the foregoing considerations, there are several mysteries to be explored in conjunction with the relationship between glial and neuronal functioning. For instance, if one were to hypothesize that glial cells and neurons interacted to give expression to cognitive functioning, how – if at all -- do the two kinds of cells communicate with one another?

Neurons communicate with each other through a combination of electrical and chemical signals. The electrical component for a given neuron is a function of ionic currents set in motion by, among other things, the impact of electrical and chemical signals on a given neuron from adjacent neurons, while the chemical signaling component involves, among other possibilities, the activity of neurotransmitters (e.g., serotonin, dopamine, GABA – gamma amino butyric acid) that are released from tiny packets or vesicles located near the axon terminals or synaptic boutons found toward the end of tube-like processes (axons) that carry information away from the soma or body of a neuron.

Every resting neuron has an electrical potential running across its membrane that is created by the charge differential existing between, on the one hand, the ions found along the interior portion of a neuron's membrane and, on the other hand, the ions located along that neuron's exterior membrane. The aforementioned electrical potential is variable but often runs in the vicinity of -70 millivolts.

The net, interior, ionic charge found in a resting neuron is negative relative to the exterior of the cell. The net, exterior, ionic charge tends to be positive.

Left to themselves, ions (such as potassium) tend to diffuse out of the neuron (i.e., going from an area of relatively high concentration to an area of relatively low concentration of potassium ions) via certain membrane channels that have been opened up by conformational changes in membrane proteins, while ions (such as sodium and chloride) tend to diffuse into the interior of the neuron via membrane channels created by conformational changes in still other kinds of membrane proteins. However, the existence of the aforementioned resting electrical potential running across the membrane of a neuron tends to resist the inclination of ions to diffuse along their respective concentration gradients.

| Explorations |

When a resting neuron receives electrochemical signals from other neurons (via the cellular extensions – known as dendrites – that send information toward the soma or cell body of a neuron), the resting neuron will either respond to those signals by depolarizing its resting membrane potential or the neuron will continue on in its default mode. If the neuron depolarizes, a series of events occur that, among other things, sequentially open and close various membrane channels that affect the flow of ions into and out of the cell all along the axon process, resulting in an electric current being sent down the length of the axon toward the axon terminal/synaptic bouton.

Once the action potential (depolarization) takes place, the generated electrical signal induces vesicles in the axon terminal to release various neurotransmitters that are contained in those packets. The released neurotransmitters diffuse across the synaptic, fluid filled spaces that border the neurons, and, then, the neurotransmitters go on to attach to the dendrite portions of other neurons, and, these post-synaptic neurons, in turn, will either respond to, or ignore, the incoming signal.

How a neuron "decides" whether, or not, to respond to incoming signals is not known ... although it seems to have to do – at least in part – with whether, or not, certain thresholds are exceeded. How the neuron 'knows' when those thresholds have been exceeded is not known.

What the individual and collective electrochemical signaling dynamics of neurons have to do with cognitive functioning (e.g., consciousness, language, thinking, creativity, etc.) is not known ... although scientists have been trying to figure this out for more than a hundred years. Furthermore, how such a system of signaling came into being is not known.

Glial cells operate quite differently than neurons do. Unlike neurons, glial cells do not undergo depolarization, and, therefore, there is no action potential-like electrical signal involved in the dynamics of glial cells.

Glial cells come in four varieties (and neurons also give expression to different shapes, sizes, and functions). One of those four kinds of glial cells is known as a Schwann cell.

There are three varieties of Schwann cells. These are referred to as: Myelinating, nonmyelinating, and terminal Schwann cells.

Whether, or not, the foregoing three types of cell are actually all variations on some sort of basic underlying Schwann cell-type is uncertain. This is because none of the three kinds of cells are shaped like one another, and, as well, they have completely different functions from each other.

Historically, all of the foregoing cells were referred to as Schwann cells in order to identify them as being something other than a neuronal form of cell. However, given the differences among those cells, they might constitute entirely different classes of glial cells, and, if so, then, there are, possibly, as many as seven – not four -- kinds of glial cells.

Notwithstanding the foregoing considerations, myelinating Schwann cells interact with certain kinds of neurons in the peripheral nervous system by either attaching to the latter or by enveloping neurons. In either case a kind of electrical insulation forms around the neurons.

The resulting sheath is referred to as myelin. The process of surrounding neurons in the foregoing ways is known as myelination.

Thus, myelinating Schwann cells and certain kinds of neurons have the potential to develop a close physical association with one another ... although not all neurons become myelinated, or if they do become myelinated, this does not necessarily happen at the same time as might be the case with other neurons. However, with respect to those neurons that do become myelinated, one might ask whether, or not, such a physically contiguous relationship enables any sort of information to be exchanged between the two kinds of cell, or is the relationship between them more like that of a car and a garage in which the latter has a functional relationship with the former, but no exchange of information appears to take place between the car and the garage (unless, of course, an electronic garage door opener has been installed and can be activated by a remote control device from, say, within the car)?

Dr. R. Douglas Fields and his lab technician, Beth Stevens (who later became his graduate student), wanted to explore whether, or not,

| Explorations |

337

some sort of communication took place between neurons and the Schwann cells that attached to neurons or enveloped neurons. So, the two researchers devised an experiment for determining whether, or not, there might be some form of signaling process that involved both kinds of cells under certain circumstances.

Aequorin is a photoprotein that is secreted by certain kinds of jellyfish and produces a blue light when it becomes attached to calcium. Dr. Fields incorporated the basic idea of the aequorin-calcium dynamic into his experiment by using a synthetic dye that was calcium sensitive.

First, DRG neurons – or Dorsal Root Ganglions – were bathed in the foregoing synthetic calcium sensitive dye. Subsequently, the neuron would be stimulated with a weak electrical current via an implanted electrode.

When the cell was stimulated in the foregoing fashion, the cell would depolarize. During the process of depolarizing, various membrane channels sequentially opened up, permitting calcium ions to flow into the cell.

The calcium ions interacted with the synthetic dye within the cell. This resulted in flashes of light.

Next, Schwann cells were introduced into the culture containing calcium ions together with the DRG neurons that had been bathed in a synthetic calcium sensitive dye. As occurred in the previous step of the experiment, the neurons were given a weak electrical charge to induce an action potential that, in turn, caused the opening of membrane channels in the DRG neurons.

Once again, as calcium ions flowed into the DRG neurons and interacted with the calcium sensitive dye in the neurons, flashes of light occurred. The more calcium ions that entered the neuron, the brighter the light from the neurons became and, as well, transitions in the color of the light would take place.

A short while later, the light emanating from the Schwann cells also began to change in color. Apparently, the Schwann cells were responding to the electrical signaling that was taking place in the DRG neurons, and, as a result, the Schwann cells were induced to open their membrane channels that, in turn, increased the flow of calcium ions

| Explorations |

into the interior of the Schwann cells, and, therefore, led to an increased brightness in the light being given off through the interaction of calcium with the synthetic calcium sensitive dye.

Some sort of signaling process appeared to be taking place between the firing of the DRG neurons and the presence of the Schwann cells. What, exactly – if anything – was meant by such signals or how the Schwann cells were picking up on those signals was unknown, but, evidently the Schwann cells (glial cells) were, in their own way, responding to the electrical activity of the DRG neurons.

However, whether, or not, the possibility of signaling is reciprocal is unknown. That is, while the Fields/Stevens experiment appeared to demonstrate that Schwann cells have some sort of 'awareness' with respect to the electrical activity of nearby neurons, their experiment did not show whether, or not, neurons were sensitive, in some fashion, to the activity taking place in glial cells.

Notwithstanding the foregoing considerations, glial cells have been shown to respond to neuronal activity in other ways. For example, glial cells help regulate what takes place in the synaptic fluid-filled spaces (roughly 25 billionths of a meter) that separate presynaptic neurons (the neurons from which neurotransmitters are released) and postsynaptic neurons (the neurons to which neurotransmitters become attached following their release from the axon bulb of the presynaptic neurons).

If the release of neurotransmitters into the synaptic areas plays a central role in the brain's system of communication, then presumably, there must be some means of making sure that the synaptic messages don't become entangled with one another or don't interfere with one another, and, in the process, introduce confusion into the information that is being communicated. In other words, once a presynaptic neuron releases its neurotransmitter message, then, there needs to be a means of resetting the synaptic blackboard back to a blank state so that the next message can be received.

The resetting mechanism comes in the form of astrocytes that constitute a second kind of glial cell (You already have been introduced to another form or kind of glial cell – namely Schwann cells). Astrocytes are found bordering the synaptic regions separating neurons.

| Explorations |

The membranes of astrocytes contain proteins that act like pumps that suck out the neurotransmitters that continue to mill about in a given synaptic area bordered by such cells. Once astrocytes remove neurotransmitters from a synaptic region, the glial cell modifies the neurotransmitters into an inert (or non-communicating) form, and, then, returns such inert neurotransmitters back to the neuron axon terminal where the neurotransmitters are re-configured and re-packaged so that they, once again, become active and ready for subsequent release into synaptic space to deliver some other message.

If astrocytes are too quick to remove neurotransmitters from a synaptic region, the intended neuronal message might not be delivered at all, or if delivered, the message might be too faint to be understood or to have the right kind of impact on the postsynaptic neuron. On the other hand, if astrocytes permit neurotransmitters to linger on in a given synaptic region, successive messages will become conflated and garbled.

In addition to removing neurotransmitters from synaptic spaces, astrocytes also provide energy for neuronal activity by metabolizing lactate molecules and generating ATP derivatives from that process. This energy is provided to meet the needs of neurons under various circumstances.

Although only a very small portion of brain activity has been described in the opening pages of this chapter, let's briefly reflect on the information that has been provided thus far. First, by means of a set of specialized membrane proteins, neurons are able to regulate the influx and efflux of ions into, and out of, such cells, and, in the process, an action potential – or electrical current – is initiated.

The action potential causes vesicles in the axon bulb or terminal of the presynaptic neuron to break open and release the neurotransmitters contained within those packets. The freed neurotransmitters diffuse across the synaptic space (approximately 25 billionths of a meter) and attach to certain membrane proteins on the postsynaptic neuron.

Next, astrocytes bordering the synaptic region into which the neurotransmitters have been released pump out the molecules that remain in the synaptic area ... but the pumping is done in a manner that does not occur either too quickly or too slowly. Moreover, the

| Explorations |

astrocytes help regulate neuronal activity by providing energy as necessary.

In addition, astrocytes deactivate the neurotransmitters that have been pumped out of the synaptic region on which the glial cells border and then those cells return the deactivated neurotransmitters to neurons. The neurons to which the neurotransmitters have been returned re-activate the molecules, and, in addition, re-package them within vesicles that are located in the axon bulb of the neuron.

From an evolutionary point of view, one wonders how the appropriate sequences of DNA base pairs came into being that encoded for all of the foregoing capabilities involving, among other things: (1) Specialized membrane proteins whose dynamics help underwrite the generation of an electrical current; (2) neurotransmitter-containing axon bulb vesicles that could be opened as a result of an action potential running down the axon process of a neuron; (3) a set of neurotransmitters that could have an array of effects on the postsynaptic neurons to which they become attached following diffusion across a synaptic space; (4) astrocytes that supply energy to neurons as needed and that also have membranes containing proteins that pump out excess neurotransmitters from a synaptic space, and, as well, have the capacity to deactivate neurotransmitters and, then, ship them back to neurons; (5) neurons that re-activate deactivated neurotransmitters and re-package them to form axon bulb vesicles. Evolutionary biologists not only fail to understand how the encoding for any of the foregoing capabilities came into being, but, as well, evolutionary biologists do not know how any of that encoding came to have meaning within the context of brain activity so that appropriate messages could be sent and 'understood' in order to give expression to a functioning brain.

In addition to the two kinds of glial cells already touched upon – namely, astrocytes and Schwann cells -- there are two other editions of glial cells – microglia and oligodendrocytes. Microglia cells help to protect the brain from disease or injury, as well as assist the brain – to varying degrees -- to recover from the effects of the foregoing sorts of problems, while oligodendrocytes help to myelinate neurons within both the spinal column and the brain (as indicated previously, Schwann cells tend to operate primarily in conjunction with the peripheral nervous systems – that is, the nerves and ganglia found outside the brain).

However, despite what biologists do know – in considerable detail – concerning the physiology of cellular dynamics (both in relation to neurons and glial cells), none of those researchers have been able to <u>causally</u> connect such cellular dynamics to phenomena involving consciousness, intelligence, language, creativity, and so on. In other words, although scientists might know a great deal about how the brain functions at a cellular level, none of what is known in that respect has been woven together in a way that shows how such cellular dynamics are capable of underwriting a viable account of just how the brain (allegedly) generates consciousness, intelligence, language, creativity, and so on.

Possibly one way of engaging the foregoing unknowns is to hypothesize that quality is a function of quantity. For example, researchers have given variable responses concerning the relative, quantitative ratios of non-neuronal cells (i.e., glial cells) to neuronal cells that might exist within the nervous system.

Some individuals believe glial cells outnumber neurons by a factor of 10. Other researchers suspect that the ratio between the two might be closer to 100 to 1 in favor of glial cells, while still other scientists maintain that the ratio between the two classes of cells might be fairly even.

Finally, certain researchers contend that the ratio between glial cells and neuronal cells depends on the part of the nervous system one is considering. This variability ranges from: Approximately, four astrocytes to every neuron in the frontal cortex of a human being (interestingly, dolphins and whales, exhibit a 7 to 1 ratio in this region of the brain), to: A hundred or more myelinating glial cells to each neuron in the case where just one axon might be sheathed or myelinated by many glial cells.

Irrespective of how one calculates the ratio of non-neuronal to neuronal cells within the nervous system, determining the relative ratio of the two classes of cells doesn't seem to advance understanding any further with respect to how the interaction between non-neuronal and neuronal cells generates higher cognitive functions such as consciousness and intelligence. While considerable evidence exists which indicates that glial cells certainly assist, support, regulate, protect, repair, complement, and help shape the dynamics of neuronal activity, nonetheless, none of what is currently known about glial functioning demonstrates how that functioning is capable of generating – on its own or in conjunction with neuronal dynamics – the higher cognitive functioning of human beings.

For example, let's return to Einstein's poor brain. Earlier in this section, information was given indicating that Dr. Diamond and her colleagues discovered that the inferior parietal cortex in the dominant hemisphere of Einstein's brain contained many more glial cells than did the inferior parietal cortices in any of the control subjects.

The higher numbers of glial cells in Einstein's brain were probably mostly astrocytes. Some number of oligodendrocytes (myelinating glial cells in the brain and spinal column) and, possibly, a smaller number of microglia cells were also likely to be present among the increased number of glial cells in Einstein's brain.

As the earlier discussion alluded, microglia are part of the immune system of the central nervous system. Those kinds of cells are estimated to constitute 10-15% of the total glial population.

Additional oligodendrocytes might help the electrochemical dynamics of neurons take place more quickly and/or more efficiently. However, understanding how greater efficiency in the dynamics of electrochemical signaling enhances a person's capacity for genius, complex thinking, imagery, and abstraction is not self-evident.

Microglia that are journeying to the site of infections in the brain do have the capacity (in the form of certain kinds of enzymes) to slice their way through a morass of neurons by dissolving the matrix proteins that hold neurons together. These same protein-dissolving enzymes are also used by microglia to help rewire the synaptic circuitry by disconnecting neurons from such synaptic spaces as part of the process of developmental transitioning or as part of a repair mechanism for injured brain circuitry.

Nonetheless, while the presence of microglia in the inferior parietal cortex might help to keep the brain healthy or might assist in the rewiring of certain synaptic circuitry under various circumstances, once again, it is not self-evident how having additional microglia in the inferior parietal cortex of the brain will generate the sort of capacity for imagery, complex thought, and abstraction that many people consider to be at the heart of genius.

Schwann cells -- one of the four kinds of glial cells -- operate in the peripheral nervous system outside the brain. So, this leaves us with astrocytes as the last remaining candidate among glial cells as a possible source of genius.

As discussed previously in this chapter, astrocytes do supply energy to neurons. Moreover, as previously outlined, astrocytes also play a key role in regulating the synaptic regions that border neurons by both controlling the length of time neurotransmitters remain in a given synaptic region as well as by removing neurotransmitters from those fluid-filled spaces, deactivating those molecules, and, then, returning them to neurons for further processing.

In addition, astrocytes regulate the concentration of certain ions that congregate along the outer membranes of neurons. More specifically, potassium ions are released by neurons into the extracellular fluid surrounding the neuron when the latter depolarizes and generates an action potential or electrical current along its axon process.

In order for the neuron to return to its resting membrane potential and, thereby, be in a position – when properly stimulated -- to generate another action potential, the potassium that has been released into the extracellular fluid surrounding the neuron must be removed from the vicinity of the outer membrane of the neuron. Astrocytes perform this function by absorbing many of those potassium ions.

In fact, astrocytes are connected to one another through a network of gap junctions or transmembrane protein channel ways constructed from connexins which constitute a family of structural proteins (connexin structural proteins form these channel ways in vertebrates but innexin proteins – quite different from connexin proteins -- form those channel ways in invertebrates). Among other things, potassium ions -- which have been absorbed from synaptic regions -- flow through the aforementioned network of gap junctions.

Since astrocytes do not function like neurons (i.e., there is no action potential), the excess potassium ions do not interfere with the functioning of astrocytes. Moreover, there are certain astrocytes that have specialized features enabling them to clamp onto small blood vessels and transfer potassium ions into the blood stream that have been flowing through the network of gap junctions of connected astrocytes and, in the process, remove excess potassium ions from the brain.

Without astrocytes performing their removal services in conjunction with potassium ions and neurotransmitters, neurons would not be able to, respectively, recharge or send and receive clear messages. Nonetheless, once again, one is still not quite sure how the presence of additional astrocytes (even a lot of them) will generate or enable a greater capacity for abstraction, imagery, or more complex thought.

In passing, one might hypothesize that while astrocytes do not seem to be responsible for complex cognitive functioning, the action of SSRIs (selective serotonin uptake inhibitors that were discussed in the first chapter) might interfere with the capacity of astrocytes to remove potassium ions and neurotransmitters (such as serotonin) from synaptic regions and, as a result, the brains of some people might respond to the excess concentrations of potassium and neurotransmitters as if they were being poisoned, and, thereby, help to bring about a condition involving some aspect of the phenomenon of 'medication madness' that has been addressed by Dr. Peter Breggin and that was discussed in Chapter 1 of the present book.

Let's consider another dimension of astrocyte dynamics. For example, when a woman becomes pregnant, the neurons and synapses that regulate lactation undergo a reconfiguring as a result of glial cell activity.

Something of a mystery is involved in trying to understand how glial cells 'know' when, where, and how to reconfigure or rewire the neuronal/synaptic circuits responsible for lactation. Something of an even bigger mystery is involved in trying to understand how living organisms came to acquire the capacity to induce astrocytes to perform this kind of magic in a functional way and at the right time and place

| Explorations |

There are still other mysteries. During pregnancy, oxytocin (consisting of just nine amino acids) is produced by, and released from, specialized cells (known as magnocellular neurons) located in the hypothalamus.

The axons of these hypothalamic magnocellular neurons extend from the hypothalamus to the pituitary gland. At an appropriate point, the oxytocin is released from the axon terminals of magnocellular neurons and diffuses into the extracellular fluids which lap against capillaries that absorb the relatively small peptides and, then, deliver those molecules to the blood stream that takes the oxytocin for a ride before distributing them to appropriate places in the body ... although how the criteria for what constitutes "appropriateness" arose and how the capacity to recognize when such appropriateness is at hand constitutes, yet, another mystery.

Oxytocin helps to induce the smooth muscles of the uterus to contract during birth. Moreover, oxytocin also helps to induce the flow of milk in mammary glands.

In addition, the presence of oxytocin also is correlated with the enhanced sense of bonding that a mother feels toward her baby. Experiments have been done in which the activity of oxytocin is blocked in rats, and the rats that are treated in this fashion tend to shun the babies that are born to them, while rats that are not pregnant, but have been injected with oxytocin, will become motherly to any baby rats that are placed in the vicinity of the non-pregnant mothers that have been treated with oxytocin.

Astrocytes play a role in the regulation of the flow of oxytocin. More specifically, the cells accomplish this by, among other things, reconfiguring their shape in and around the axon terminals of the magnocellular neurons and, thereby, permit the specialized neurons to freely release oxytocin to be absorbed, first, by capillaries, and, then, be fed into the blood stream for subsequent distribution.

How the oxytocin peptide came to be coded for by magnocellular neurons is not known. How the same oxytocin molecule came to mean three different things in three different circumstances (lactation in the mammary gland, contraction in the uterus, and a feeling of enhanced bonding of a mother for her baby) is not known.

| Explorations |

What induces astrocytes to reconfigure themselves at the appropriate time and place in order to change neuronal and synaptic dynamics is not known. How such a capacity for integrated functioning arose is not known.

As previously noted, astrocytes have important roles to play in monitoring and regulating neuronal and synaptic dynamics. Beyond what already has been said about such processes, there are several additional ways in which astrocytes impact neuronal and synaptic functioning.

First, Stéphane Ouellet, a French neuroscientist, has demonstrated that voltages decrease in certain synaptic regions of the hypothalamus when astrocytes undergo reconfiguration with respect to some of the properties of such cells These reconfigurations involve transitions in shape as well as the manner in which various projections of astrocytes extend into, and withdraw from, various synaptic spaces.

Secondly, just as neurons release neurotransmitters, so too, astrocytes release a number of gliotransmitters that are capable – each in its own way -- of modulating some of the membrane receptors of neurons. The release of gliotransmitters affects what transpires both within certain neurons as well as affects what takes place in the synaptic regions bordered by the neurons that are being impacted by gliotransmitter activity.

Glial cells are implicated in all kinds of regulatory dynamics involving neurons and synapses. These regulatory activities range from: Pregnancy, birth, and mothering behavior, to: Sleep, fine motor movement, gender blindness and thirst. However, none of the foregoing sorts of regulatory activities can be tied – in a concrete, demonstrable, causal way – to the emergence of genius, or a heightened capacity for: Abstraction, complexity of thought, or the quality of imagery that are manifested in mental phenomenology.

Clearly, astrocytes are affecting – if not helping to regulate -- neuronal activity and synaptic dynamics. What is less clear is how astrocytes are being induced to affect/regulate neuronal activity and synaptic dynamics in one way rather than another, and what is even less clear – to the point of being downright murky -- is how all of this integrated, regulatory capability came into being in the first place.

| Explorations |

347

Naturally, when the dynamics of glial cells are compromised, there are ramifications for the rest of the brain and for mental functioning. For example, there is a protein known as GFAP – glial fibrillary acidic protein – that is found in astrocytes, but this protein is also given expression in various other kinds of cells as well.

The functional role that GFAP plays within those cells is not fully understood. At a minimum, GFAP appears to lend structural support to such cells, and GFAP is found in all healthy astrocytes.

However, in conjunction with certain kinds of pathological conditions (e.g., Alexander disease), the quantity of GFAP in astrocytes proliferates. In turn, an excess amount of GFAP is correlated with the emergence of a glut of Rosenthal fibers within astrocytes that are somewhat similar to the fibrillary tangles found in the neurons of individuals with Alzheimer's.

In the 1947 clinical case in London, England that had led to the naming of the diagnostic condition that came to be known as Alexander disease, the postmortem examination showed that the brain of the patient (a fifteen-month old male baby) had degenerated extensively due to the presence of rod-shaped bodies (Rosenthal fibers) within the astrocytes of the baby's brain. Over a period of some eight months when the child was alive, the proliferation of Rosenthal fibers led, in succession, to a substantial enlarging of the baby's head, a deterioration of cognitive functioning, very high fever, convulsions, and, finally death.

Obviously, while the presence of a certain amount of GFAP within astrocytes is a good thing, too much of that protein is problematic. Under certain conditions of pathological stress, the production of GFAP is increased, and this seems to open the door for additional problematic events (such as the appearance of Rosenthal fibers) to enter the picture.

As indicated previously, the role or roles that GFAP plays within healthy astrocytes is not fully understood. Nonetheless, when something goes wrong with the metabolic pathways through which GFAP is generated, trouble ensues.

The fact that GFAP can be shown to play a role in undermining healthy cognitive functioning does not necessarily mean that the presence of GFAP in the right amounts is responsible – at least in part –– for such capacities as abstraction, imagery, and complex thinking, anymore than a properly functioning radio is responsible for the content of the programming that an effectively operating radio enables a person to hear. The appropriate amount of GFAP within astrocytes helps those cells to operate properly, just as, among other things, an appropriate number of, say, transistors helps enable a radio to function properly.

Notwithstanding the foregoing considerations, in 2002 a group of Japanese scientists discovered evidence that GFAP appeared to play a more varied role than just lending cellular structural support for astrocytes. Nobufumi Kawai and a number of research associates experimented with mice by removing the gene that coded for GFAP in the astrocytes of those mice.

The foregoing experiment left neuronal functioning intact. Nonetheless, the memory of the mice that were missing the GFAP gene seemed to be adversely affected, and this was an experimental result that tended to conflict with the widely accepted idea that memory was a function of neuronal activity.

The possibility that astrocytes might play a much larger role in the functioning of memory than previously had been thought was further strengthened by a project somewhat similar to the foregoing one, but this experiment was carried out by a different set of Japanese researchers led by Hiroshi Nishiyama. This latter research group found that when they removed the gene known as S100 from mice, these experimental mice were able to run a maze more quickly than mice that were not genetically engineered in this same fashion.

Apparently, the mice without the S100 gene had become smarter in some way. Perhaps, their capacity for remembering had been enhanced to a certain degree.

On the other hand, maybe the genetic modification that involved the removal of the S100 gene didn't either improve memory or make those mice smarter. Possibly, the removal of the gene permitted the mice to bypass a processing step that would normally have slowed them down slightly.

The S100 gene gives expression to a calcium-binding protein. Perhaps, the missing gene didn't necessarily make the mice smarter or provide them with improved memories but, instead, the missing gene might just have allowed certain aspects of brain functioning to take place more efficiently, and, in the process, permitted the maze to be completed more quickly.

What is actually taking place in the brain is hard to know without studying the S100 gene and determining what, precisely, its role (or roles) is (are) in astrocyte functioning. Furthermore, whatever might have been gained in terms of how quickly a maze was completed might also be counterbalanced by whatever could have been lost with respect to overall functioning -- losses that might not show up immediately – due to the absence of the S100 gene.

Astrocytes do have the capacity to both excite and inhibit neuronal activity via gliotransmitters that are released. Given the right set of neuronal and synaptic conditions, exciting or inhibiting certain neurons via gliotransmitters could both lead to speeding up the running of a maze, and, similarly, the absence of the GFAP and SA100 genes could have inhibitory or excitatory effects upon neuronal and synaptic functioning that, respectively might undermine or speed up functioning.

Yet, none of foregoing possibilities necessarily has anything to do with the generation of mental functioning such as association, abstraction, and so on. Rather, the impact of the missing genes might only be indirect as far as mental functioning is concerned.

That is, speeding up biological processes in the brain, or helping to enhance/stabilize those processes, or undermining such dynamics in some way could all impact the time it took to run a maze without necessarily requiring one to suppose that an organism's capacity for intelligence or memory had been altered in order to be able to explain changes in the time it took to complete a maze. The foregoing possibility is similar to the way in which changes in the architecture of a radio receiver might impact the clarity of the signal that is being received without necessarily having anything to do with the content of that signal.

Aside from the GFAP molecule, both glial cells and neurons use other kinds of molecules (such as glutamate and ATP) in order to

| Explorations |

transmit signals throughout the brain. For example, when cellular vesicles containing ATP are induced to release their contents -- through the presence of glutamate molecules that are binding to certain membrane proteins -- ATP will, in turn, become attached to certain astrocyte membrane proteins and, thereby increase the flow of calcium atoms within those glial cells. This, in turn, will lead to the further release of, among other molecules, ATP ... and so on.

Aside from serving as a source of energy, ATP (adenosine triphosphate) also is a source of adenosine. In other words, when ATP is stripped of its phosphate groups, adenosine remains, and on its own, adenosine can serve as an inhibitory neurotransmitter or signal.

For instance, when a neuron fires, sometimes that neuron might release glutamate into a given synaptic region. The presence of glutamate in such an extracellular space might induce astrocytes bordering that space to release ATP.

After being released, ATP might be stripped of all of its phosphate groups, leaving just adenosine. As previously noted, astrocytes are connected to one another through a network of gap junctions or transmembrane protein channel ways, and such gap junctions give astrocytes the potential (e.g., via the flow of, say, adenosine through those junctions) to impact on (in an inhibitory manner) the dynamics of neuronal and synaptic activity in relatively distant localities.

Moreover, in 2005, Philip Haydon and a number of research associates showed that when astrocytes are induced to increase the flow of calcium due to transitions in the synaptic activity associated with hippocampal neurons, the aforementioned calcium ions will flow through the gap junctions formed by networks of astrocytes and subsequently induce distant astrocytes in that network -- through the release of certain gliotransmitters at those sites -- to strengthen the synaptic circuits associated with portions of those hippocampal neurons.

The notion of long-term potentiation (LTP) is considered to go to the heart of the modern theory of memory and learning. Long-term potentiation refers to the process of strengthening synaptic circuitry through the manner in which neurotransmitters and gliotransmitters cause voltage changes in synaptic spaces ... changes that result in lasting patterns of reconfigured circuitry, and the synaptic circuitry

| Explorations |

that has been induced to persist (i.e., be strengthened) is said to give expression to the memory of something that has been learned.

Although astrocytes have the capacity to strengthen or inhibit synaptic circuits -- both locally and in, relatively speaking, more distant locations – through the release of ATP, glutamate, and calcium ions, nevertheless, determining what, exactly, is being strengthened or inhibited is not necessarily a straightforward matter. All of the aforementioned glial, synaptic, and neuronal activity can be correlated with various kinds of sensory and cognitive functioning, but whether, or not, such strengthening and inhibiting of synaptic circuits is generating cognitive functioning (in the form of abstraction, imagery, memory, and association) is not necessarily a foregone conclusion ... anymore than properly functioning radio circuitry can said to be responsible for the signal content to which such circuitry gives audible expression.

Even if it were clear (which it is not) that the activity of synapses, astrocytes, and neurons gave expression to mental phenomenology, there would still be at least one outstanding set of mysteries that would need to explained. More specifically, what is organizing, coordinating, and integrating the flow of all the neurotransmitters, gliotransmitters, calcium ions, and other brain molecules so that such a flow of materials will strengthen or inhibit one specific idea rather than some other idea, or will strengthen or inhibit one particular image rather than some other sort of imagery, or will strengthen or inhibit this or that association rather than some other kind of association, or will give expression to one type of genius rather than some other manifestation of genius?

In other words, how do the astrocytes know which synaptic circuits to strengthen or inhibit in order for an organism to be able to learn or remember one kind of thought, image, or association rather than some other thought, image, or association? And prior to the process of strengthening or inhibiting such circuits, what establishes those circuits to begin with as giving expression to a specific idea, association, image, or abstraction that might, or might not be subject, subsequently, to strengthening or inhibiting?

For someone to claim that glial cells play a role in the strengthening and inhibiting of synaptic circuits is one thing, and there is considerable evidence to support such a claim. Nevertheless, for someone to claim that glial cells -- by themselves or in conjunction with neurons -- construct synaptic circuits that constitute ideas, imagery, and abstractions might be quite another thing, and, in fact, there is little evidence to demonstrate the truth of such a claim.

Signaling is occurring, and communication is taking place, and information is being processed in conjunction with the interaction of glial cells, neurons, and synaptic spaces. However, the precise nature of what is being signaled, communicated, or informationally processed is not really known even though it all can be correlated, to one degree or another, with various kinds of sensory processing and cognitive functioning.

Consider the following. There is a form of brain scanning technology known as diffusion tensor imagining (DTI) that is capable of assisting researchers to differentiate among, and follow the pathways of, myelinated axons amidst the jungle of white matter tracts in the brain where only axons and glial cells (consisting of oligodendrocytes and astrocytes) exist.

DTI technology keys in on the behavior of water in the brain. The DTI scanner sends out magnetic impulses, and water within the scanned areas begins to oscillate in response to those impulses.

As a result, the affected water radiates radio waves that are picked up by the DTI scanner. These electromagnetic signals are translated by the scanner into the form of colored representations of water's behavior in the brain.

Water can flow along myelinated axons, or it can flow across those axons. The more tightly packed myelinated axons are (and this packing includes the presence of astrocytes), the more likely it is that water will flow <u>along</u> those axons rather than <u>across</u> them.

Research has shown that the more water flows <u>along</u> axons (indicating that they are tightly packed), the more intelligent a person is. In color-coded terms, the redder that the DTI-representation of water's movement in the brain is, the higher the IQ of the individual being studied will be, while the bluer or cooler the DTI-representation of water's movement in the scanned areas of a person's brain is, the lower the IQ of that individual will be (indicating that more water is moving <u>across</u> axons rather than <u>along</u> them, and, therefore, also indicating that myelinated axons are not as tightly packed).

Does the foregoing research indicate that intelligence is caused by the manner in which, and degree to which, astrocytes and oligodendrocytes pack in and around axons? Not necessarily.

Radios can be built with different qualitative capabilities – from being fairly simple to being far more sophisticated. Among other thing, the kinds of signals that can be detected, the precision with which those signals can be differentiated, and the character of the sound that can be produced in conjunction with those signals depends on the quality of the radio's construction.

However, the signals that are being received by a given radio are quite independent of that device. The quality of the radio will determine to what extent, and in what ways, those signals can be detected and translated into audible sounds, but the radios do not generate the signals being received.

Similarly, one might liken the packing of myelinated axons to radio quality. The more tightly packed a white tract of the brain is, the better will be the quality of its capacity to receive and translate incoming signals, but, nonetheless, a distinction needs to be made between a receiving device and the signals being received through such a device.

Normally speaking, one doesn't refer to a radio as having a high IQ just because it is capable of receiving certain kinds of signals. Consequently, it might not necessarily be the case that tightly packed myelinated axons in white tract areas of the brain are the <u>source</u> of intelligence even as those areas might have the capacity for receiving and modulating a wider and more precise array of incoming signals than white tract areas that are less tightly packed.

Densely packed white tract areas of the brain consisting of axons, oligodendrocytes, and astrocytes are correlated with higher IQ. Nonetheless, there is no causal evidence indicating that the materials making up those densely packed areas are responsible for intelligence ... even though those biological materials might play some sort of supporting or subsidiary role in relation to the manifestation of intelligence.

| Explorations |

The degree of myelination issue is also associated with another facet of higher cognitive functioning. In human beings, the last segments of the brain to become fully myelinated are in the forebrain, especially those aspects of the forebrain that are associated with impulse control, complex processes of reasoning, and considered judgment.

Can one conclude that myelination is responsible for impulse control, complex processes of reasoning and good judgment? Once again, the answer is: Not necessarily.

A radio that possesses uninsulated wires will tend not to function as well as a radio that possesses wires that are insulated. But while those wires might have a role to play with respect to the quality of reception, they have nothing to do with generating the signal that is being received.

A wide variety of neurological disorders – perhaps most of them -- are due to disruptions in glial functioning as a result of the presence of toxic substances, disease processes, and infections of one kind or another. The fact that cognitive impairment emerges due to the presence of dysfunctional glial cells does not necessarily mean that glial cells are responsible for cognitive functioning since it could be the case that dysfunctional glial cells merely interfere with independently produced cognitive processes, or glial cells might lend support to independently produced cognitive functioning when glial cells operate properly.

Nonetheless, in neither of the foregoing cases are glial cells necessarily the source of cognition even as they play supporting roles with respect to the visibility of that cognitive functioning in consciousness. This would be similar to the manner in which the components of a radio operate in relation to certain kinds of electromagnetic signals that are generated outside of that device.

Human beings who suffer from clinical depression, schizophrenia, and childhood neglect all show deficiencies in the development of white matter (glial cells) within the brain. On the other hand, animals such as rhesus monkeys and rats that have been reared in what are considered to be experientially enriching environments (a somewhat arbitrary notion) tend to show evidence of increased white matter -- or glial cells -- in, respectively, the corpus callosum and visual cortex.

| Explorations |

355

Once again, one should not automatically conclude that glial cells are responsible for higher cognitive functioning any more than better components in a radio are responsible for the character of the radio wave content that is being received. Nevertheless, the number and kinds of glial cells that are present might appreciably affect the performance of cognition, just as the number and kinds of components that are present might appreciably affect the quality of a radio's performance with respect to the signals that are being received from outside the radio.

Many people have assumed, on the one hand, that the individual and collective activity of glial cells, neurons, and synaptic circuits and, on the other hand, cognitive/mental functioning are one and the same. However, just as there is a difference between a radio and the ordered program content the radio receives (in the form of radio waves) and renders audible through the radio's circuitry and its speakers, there also might be a difference between the receiving capacity of brain activity/circuitry and the source of the content of the mental programming that is strengthen, inhibited, or otherwise modulated by that brain activity/circuitry in order for such programming to be rendered 'visible' to human consciousness.

Let's restate the foregoing ideas in a slightly different way. A great deal of brain activity can be tied to the monitoring (i.e., receiving signals in relation to certain kinds of biological, homeostatic functioning) as well as the regulating and modulating of bodily functions (in response to received signals) that are responsible for keeping an organism alive. Moreover, a great deal of additional brain activity can be tied to the receiving and modulating of sensory signals (e.g., visual, auditory, aromatic, tactile, and proprioceptive) that also play a role in helping to keep an organism alive.

Why not also suppose that a great deal of the remaining activity of the brain involving both neurons and glial cells (especially astrocytes and oligodendrocytes) also involves the effective monitoring (receiving) and modulating of other kinds of stimuli that are impinging on human beings? This latter kind of stimuli might consist of informational content (for example, such data might involve imagery, ideas, or symbolic abstractions) that are different from the kind of data that is processed through the usual sensory channel ways.

In short, much of the activity of the brain entails the monitoring (receiving) and modulating of a variety of signals from different sources that occur both within and without the body. Consequently, why suppose that the dynamics of neurons and astrocytes in, say, the inferior parietal cortex (the alleged, possible locus of genius) operate any differently. In other words, why not suppose that cells -- for example, in the inferior parietal region of the brain – receive, monitor and modulate certain kinds of incoming stimuli (for example, ideational or symbolic vectors) that are not sensory in the usual sense?

There is no direct, causal evidence indicating that the interactional dynamics of astrocytes and neurons generate abstraction, imagery, or complex thinking. The data is correlational in character.

However, what if we were to consider the brain as being, primarily, a very complex receiver and modulator of signals? Under such circumstances, claiming that neurons and astrocytes interact – e.g., in the inferior parietal cortex -- to receive and modulate signals of certain kinds (e.g., ideational or symbolic) becomes consistent with the activities of other facets of the brain that are dedicated to the receiving, modulating, and regulating of signals of one kind or another that are being communicated to, and received by, the brain.

Throughout history, human beings gradually have become aware that more and more kinds of signals are acting on us ... from: gravitational influences and electromagnetic radiation, to: weak forces, strong forces, and, possibly, even dark matter/energy. What if there are other, currently unknown, forces flowing through us that are detected and received by certain sections of the brain, just as, say, the sensory cortex detects and receives various kinds of vibrational energies that flow to and through us from certain dynamics of the physical environment?

From second to second, all manner of ideas, intentions, intuitions, insights, images, and emotions appear on the screen of consciousness. We have been led to believe – by many scientists and philosophers -- that we are the authors of such phenomenological occurrences, but what if this is not the case ... either partly or completely?

We don't know how ideas, intuitions, imagery, or emotions are possible. The etiology of the phenomenological contents coursing

| Explorations |

through consciousness is elusive and has been since human beings first began to focus on such matters.

Currently, many people believe that the brain somehow generates those ideas, intuitions, and so on. But, maybe, the brain doesn't generate such content (or, maybe, the brain generates only a fraction of that content) and, instead, merely receives it and frames it and modulates it as those kinds of signals flow through us from who knows where and according to who knows what kind of dynamics.

The foregoing possibilities seem relatively alien because we have been induced (via education, other forms of socialization, or some set of self-serving motivations) to filter experience according to certain ideological inclinations toward receiving, framing, and modulating the mental/emotional currents running through us. But, every generation has its mythologies (even so-called scientific ones), and a person often has to struggle against the tidal forces of those mythologies in order to continue to search for the actual truth of things.

| Explorations |

Mirror Neurons

For much of human history, the only way to explore the issue of other minds was through philosophical reflection. Beginning in the early 1980s, the foregoing situation began to change ... maybe.

In 1981 the neurophysiologist Giacomo Rizzolatti -- along with a group of fellow researchers in Parma, Italy – was studying the F5 area of macaque monkeys. This region of the brain is embedded in the premotor cortex which is a facet of the neocortex that is considered to be responsible for organizing and implementing actions.

Despite the fact that the F5 area consists of millions of neurons, it's focal concerns seem to be fairly narrow. More specifically, the neurons and synapses of F5 encompass actions of the hand -- such as selecting, transporting, holding, and pulling.

The F5 cells being studied by Rizzolatti and his colleagues were referred to as motor cells. Those cells specialized in the initiating of movement and, at the time, such cells were considered to be quite independent of cognitive functioning involving, say, sensory processing that was believed to be handled by other kinds of specialized neurons.

As sometimes happens in the lab, several fortuitous incidents occurred in Parma that began to alter the way researchers thought about how the brain operated. First, one of Rizzolatti's research associates – Vittorio Gallese – was reaching for something in the laboratory and a computer connected via electrodes to one of the macaque monkeys that was being studied began to register data, and during a separate occasion, another of Rizzolatti's colleagues – Leo Fogassi – reached for, and, then, grasped a peanut, and, once again, the computer hooked up to a macaque monkey began to chatter.

At the time, no one in the laboratory understood what was taking place. However, over time (several decades) the Parma researchers came to the conclusion that F5 cells were not only capable of initiating movements of the hand, but, as well, those cells were able, somehow, to perceive when such movements were taking place in other organisms (such as humans) even though the hands of the macaque monkeys were not involved in those movements.

| Explorations |

In addition, over a period of time, the Parma group discovered there were other regions of the premotor cortex that involved motor activities different from hand movements that behaved in a similar fashion to the F5 region. In other words, if a macaque monkey observed the actions of a human being moving, say, his or her leg, then motor neurons in the region of the motor cortex of such macaque monkeys that were capable of initiating those kinds of actions would fire even though the macaque monkey was not moving that part of the body.

The Parma researchers were also exploring a subset of neurons in the F5 region that seemed to become active when an object was close enough to be selected, held, and grasped. Thus, movement – either on the part of the monkey or in relation to the activities of a human being – did not have to be taking place in order for such neurons to fire ... it was enough that an object was sufficiently accessible for that object to be able to induce such neurons to fire.

The neurons that exhibited an inclination toward a certain kind of activity (such as grasping) came to be known as canonical neurons. Moreover, the process of inducing those neurons to fire is known as canonical neuron activation.

Thus, in three different circumstances, there were neurons in the F5 region of the premotor cortex that tended to fire. (1) When objects were sufficiently close to a macaque monkey to be grasped, then certain canonical neurons in the F5 region might fire even if the monkey didn't reach for the object. (2) If a macaque monkey saw the hand of a laboratory researcher reach for or pick up an object, then, neurons in the F5 region tended to fire. (3) Finally, if the macaque monkey used its hand to reach for, grasp, or hold an object, then neurons in the F5 region also fired.

Another group of neurons in the F4 region of the premotor cortex tended to fire when movements of the monkey's face, neck, or arm were involved. However, the neurons in that region also fired when the foregoing areas of the body were merely touched even though no movements of those parts of the monkey's body were involved, and, thus, once again, neurons that previously had been thought of in narrow terms of just helping to initiate specialized motor functioning seemed also to be connected, in some way, with the capacity to respond to sensory stimulation as well as motor movement.

In short, the Parma discoveries concerning the F4 and F5 regions of the premotor cortex appeared to indicate that data concerning sensation and movement were closely linked with one another. In fact, sensation, perception, understanding (of a sort), and movement were all being fused together in some fashion in those two regions of the premotor cortex.

The foregoing research makes a distinction between canonical neurons and mirror neurons. F5 canonical neurons are active in situations when, say, graspable objects are nearby but are not grasped, whereas mirror neurons are active when a macaque monkey sees someone else grasp an object but is not doing so itself.

Nonetheless, both kinds of motor neurons are involved in a process of perceptual reflection in relation to the environment. Canonical neurons reflect what is graspable in the environment, whereas mirror neurons reflect the kind of action that is taking place through another organism in that environment.

Canonical neurons reflect nearby objects that constitute possible candidates for grasping. Mirror neurons reflect actual movements of a hand (someone else's hand) in conjunction with objects that might be nearby or far away.

Moreover, there are different sets of canonical neurons and mirror neurons within the premotor cortex that are involved in reflecting different kinds of movement possibilities (in the case of canonical neurons) and different kinds of observable movements in other organisms (in the case of mirror neurons). For example, different neurons in F5 will fire when the grasping of a large object is involved than when the object to be grasped is relatively small (and vice versa).

Sometimes the same mirror neurons in the F5 region fire irrespective of whether the monkey itself seeks to grasp something or observes another monkey or human grasp that same something. These neurons are referred to as 'strictly congruent mirror neurons'.

However, there are other kinds of mirror neurons that fire when the movements performed or observed are only similar to one another

| Explorations |

rather than being identical. These neurons are referred to as 'broadly congruent mirror neurons'.

Given the foregoing perspective, one might wonder about how the DNA coding came about that gives differential expression to canonical neurons and mirror neurons. One also might wonder about how the DNA coding came about that gives differential expression to neurons that respond to large objects but do not respond to smaller objects (and vice versa).

In addition, one might wonder about how the DNA coding came about that gives differential expression to strictly congruent mirror neurons and broadly congruent mirror neurons. Finally, one might wonder about how the DNA coding came about that gives differential expression to the kinds of movements that are monitored in F4 regions rather than F5 regions (and vice versa).

Beyond the foregoing considerations, one might also wish to pose questions about the actual dynamics of any given instance of a mirror neuron or a canonical neuron in action. For example, how do such cells "know" when to fire?

What organizes the set of excitatory and inhibitory signals to form a synaptic circuit that gives expression to mirror neuron activity rather than canonical neuron activity (or vice versa), and how does this underlying source of organization acquire the capacity to 'know' how to accomplish this? What organizes the set of excitatory and inhibitory signals to form a synaptic circuit that gives expression to strictly congruent mirror neuron activity rather than broadly congruent mirror neuron activity (or vice versa), and how does this underlying source of organization acquire the capacity to 'know' how to accomplish this?

How do we know that a mirror neuron or a canonical neuron actually perceives that for which it is firing rather than merely being informed by some other mode of understanding/awareness that is actually monitoring those movements and merely relaying appropriate information to such neuronal groups? How are synaptic circuits associated with mirror neuron or canonical neuron activity translated into phenomenological representations?

| Explorations |

None of the foregoing questions and considerations is intended to find fault with the idea that macaque monkeys and human beings have the capacity to perceive possible movements in relation to nearby objects or to be aware of the movements of other organisms that are visible. Instead, the issues being raised in the foregoing several paragraphs all have to do with trying to understand the identity and nature of that which is responsible for the sorts of capacities being discussed.

Are neuron groups mirroring the movements of other organisms? Or, do neuron groups merely serve as physiological markers indicating that such mirroring activity is taking place in some other fashion just as the audible sounds arising from speakers serve as physical/material markers that signals are being organized and sent out from elsewhere and, then, received by a radio?

Does understanding arise from the pattern of neurons that are firing? Or, is the pattern of neurons that are firing a function of, or follow from, an existing understanding of some kind?

A graduate student working in the lab run by Giacomo Rizzolatti at the University of Parma conducted a series of experiments that appear to shed some light on the foregoing considerations. The name of the graduate student is **Alessandra** Umiltà.

Ms. Umiltà first set a baseline for comparison by running an experiment that already had been done. In other words, she charted the activity of mirror neurons in F5 when a monkey observed a person grasping an object.

In a second experiment, **Ms.** Umiltà had an associate make a hand movement as if that person was grasping an object ... but there was no object present to grasp. The monkey's mirror neurons in F5 did not respond to that movement.

Next, **Ms.** Umiltà placed an object on a table, and, then placed a screen between the monkey and the object that prevented the monkey from being able to see the object that had been placed on the table. Once this had been done, she had a colleague reach behind the screened- object as if to grasp it.

| Explorations |

Did the mirror neurons in the monkey's F5 region respond to the foregoing movements of Ms. Umiltà's associate? Some of them did, and some of them did not ... the split was roughly 50/50?

In the final experiment, the table in front of the monkey was initially bare. Subsequently, a screen was placed on the table, but there was no object being blocked by the screen.

An associate of Ms. Umiltà once again reached behind the screen as if reaching for and grasping an object. However, the mirror neurons of the monkey did not respond to the hand movements of the assistant.

In the latter two experiments, the monkey could not see what was taking place behind the screen. In the earlier experiment, there was a graspable object behind the screen, whereas in the latter experiment there was no object behind the screen.

In the next to last experiment (outlined earlier), roughly 50% of the mirror neurons in F5 fired when Ms. Umiltà's associate reached behind the screen where there was an object. When the final experiment of the series was conducted, none of the mirror neurons responded to the associate's hand movements going behind a screen.

A strong case might be made for the idea that understanding was informing F5 mirror neuron activity rather than the other way around. When the monkey understood that an object was behind the screen, then roughly 50% of the neurons fired because there was no way to determine whether, or not, there was any grasping of an object that was taking place behind the screen.

This indeterminacy (an epistemological condition) was reflected by the fact that roughly half of the mirror neurons did fire. However, when the monkey was observing a scene in which it understood that no object was on the table other than the screen, then this understanding informed the monkey's F5 region and, as a result, no mirror neurons fired when the associate's hand went behind the screen.

The monkey's F5 neurons were mirroring its phenomenological understanding of the experimental conditions. The monkey's F5 mirror neuron activity was responding to the monkey's state of understanding concerning the context in which hand movements were taking place.

| Explorations |

365

Is it possible that the F5 neuron activity was generating understanding in of itself? Yes, it is, but there are a variety of questions swirling about that sort of an approach to things.

For example, how do synaptic circuits know how to reconfigure themselves to establish an understanding that reflects the presence of an object rather than the absence of an object (or vice versa)? And, if synaptic circuits do not know how to reconfigure themselves in this fashion, then, what is it that does know how to reconfigure synaptic circuits in the F5 region so that those circuits will reflect what is transpiring on, say, a given table in the laboratory?

How do synaptic circuits know how to reconfigure themselves to differentiate between a context in which an object exists behind a screen that someone might or might not be grasping and a context in which an object does not exist behind a screen? How do synaptic circuits inform neurons not to fire when an object is not present but induce them to fire when an object is present? How do synaptic circuits understand the meaning or significance of their own circuitry, and how did synaptic circuits acquire the capacity for such understanding and self-awareness?

If one were not using neuronal activity and synaptic circuitry in the F5 regions as a way of trying to explain how certain kinds of knowledge and understanding are possible, one still would be confronted with variations on the foregoing questions. No matter how one proceeds methodologically, one would like to be able to understand the nature of the processes through which macaque monkeys and human beings are able to perceive, know, and understand a given set of circumstances, but be that as it might, trying to claim that F5 neurons and related synaptic circuitry account for perception, understanding, and knowledge is not a self-evident or slam dunk sort of hypothesis.

There are a lot of questions that need to be answered in relation to a neuronal/synaptic circuit account of understanding, and, currently, none of those questions has been addressed in a satisfactory manner. No one knows how neuronal activity and the reconfiguration of synaptic circuitry in, say, the F5 region of the premotor cortex produces knowledge, understanding and perception with respect to mirror/reflection dynamics involving hand movements, and no one knows what the organizing principles are that shape neuronal activity and synaptic reconfigurations concerning those movements, and no one knows how neuronal activity and synaptic reconfigurations generate phenomenology in conjunction with those movements, and no one knows how the DNA coding that underwrites such activity and reconfigurations came to have the capacity to give expression to an array of states of differentiated understanding in the form of neuronal activity and synaptic reconfigurations of one kind rather than another kind in relation to hand movements.

The firing of mirror neurons in the F5 region and the reconfiguring of synaptic circuits associated with those neurons clearly have roles to play with respect to the dynamics of perceiving and understanding hand movements. However, the roles played by such neuronal activity and synaptic reconfigurations might be entirely secondary and supportive rather than primary and generative ... just as the capacity of a radio is entirely secondary and supportive to the primary and generative character of the signals being received by that radio.

The neuronal activity and synaptic reconfigurations taking place in the F5 region might be the physical/neurological markers indicating that organizing signals are being received from elsewhere ... like a radio receiving signals from a radio station. Those organizing signals carry all of the information that shapes and orients neuronal and synaptic activity in the F5 region, and like a radio, the neuronal activity and synaptic reconfigurations translates that organizing signal being received from outside the F5 region in a manner that permits the latter part of the brain to reflect the presence of such signals.

Thus, mirror neurons do reflect something. However, the something being reflected is not the external context of, for example, hand movements in relation to objects on a table, but, rather, what is being reflected in the F5 region is the presence of an organizing signal from beyond the horizons of the F5 region that gives expression to an understanding of what is transpiring in the laboratory concerning objects, screens, a table, and moving hands, and, as such, neuronal activity and synaptic reconfiguration in the F5 region are reflecting the presence of that understanding rather than generating it.

| Explorations |

Consider an experiment by Leo Fogassi, one of the members of the Parma laboratory. Dr. Fogassi was interested in whether, or not, mirror neurons were capable of distinguishing between different kinds of intentions that were associated with hand movements that were roughly the same.

In one experimental trial, a monkey would reach for an <u>edible</u> item placed relatively near to the monkey, grasp that object, and, then, deliver the edible item to the monkey's mouth. In another experimental trial, the monkey would reach for an <u>inedible</u> object located where the previous edible item had been placed in the earlier trial, grasp the inedible item, and, then, deliver that object to a container.

In each trial, the monkey would: See, reach for, grasp, and, then, deliver an object to a receptacle (either a mouth or a container). In both experimental trials, the monkey would receive something edible – either in the form of an edible object being grasped and delivered to the monkey's mouth, or in the form of an edible reward that would be given to the monkey following the delivery of an inedible object to a container.

Approximately $1/4^{th}$ to $1/3^{rd}$ of the neurons being recorded fired irrespective of experimental trial conditions – that is, irrespective of whether, or not, a monkey was delivering an edible object to its mouth or the monkey was delivering an inedible object to a container. However, nearly three-quarters of the neurons being monitored responded with greater intensity when the monkey was delivering food to its mouth, while only approximately $1/4^{th}$ of the neurons being monitored fired more intensely when the monkey was delivering an inedible object to a container ... despite the fact that such an action would lead to being rewarded with an edible item.

In a follow up series of experiments, a human being sat in front of a monkey and performed movements similar to what the monkey had done in the earlier set of experiments. In other words, a human being would either: Grasp an edible object and, then, deliver that object to his or her own mouth, or the human being would grasp an edible object and place it in a container.

The only difference associated with the two actions of the human being was the presence of a container. In those experimental trials in which a human being would grasp and, then, eat an edible item, no container would be present, but in those experimental trials in which a human being would grasp and, then, place that edible item in a place other than his or her mouth, a container was present.

The foregoing experimental trials reflected what took place in the earlier trials involving a monkey doing what, now, was being performed by a human being. That is, the same set of neurons that fired intensely when a monkey grasped an edible item and placed that item in its mouth were also firing intensely when the monkey observed a human being doing the same thing, while the same set of neurons that fired intensely when a monkey grasped an item in order to place that object in a container also fired intensely when the monkey observed a human being doing the same thing.

According to some individuals, the foregoing set of experiments conducted by Leo Fogassi lent support to the hypothesis that mirror neurons gave expression to the brain's capacity for being able to understand the mental states of other organisms (e.g., monkeys or human beings). However, as noted previously, the activity of certain neurons in the F5 region does not necessarily generate such understanding as much as the activity might just reflect the presence of the epistemological or hermeneutical orientation of that kind of intentionality that might be generated through some other dynamic outside of the F5 region.

Intention is a state of vectored understanding. The dynamics of mirror neurons do not necessarily generate intentionality as much as that activity might reflect the presence of an intentionality that has arisen in some other fashion (within or outside of the brain), and, if so, the neuronal activity of mirror neurons in the F5 region is being shaped by the presence of that kind of understanding rather than generating it.

Once again, if one is going to entertain the hypothesis that mirror neurons are responsible for the neurological capacity to understand, say, the mental state of a human being or monkey, then there are a gaggle of questions that need to be answered in relation to the issue of just how the dynamics of mirror neurons are able to generate differential states of intentionality concerning, in this case, edible objects and containers. For instance, how do mirror neurons 'know' when, and under what circumstances, to become intensely active in conjunction with edible food items destined for the mouth rather than objects that are destined for a container? How do neurons in the F5 region of the premotor cortex in a monkey 'know' how to be equally active irrespective of whether the monkey is eating an item or watching someone else eating something? Why do approximately 1/4th to 1/3rd of the F5 motor neurons fire irrespective of whether an object is delivered to the mouth or to a container?

How do states of intense mirror neuronal activity translate into a phenomenological representation of that state of activity, and if there is no phenomenological understanding concerning the activity of those mirror neurons, then, in what sense can one say that mirror neurons are differentiating between various kinds of intentionality? How do mirror neurons acquire their capacity to focus on – and reflect -- one set of movements rather than some other set of movements?

Some fifteen years before mirror neurons were discovered, Andrew Meltzoff, an American developmental psychologist, discovered in the 1970s that even very young infants (as little as 41 minutes old) had the capacity to imitate the actions of other human beings. Steps were taken in the experiments of Dr. Meltzoff -- such as closely monitoring the life of the infant right up to the point of the experiment -- to ensure that the infant would not be exposed to the external actions that Dr. Meltzoff and his colleagues wanted to see how, or if, the infant might respond to such actions.

Demonstrating that infants could imitate the behavior of other individuals caused quite a stir. Prior to the work of Dr. Meltzoff, much of developmental psychology was dominated by the work of Jean Piaget who maintained, among other things, that children learned to imitate during the second year of life.

The revolutionary facet of Dr. Meltzoff's experiments was not just the time when children first started to exhibit imitative behavior, but even more revolutionary was the nature of the relationship between learning and imitation that was being proposed. Piaget believed that the capacity to imitate was acquired through a process of learning, whereas Meltzoff's experiments indicated that the capacity to imitate was the process through which infants/children learned.

| Explorations |

The capacity to imitate has been linked to language learning, socialization, acculturation, and the development of conceptual understanding. Many psychologists now believe that the notion of mirror neurons fits in quite well with the idea of imitation, and, from such a perspective, mirror neurons have been hypothesized to serve as a neurological basis through which certain facets of language learning, socialization, acculturation, and conceptual development are made possible.

For example, fMRI (functional magnetic resonance imaging) studies have been done which demonstrate that there are regions within the human brain that are anatomically comparable to regions in the brain of macaque monkeys as far as the presence of mirror neurons are concerned. These similarities in anatomical structure involve the F5 premotor cortex regions of the frontal lobe that have been discussed throughout this section of the third chapter, as well as mirror neurons that are located in an area known as PF in the parietal lobe.

One of the regions containing mirror neurons in the frontal lobe of human beings is Broca's area ... an area involved in the production of speech. This fact has led some psychologists to propose that speech/language is, in part, a function of mirror neurons ... for instance perhaps mirror neurons in Broca's area underwrite the ability of infants and children to imitate the speech sounds heard from other human beings.

Imitation is a fairly complex process. It presupposes the ability to be aware, to some degree, of the environment as well as a capacity to focus in on some particular facet of that environment, and, thereby, be able to differentiate one part of the environment from other aspects of that same environment.

In addition, imitation requires the presence of some level of interest or motivation that directs focus toward one dimension of the environment rather than some other dimension of that environment. Moreover, a form of interest or motivation must be present that is capable of sustaining attention for as long as are necessary with respect to whatever purposes are being served by the act of imitation.

Finally, if imitation is to serve as a means of learning, then, what is imitated must be remembered. Consequently, a capacity to forge a link of some kind between the activity of certain mirror neurons (the alleged process of imitation) and the memory of what is being imitated must be present.

How do mirror neurons accomplish all of the foregoing? What are the concrete molecular dynamics that make such capacities possible?

How did mirror neurons acquire the capacity to accomplish all of the foregoing? How did DNA come to acquire the organizational wherewithal to give expression to such capabilities?

There is experimental evidence indicating that the firing of mirror neurons in both macaque monkeys and human beings can be correlated with certain kinds of imitative behavior. Beyond such correlations, however, there is very little evidence indicating how the molecular dynamics of mirror neurons and associated synaptic reconfigurations (along with the underlying DNA coding) is capable of explaining the nature of imitative behavior.

One should not construe the foregoing considerations to mean that I believe that no compelling account of imitative behavior as a function of mirror neurons is possible. Someone, someday, might come up with the evidence to prove such an explanatory model, but that kind of evidence does not currently exist.

At the present time, the causal link (as opposed to the correlational link) between mirror neurons and imitative behavior is just an unproven hypothesis. We don't know whether the capacity to imitate somehow informs mirror neurons to fire in one pattern rather than another (much like an incoming radio signal from an external source informs a radio to give auditory expression to that signal in one way rather than another), or whether the activities of mirror neurons themselves give expression to the process of imitation ... and if so, then how.

Over the last 140 years, there has been a concerted effort by many scientists to force-fit mental functioning (such as the capacity for imitation) into a reductionistic framework in which mental phenomenon are explained as a function of the dynamics of neurons, synapses, and molecules. As has been pointed out in the first two sections of this chapter (i.e., Glial Mysteries and Mirror Neurons), as alluring as such a reductionistic framework might be, nailing things

| Explorations |

down has proven to be quite elusive, and in place of an explanatory account we only have a lot of unanswered questions (some of which have been asked in the foregoing discussions.

A great deal of evidence has accumulated – and at an accelerating pace – during the aforementioned 140-year period concerning the neurophysiology of the brain. Nonetheless, very little, if any, of that data has accomplished much more than give rise to some interesting and intriguing speculations (e.g., mirror neurons) concerning how mental phenomenology is generated as a function of neuronal, glial, and synaptic activity. To be sure, the dynamics of neurons, glial cells, and synaptic circuitry all have their roles to play, and on a physiological level a great deal is understood about how those kinds of processes work in relation to neuronal, glial, and synaptic functioning, but what is still missing from all that data is a plausible account of how those physiological processes generate mental activity and phenomenology.

The idea that the interacting dynamics of neurons, glial cells, and synaptic circuits cause: Consciousness, thought, language, reason, understanding, intelligence, creativity, and so on is not the best available scientific theory that we have to explain the phenomenology of the mind. At the present time, such a theory is no more scientific than is the notion that all of life can be accounted for through evolutionary principles since the evidence necessary to prove that kind of an account has not been discovered yet ... although such evidence might be discovered somewhere down the empirical road.

The truth of the matter is that, currently, we do not understand what makes the phenomenology of mind possible. We do know that physiological diseases, infections, seizures, and ablations can interfere with that phenomenology just as a defective radio can interfere with the reception of signals from a radio station or radio tower, but a properly operating, neurophysiological system does not necessarily mean that such a system is responsible for the presence of consciousness or thought anymore than a properly operating radio necessarily means that the radio is responsible for the signals it is receiving.

Memory

Daniel Tammet has been described as a prodigious savant – that is, an individual who, at a very early age, exhibited extraordinary intellectual, musical, and/or creative gifts. At any given point in history, there are only a very limited number of these kinds of individual who are known to exist (In today's world of more than seven billion people there are estimated to be between 50 and 100 individuals who cognitively operate in this manner).

In 2004 Mr. Tammet set a European record for being able to recite the first 22,514 numbers of π (3.14159 ...). This number is irrational (i.e., it cannot be expressed as a common fraction), and the number-sequence that gives expression to it does not involve any discernible, repeating patterns.

Mr. Tammet did not just spontaneously spout the record, 22,514 numbers. He spent a number of weeks preparing for that feat.

During the period leading up to his achievement, he focused on training an intriguing mental capacity he possessed. More specifically, he sees numbers as flowing, complex, colored, lit, textured, audible, multidimensional forms, and he used this ability to teach himself how to navigate his way through the numerical sequences of π.

In fact prior to the public demonstration of his facility with the numbers of π, Mr. Tammet composed a symphony of numbers made up of notes and chords of colors, shapes, lights, sounds, and complex dimensional forms. As he performed his musical composition in the privacy of his mind, he was led through the number sequence that gives expression to π (or, at least, the first 22,514 of those digits).

Consequently, in effect, Mr. Tammet was remembering more than numbers. He was remembering colors, shapes, sounds, textures, currents, meanings, and multidimensional forms ... which makes his feat of memorization even more impressive than just being able to recall several tens of thousands of measly numbers.

In effect, Mr. Tammet had constructed a mnemonic technique for remembering the numbers. He was remembering how to remember.

Memory involves learning. Learning involves memory.

| Explorations |

He had to learn a symphony of sounds, textures, colors, lights, shapes, and multidimensional forms. Once he had learned -- or taught himself -- the multimedia symphony, he could remember the number sequence of π.

Learning involves grasping the character, nature, properties, or structure (or an aspect thereof) to which a given experiential context appears to give expression. Memory involves anchoring what has been learned in a way that renders the latter accessible to awareness under various circumstances.

The multimedia symphony constructed by Mr. Tammet served as an anchoring process. When he ran through the symphony, the numbers flowed into awareness.

Mr. Tammet has little difficulty – relative to the rest of us -- remembering a numerical sequence that is 22,514 digits long. Nevertheless, he has quite a bit of trouble identifying (i.e., remembering) the faces of some people he has known for years.

Why does his mnemonic technique work for numbers but not for faces? Mr. Tammet doesn't appear to know the answer to such a question for if he did he likely would have provided an account for such differential abilities, but based on my reading of his book: *Embracing the Wide Sky*, he either doesn't know the answer to the foregoing question or, for his own reasons, he has decided to keep that answer under wraps.

Why does Mr. Tammet perceive numbers through colors, shapes, textures, sounds, and multidimensional forms? What makes such a capacity possible?

Mr. Tammet doesn't know the answer to either of the foregoing questions (at least not yet). Moreover, no one else knows the answer to those sorts of questions either.

Do Mr. Tammet's perceptions of numbers take place within his mind or within his brain or both? Does the memory of what is perceived in conjunction with, say, numbers reside in his mind or in his brain or in both?

Mr. Tammet doesn't know the answer to such questions. Furthermore, no one else knows the answer to those kinds of questions either.

| Explorations |

Do the dynamics of Mr. Tammet's brain give expression to the phenomenology of his mind? Or, does the mind somehow send signals that are received by the brain and -- like a radio -- the brain, then, translates those mental signals into discernible patterns involving neuronal, glial, and synaptic activity.

Mr. Tammet does not know the answer to the foregoing questions. And, at the present time, no one else knows how to answer those questions either.

There are certain individuals who have memories that are just as impressive as that of Mr. Tammet even as the memories of these other individuals appear to operate somewhat differently than does the memory of Mr. Tammet. For instance, the Russian neuropsychologist, Alexander Luria released a book in 1968 entitled: *The Mind of a Mnemonist: A Little Book about a Vast Memory* that discussed one of his patients – referred to as 'S' – who had the capacity to remember incredible amounts of information (often seemingly quite meaningless data) to which the patient had been exposed for only a relatively short period of time, and when tested many years later 'S' could, without review, recall the material in question (remember, Mr. Tammet spent a number of weeks creating a mixed-media symphony in order to remember 22, 514 digits of π).

There are other individuals who exhibit a capacity that is known as 'highly superior autobiographical memory (HSAM). If you give them a date, they can tell you what day of the week it was, and, as well, they can proceed to relate a variety of facts about that day concerning their own lives as well as some of the news of the day that occurred on that occasion.

People who demonstrate the HSAM capability do not have photographic memories. Thus, unlike 'S' above, they cannot be given a list of words or data to memorize and, then, many years later reproduce that list upon demand, but, on the other hand, such individuals don't seem to have exerted any kind of special effort to remember the things that they can remember in a largely errorless fashion many years later.

MRI anatomical studies have been done in conjunction with HSAM individuals. For example, the uncinate fascicle white tracts in the brains of HSAM individuals – these white tracts consist largely of glial cells and axons that pass information between the frontal and temporal cortices -- seem to be better connected than are the uncinate fascicle tracts of individuals without the HSAM capacity.

The foregoing finding has been suggestive since clinical work has indicated that damage to the uncinate fascicle has been correlated with impairment of autobiographical memory. However, conceivably, the more enhanced connections of HSAM individuals might be a result from the activity of such a capacity (similar to the way muscles get larger and better toned through exercise) rather than the cause of the HSAM capacity. Moreover, even if those white tracts are the cause of HSAM, nonetheless, precisely how the uncinate fascicle white tracts of HSAM individuals make such a capability possible is not known at the present time.

Another kind of memory phenomenon is known as "flashbulb memory". Flashbulb memories" involve allegedly very clear and accurate remembrances of events that tend to be emotionally laden.

As I am writing these words, the anniversary of the death of John Kennedy is just three days away. Around the time that President Kennedy was assassinated, I was playing squash at the Cambridge YMCA.

After finishing the game, I remember walking up the stairs toward the street-level common room where a fairly large number of people were watching television. I asked what was going on and was informed that the President had been shot.

I don't remember with whom I had been playing squash. I don't remember if I won or lost the game. I don't remember who answered my question, and I don't remember what happened after my question was answered.

I do remember walking up those stairs and seeing people watching the television. It was a flashbulb-like memory.

Is my foregoing recollection correct? Possibly, but it also might be a false memory.

Many people suppose that flashbulb memories are unusually clear and accurate. However, this is not always the case.

| Explorations |

One person who has studied this sort of memory is Dr. Heike Schmolck. One of her experiments involved exploring people's recollection of the O.J. Simpson verdict.

After locating individuals who had watched the giving of the Simpson verdict on television, she asked her subjects a series of questions concerning the verdict. The same questions were asked of the same people: Three days after the verdict, fifteen months following that event, and, again, 32 months later.

Dr. Schmolck discovered that after 15 months had passed, only 50% of her subject's responses reflected their original descriptions and approximately 11% of those responses entailed serious discrepancies relative to their original descriptions. 17 months later (at the 32 month mark), the degree of agreement between the latest memories of her subjects and the earliest accounts of those subjects (three days after the Simpson verdict had been delivered) degraded another 21% (to 29%), and 40% of the 32-month responses involved serious discrepancies relative to their original responses.

The foregoing study certainly indicates that memories tend to fade over time. Nonetheless, I am not certain that Dr. Schmolck's study is about flashbulb memories ... although some of her subjects might have had flashbulb memories concerning their recollection of witnessing the Simpson verdict.

Dr. Schmolck maintains that oftentimes our memories become corrupted in one way or another over time. Furthermore, she indicates that the longer the period is between some given event and the recall of that event, the more likely it is that some facet or facets of our memory have been re-configured by our brain.

Given the extent to which memories fade, degrade and become corrupted, one wonders if one should refer to such phenomenological entities as 'memories' at all. Determining where the truth of memory ends and its corruption begins is not necessarily an easy thing to establish.

A few years ago, my wife and I took a trip back to the town of Rumford, Maine were I had lived, for the most part, up until the age of 11. We visited the street where I grew up.

| Explorations |

I remembered how shocked I was concerning the length of the street -- where my family's house had been located – before it forked and divided up between a road that curved down toward a local variety store and the other fork that continued on toward the end of the neighborhood development. I remembered the pre-fork portion of the street (the portion that went by my childhood house) as being much longer than it appeared during the visit.

Last summer my wife and I, once again, traveled back to Rumford. As was the case during the last trip, we visited the street where my childhood home had been, and, this time I was shocked over how much longer the street seemed to be relative to my experience when my wife and I had visited my childhood town a few years earlier.

Which, if either, of the foregoing memories concerning the length of the street is correct? Was the portion of the street prior to the fork relatively longer or was it relatively shorter, or was it somewhere in between?

I have a memory of the street in question as being somewhat longer. I also have a memory of that street being much shorter.

Moreover, I have a memory of being shocked on both occasions. The memories of my sense of shock were sort of like flashbulb memories that are still fairly vivid, but I remain uncertain about the actual length of the street that runs by my childhood home ... the portion of the street that is prior to the infamous (for me) fork in the road.

We have beliefs and opinions about some of our memories. Sometimes, those memories are more a function of beliefs than they are of things remembered ... that is, sometimes we remember what we believe about the past rather than remembering the actual nature of the past about which we harbor beliefs.

Studies have been done concerning memory that indicate many people tend to retain the gist of events from their past but, over time, they tend to lose sight of many of the details of those events. One wonders how synaptic circuits differentiate between the gist of something and the actual details of that same something, and one wonders whether one can label beliefs -- about what we consider the gist of an event to be -- as 'memories' rather than merely being beliefs.

| Explorations |

Confabulation is a process of fabricating or distorting one's understanding about the past and treating that understanding as an actual memory rather than an invented narrative. The fabrication is done without any overt intent to deceive other people ... although, certainly, the first casualty of confabulation is the person who is doing the confabulating since like false beliefs concerning past events, the process of confabulation distances an individual from the nature of reality.

Jean Piaget -- who played an influential role in assisting the field of developmental psychology to work toward becoming a scientific discipline -- had a vivid childhood memory of being the subject of an attempted kidnapping. His account is quite detailed.

He remembers an assailant lunging out from some bushes that were near where he and his nanny were walking. He remembers that his nanny struggled (successfully) with the assailant and was scratched by the latter individual in the process.

Piaget remembers the policeman who interviewed them after the incident. He remembers the faces of the people who were milling around the vicinity where he and his nanny were standing shortly after the event.

It was an intriguing story, and therein lays the problem. The story had been made up by Piaget's nanny and was not an actual recollection of a past event.

The nanny did not confess the truth concerning the alleged attempted kidnapping until many years later and only after undergoing a religious conversion that induced her to come clean about her past. Yet, in the meantime – and this is the most interesting aspect of the incident -- Piaget seemed to have remembered the entire affair in considerable detail as an actual event and not as a story invented by his nanny.

When he was a child, Piaget and his nanny developed a consensus 'reality' concerning the alleged kidnapping incident. The nanny knew that the event was fabricated, but Piaget confabulated a 'memory'.

Sometimes (for example, consider the previously discussed issues of: HIV causes AIDS, SSRIs, Antineoplastons, and the theory of evolution), scientists seem more like they are involved in the process of confabulation than they are engaged in the process of science. They appear to sincerely believe (to give them the benefit of a doubt) that the narratives they are spinning constitute accurate reflections or memories of the available evidence when, on closer examination, their narratives seem more like confabulations involving that evidence.

Like Piaget and his nanny, sometimes scientists become committed to various editions of a consensus reality that has been cobbled together from mutually agreed upon fabrications of the data. Like Piaget and his nanny, sometimes such confabulations take on the appearance of reality because those appearances serve the interests of the individuals who have created such a worldview and not because those appearances give expression to the truth concerning the reality to which a given confabulation, or consensus reality, or worldview problematically alludes

Claiming that memory is a function of neurophysiology might be a modern form of confabulation or a form of consensus reality that is rooted in something other than the truth of things. If nothing else, there are many lacunae in the account (narrative) being given by scientists in relation to the phenomenon of memory.

For more than fifty years prior to his death in 2008, Henry Molaison was known only through the initials HM. The use of initials was intended to keep his identity hidden from the general public because, in his own modest way, HM became quite famous in the world of psychology.

In 1953, at the age of 27, Henry Molaison had surgery that was intended to treat a severe, potentially terminal form of epilepsy that had been creating havoc in Henry's life. During that surgical procedure the hippocampal region of his midbrain was removed.

The surgery cured his epilepsy, but he paid a price for this newly discovered relief. He lost the ability to establish new memories that lasted for more than a very, very short period of time.

HM could remember a great many things that had happened prior to his surgery (notwithstanding, of course, the troubles we all have in relation to recalling the past). However, HM could not translate present experience into long-term memories or learning.

If someone came into HM's room, introduced himself, or herself, to HM, provided some information to HM, left the room, and, then, re-entered the room a few minutes later, HM would have forgotten having been introduced to the individual and would have forgotten that a conversation had taken place prior to the 'stranger' having re-entered the room.

Under certain conditions, HM could learn new things – say a person's name. However, he wasn't able to anchor what had been learned in the form of a, more or less, permanent memory, and, therefore, he couldn't remember experiential events that took place in his presence beyond a few minutes.

As a result, HM suffered from anterograde amnesia. He couldn't form or recall new memories.

Prior to HM, the prevailing theory of memory maintained that experiential learning (whether episodic, factual/declarative, or procedural) was stored as memories in the two, hippocampal bodies (one hippocampus resides in each hemisphere) that are located under the cerebral cortex. As such, the hippocampus was considered to be primarily a place where memories were made, and, then, stored.

| Explorations |

However, as psychologists began to work with HM (and one wonders how the issue of informed consent was handled since HM would forget whatever he might have given consent to within a very short period of time), theories about the role of the hippocampus in relation to the phenomenon of memory began to undergo a substantial change. More specifically, the neocortex came to be seen as the place where permanent memories were stored, and one of the roles of the hippocampus was to assist the transition of short-term memories into the long-term storage facility residing within the neocortex.

In addition, many psychologists now believe – again, as a result of studies carried out in conjunction with HM -- that the hippocampus also plays a role in helping to preserve old memories. According to psychologists, as we age, little used information tends to fade because the synaptic configurations that are considered to store that information begin to break down.

Over time, HM exhibited a substantially greater degree of deterioration in remembering information that he once knew (such as the meaning and spelling of common words) than control subjects did who were similar to HM in age, education, and so on but who, unlike HM, possessed intact hippocampi. As a result, some psychologists hypothesized that the difference between HM and the control subjects could be explained as being due to the absence of hippocampi that, from time to time, might help HM refurbish or strengthen old memories as did – or, so, the hypothesis went -- normal, control subjects.

While studies can be run that indicate there are memory differentials between a person like HM who has no hippocampi and control subjects who do possess hippocampi, this set of facts does not necessarily prove that hippocampi create memories, or transition experience into long-term memories, or, over time, help to preserve or strengthen those memories. One can also show that there are performance differentials between a damaged radio and a functional radio, but, nonetheless, such differentials do not prove that radios generate the signal they are receiving.

Obviously, hippocampi play some sort of role with respect to memory. However, pinning down the nature of that role in a precise

| Explorations |

383

fashion is not necessarily a straightforward and easily understood process.

How do synaptic spaces become sufficiently aware of themselves to be able to reconfigure connections in one way rather than another? In other words, what is the nature of the process through which the hippocampus comes to 'know' or 'understand' how to recognize, arrange, and integrate meaning, value, and structural properties involving an idea, emotion, and/or experience into a pattern of neuronal firing and synaptic configurations that constitutes one kind of memory rather than another kind of memory?

How does the hippocampus 'know' what kind of synaptic configuration will constitute the memory of, for example, an emotion rather than the memory of an idea or belief or episodic experience? How do neuronal activities and synaptic configurations come to give phenomenological expression or phenomenological representation to a memory of one kind rather than another?

What are the specific dynamics that permit the hippocampus to translate short-term memories into long-term memories? How are memories transferred from the hippocampus to the neocortex?

How do synaptic configurations remember themselves? Assuming that a person does not have an eidetic memory (and very, very, very few of us do), what decides – as well as why and how -- which of the second-to-second synaptic configurations that are being generated in the hippocampus are to be transitioned into long-term memory storage?

Once stored in a relatively permanent fashion, how do synaptic configurations find their way back into awareness? What determines which stored synaptic configurations (i.e., memories) will be activated in any given instance? How does the hippocampus 'know' where to find the synaptic configurations it has helped transition into long-term memories that are stored in the neocortex in order, from time to time, to help strengthen those synaptic configurations?

How does the hippocampus 'decide' which memories are important and which are not? Why are some memories that involve apparently unimportant data transitioned into long-term storage whereas other instances of seemingly equally unimportant information are not so transitioned?

How did the hippocampus acquire the capacity to create memories? How did the hippocampus acquire the capacity to facilitate the transition of short-term memory into long-term memory? How did the hippocampus acquire the capacity to strengthen synaptic configurations in the neocortex from time to time?

| Explorations |

A number of years ago, Rodrigo Quiroga, Itzhak Fried, Christof Koch, Gabriel Kreiman, and Lela Reddy discovered something. While working in conjunction with a patient who had given consent for certain kinds of experimental research to be conducted during treatment for a neurological disorder, the foregoing researchers came across a neuron in the patient's hippocampus that responded vigorously when various photographs of Jennifer Aniston, an actress, were made visible to the patient, but the same neuron appeared to be indifferent to photographs of a number of other famous individuals.

The aforementioned researchers found a neuron in another patient that responded strongly when pictures of Halle Berry were shown to the patient and, in addition, that neuron also responded when the name of the actress was being typed on a computer screen visible to the patient.

Another neuron was discovered in one of the patients being studied that actively responded when images of Luke Skywalker were shown to the patient. Moreover, the same neuron responded to either the typed name of the science fiction character or if that name was spoken.

On the day following the discovery of the Jennifer Aniston neuron, the same experiment was repeated. In addition to once again being shown various pictures of the aforementioned actress, the patient also was shown photographs of Lisa Kudrow, a costar with Aniston in the television show *Friends*. The Aniston neuron responded to pictures of Lisa Kudrow as well.

Other individual neurons were discovered that similarly responded to related themes. For example, the neuron that previously had responded to pictures, sounds, and typed names involving Luke Skywalker also responded to images of Yoda, a fellow character in some of the *Star War* movies.

The researchers came to refer to neurons that fire in response to multiple, but related, stimuli as 'concept cells'. Each concept cell was considered to be part of a larger network of neuronal cells that give expression to a more detailed and complete representation of whatever theme or topic was being constructed through the interactive and collective efforts of the individual concept cells.

An ensemble of concept cells integrates information from the visual and auditory cortices. Other kinds of information also are integrated into the formation of a composite representation of this or that aspect of experience.

The foregoing concept neurons were found in the hippocampus. In the previous section on the patient HM, the discussion indicated that many psychologists believe – as a result of the experimental and observational data that was discovered by working with HM -- that short-term memories are created in the hippocampus and, then, converted into long-term memories that are stored in the neocortex. Consequently, if the latter theory is true, why are concept cells being found in the hippocampus, or, if we consider this issue from an alternative perspective, does the fact that concept cells are being found in the hippocampus constitute, to some degree, countervailing information concerning the theory of memory developed in relation to studies of HM?

According to some of the aforementioned researchers, the presence of concept cells in the hippocampus plays a central role in the translating of short-term memories into long-term memories that, subsequently, become warehoused in other parts of the brain. According to them, concept cells work with whatever has been triggered into awareness by the impact of sensory stimuli and, then, go about forging a long-term memory.

How do concept cells get triggered into awareness by sensory stimulation? How do concept cells 'know' what to do with the incoming sensory information that has triggered them into awareness?

Understanding how concept cells come to give expression to a concept remains something of a mystery. For example, how does a given neuron come to be associated with, or form, a particular meaning (say, Jennifer Aniston or Luke Skywalker or Halle Berry)? Does that meaning reside in the neuron, and, if so, how does this happen and what sustains that meaning in a given neuron?

The idea that neurons give expression to concepts seems at odds with another popular view held by many psychologists who contend that concepts are a function of synaptic spaces. On the latter view, neurons provide information that can induce synaptic spaces to reconfigure themselves, but when neurons have completed their task

| Explorations |

387

of generating an action potential that leads to the release of neurotransmitters into synaptic spaces, then according to the underlying theory, neurons return to their default position, and, as a result, their slate is wiped clean, so to speak, and, therefore, one has difficulty understanding how neurons give expression to concepts.

If neurons are firing in relation to certain stimuli, what, if anything, is taking place in the synaptic spaces bordering such neurons? Do the dynamics of neurons entail dimensional complexities beyond what traditional neurophysiology has been claiming for quite some time?

Is the neuron firing when shown pictures of, say, Jennifer Aniston because it is induced to fire by contiguous synaptic circuits? If so, what is the nature of that induction process?

How do synaptic circuits recognize an image being presented to a patient? Why do those circuits induce neurons to fire (if this is what happens)?

How do synaptic circuits give expression to a concept? How do synaptic circuits reconfigure themselves to give expression to one kind of concept (say, Jennifer Aniston related issues) rather than another kind of concept (say, Luke Skywalker related issues)? What organizes the reconfiguration process?

What is responsible for integrating different concept cells into a larger, more complete, and detailed ensemble or composite? What is sufficiently aware of the contents of different concept cells (and how is this awareness acquired and possible) to be able to integrate those cells into a coherent, meaningful, logical whole?

Does the brain (as a function of neuronal and synaptic activity) create the phenomenology of the mind? Or, is there some other dimension of the mind inducing certain neurons and/or synaptic circuits to fire when a patient is presented with a visual or auditory cue?

Does the causal flow of concepts run from mind to brain? Or, does that causal flow run from brain to mind? Or, does it run in both directions?

If one explores the circuitry of a radio or television set with an electrical probe, one can induce certain kinds of responses in the

| Explorations |

388

receiving device. However, the existence of such responses does not mean that a program being received by the radio or television set is generated by that circuitry.

The two (i.e., circuits and external signals) are correlated when considered from the perspective of the set. In order for a program to be made visible or audible, there must be collaboration between the signal and the set that is receiving that signal, but the signal and the receiver are different entities.

Similarly, the activities of the brain and the phenomenology of the mind are correlated. In order for the programming of understanding to be rendered visible, there must be some sort of collaboration between the mind (the station through which programming arises) and the set (i.e., the brain) that transduces that signal, but mind and brain are not necessarily coextensive with one another.

Some individuals (for example Stephen Waydo) have constructed neural networks by means of software programming. Some of these neural networks have been able to generate a means of recognizing and differentiating among a variety of unlabeled photographs and images of objects such as: planes, human faces, cars, and motorcycles.

The foregoing neural networks are described as having achieved their capacity to differentially recognize objects without being supervised by a teacher. Such descriptions seem somewhat misleading because the programming – however general it might be – that goes into stipulating the rules that govern the way in which the neural networks operate gives expression to the constant presence of a teacher (the programmer) that shapes whatever ensues once the neural network is permitted to reiteratively work out the possibilities that are entailed by the dynamics inherent in the rules governing a particular program.

In any event, the suggestion has been made that the foregoing sort of neural networks go about their activities in a manner that is somewhat akin to the way in which concept cells operate. Since no one really knows how concept cells go about their business (assuming that such cells exist), one really isn't in a position to determine whether, or not, neural networks and concept cells operate similarly to one another, and, indeed, concept cells (if they exist) might achieve the process of conceptualization in a manner that is very different from

| Explorations |

the way in which neural networks give expression to their own way of classifying the stimuli to which those networks are exposed.

| Explorations |

Recently, I watched a 'TED' talk (TED is an acronym for 'Technology, Entertainment, and Design'). Two neuroscientists -- Steve Ramirez and Xu Liu – gave the talk, and it took place in Boston, June 2013.

The presentation was based on research that led to several publications that appeared in the science journals, *Nature* and *Science*. The title of the *Nature* article is: '*Optogenetic stimulation of a hippocampal engram activates fear memory recall*,' and it was published in early 2012, while the *Science* report was entitled: '*Creating a False Memory in the Hippocampus*,' and the latter article was published in July 2013.

The ideas entailed by the foregoing articles and TED talk will be elaborated upon shortly. However, first, I would like to create a context for the critical reflection that will give expression to my comments concerning the research of the two aforementioned neuroscientists.

Toward the end of the June 2013 TED presentation, Steve Ramirez indicated that one of the purposes of their talk was to bring people up to date on the kinds of research that were taking place in neuroscience, as well as to acknowledge (even if only vaguely) the existence of various ethical issues raised by their research, and, finally, to invite people to join in the discussion with respect to their research. Steve's co-presenter, Xu Liu, also stipulated at one point near the end of the talk that their research was rooted in a philosophical principle of neuron science – namely, that, ultimately, mind is a function of physical stuff ... stuff that can be "tinkered with" and a tinkering process that is limited only by our imagination.

On the one hand, the following comments constitute my acceptance of the aforementioned invitation from Steve Ramirez during the June 2013 presentation for people to join in the conversation concerning their research. Consequently, part of my comments will address some of the ethical concerns that were alluded to by Steve Ramirez during the Boston presentation, while another aspect of my comments – perhaps the more central dimension of such comments -- will revolve around an exploration of the philosophical principle cited by Xu Liu that is at the heart of neuroscience and that,

| Explorations |

391

as indicated earlier, seeks to reduce mental phenomena to biological, material, or physical events.

Let's begin by providing an outline of the experimental model employed by Steve Ramirez and Xu Liu. Among other things, that model involves introducing mice to a few methodological bells and whistles.

Optogenetics (a word that appeared in the title of the aforementioned *Nature* article) is a term that – as the sub-components of the word might suggest – involves combining optical and genetic properties in certain ways. Essentially, microbial or viral genes are engineered to become receptive or sensitive, in some manner, to light or optical energies and, thereby, such genetic residues are enabled to, in effect, serve as a target for light sources (e.g., lasers) that will induce the target molecules to serve like switches that are capable of turning certain aspects of cellular functioning on and off when the genetically engineered concoction is injected into, say, mice and, subsequently, activated by laser stimulation.

In their presentation, Ramirez and Liu also point out that there is a biological marker or indicator present in cells that signifies certain kinds of activity have taken place in those cells. Therefore, part of the process of genetic engineering employed in the optogenetics technique is to take a molecular component that has a sensor-like capacity which is able to detect the presence of the aforementioned cellular indicator or marker signifying recent cellular activity and, then, splice that sensor component to the aforementioned molecular/genetic switch which, subsequently, can be activated and deactivated through the application of targeted laser energies.

In the case of the Ramirez-Liu experiments, the 'switch' portion of the genetically engineered component is channelrhodopsin. This is a membrane protein that controls the flow of certain ions (for example, sodium – $Na+$) into the interior of a cell. Modifying the flow of ions into a cell is possible because channelrhodopsin is a protein whose three-dimensional conformation can be altered when stimulated by, among other things, laser light and, in the process, open or close a membrane channel-way with respect to ion flow, thereby affecting the functioning of such a cell.

| Explorations |

392

To sum up, the general idea employed by Ramirez and Liu in their experiments is to identify cells that are involved in, for example, memory formation through the manner in which those cells will leave an activity signature or marker. This marker can be detected by the genetically engineered sensor-switch component and, this, in turn, will transform the cell into a target that is believed to have something to do with memory formation and that -- when deemed appropriate by the researchers – can be activated by stimulating the switch side (i.e., the membrane protein channelrhodopsin) of the generically engineered virus with laser light.

For quite some time, the hippocampus (a ridge section found along the bottom of the lateral ventricle portion of the brain – there are two such ridge sections ... one in each hemisphere) has been implicated (via an array of experimental and clinical evidence) as playing an important role of some kind with respect to memory formation. Thus, when one scans the title of the aforementioned *Nature* journal article – i.e., *'Optogenetic stimulation of a hippocampal engram activates fear memory recall'* – and understands that the term "engram" is a way of referring to a memory trace that has arisen through a hypothesized change (temporary or permanent) in brain chemistry within the hippocampus, then one is being told by the *Nature* article title that the Ramirez/Liu experiment is one which uses optogenetic methods (outlined previously) to bring about the activation (or recall) of memories involving fear.

In 2000, Eric Kandel received the Nobel Prize for research that helped establish the nature of some of the physiological dynamics that are associated or correlated with memory formation/storage in Aplysia -- a sea slug whose relatively large nerve cells made it a good candidate for trying to scientifically analyze what happens biochemically when learning or memory formation occurs in those life forms. To make a much longer story somewhat shorter, Kandel and other researchers discovered -- while studying the gill-withdrawal reflex in Aplysia -- that sensitization and habituation (which are both forms of learning and, therefore, constitute instances of memory formation) were associated with the release of certain kinds of molecules ... [e.g., c-Amp – the so-called second messenger of the cell -- serotonin (a neurotransmitter), PKA (c-AMP dependent kinase), and

| Explorations |

CREB (c- AMP response element binding protein) -- that appeared to play important roles in short-term and long-term memory formation, and, as well, the foregoing molecules seemed to be implicated in the processes that converted short-term memory into long-term memory.

The generation of the foregoing sort of cascade of biochemical molecules also was correlated with increases in synaptic complexity or connectivity. As a result, Kandel came to believe that changes in synaptic connectivity were indications that learning/memory was somehow being established through those synaptic enhancements, and, in turn, those changes in synaptic connectivity were some kind of a function of the cascade of biochemical changes that were taking place within neurons ... although many of the details were lacking with respect to the precise dynamics of that function.

Mice are more complex than Aplysia, and humans are more complex than either mice or Aplysia. Nonetheless, ever since the work of Kandel began back in the 1960s, a great deal more biochemical, physiological, cellular, and neuronal evidence has been generated that is consistent with the idea that when certain (a) biochemical changes in cellular physiology are correlated with (b) changes in synaptic connectivity that are correlated with (c) differences in behavioral activity over time, and when the foregoing three elements occurred in relatively close temporal (if not spatial) juxtaposition to one another, then the collective presence of those three elements was interpreted to indicate that learning or memory had been generated ... and, this remains the basic idea concerning the issue of memory formation irrespective of whether one is talking about Aplysia, mice, humans, or any other life form that is capable of exhibiting a capacity to learn or retain memories (short-term or long-term) with respect to on-going experience.

Naturally, the physical/material details of learning and memory might change as one moves from species to species. Nevertheless, a growing body of evidence lends support to the idea that learning/memory is entirely a function of physical/material events.

The Ramirez/Liu research that was outlined in the June 2013 TED talk is a continuation of the foregoing perspective. The two investigators took mice and surgically implanted a means of delivering laser stimulation to the hippocampus portion of a mouse's brain that

| Explorations |

also had been equipped with a genetically engineered 'sensor-switch' that could detect recent activity in cells that seemed to be involved in the formation of memories concerning fear in the experimental animals.

More specifically, the researchers placed a number of surgically altered, and genetically engineered mice into a chamber where an electrical shock was applied to the feet of the animals. As a result of this experience, certain cells in the hippocampus portions of the mice brains became active, and this activity left a biochemical footprint that was detected by the genetically engineered sensor-switch that had been injected into the mice through a viral host and, as a result, served as target candidates for subsequent laser stimulation.

The fact specific cells became active during the shocking process was interpreted by the researchers to signify that a memory had been formed. However, a number of questions can be raised concerning that kind of interpretation.

To begin with, what does it mean to say that a cell has left a marker indicating that the cell has been active recently? Active doing what?

The presumption of Ramirez and Liu is that the cellular activity gives expression to processes that are involved in learning or memory formation. However, one could ask in relation to such activity: Involved how?

How does a neuronal cell's activity generate learning or memory formation? Where, exactly, is the memory amidst such cell activity?

Is learning/memory in the cells that have been activated? If so, what is the form of the dynamic structure or process that is said to 'hold' the memory in the cells – whether considered either individually or collectively? Or, is the memory of fear to be found in the synaptic changes that follow from the changes in cell chemistry? Or, is it some combination of the foregoing two possibilities?

According to Ramirez and Liu, the process works as follows. First, the three-dimensional conformation of channelrhodopsin is induced to change. As a result, certain ions begin flowing into the interior of the cell.

In turn, the ion influx leads to a cascade of metabolic processes involving, among other things, c-AMP, serotonin, CREB, PKA, and other bio-molecules. Where is the memory or learning in all of this, and how did this cascade of cellular denizens come to signify, or be interpreted to mean, "fear"?

Kandel and others believed that the foregoing cascade of events was functionally related to changes in synaptic connectivity and that it was this transformation in synaptic connectivity and complexity that signified that learning had occurred or that a memory had been formed. So, does the memory reside in the synaptic connections, and, if so, how is the memory instantiated in those connections, and if the memory is held through those synaptic connections, what determines the holding pattern and what 'reads' that pattern to understand that it is a memory which holds one kind of learning rather another kind of learning?

What is the relationship between, on the one hand, cells that are active during memory formation (the sort of cells in which Ramirez and Liu are interested and for which they have genetically engineered their sensor-switch mechanism) and, on the other hand, changing synaptic connectivity (which people such as Kandel believed was central to learning and memory formation)? If memory is in the cells – as Ramirez and Liu seem to believe – then what is the significance of the changes in synaptic connectivity and how does what transpires in the cell shape, color, and orient those synaptic changes?

Alternatively, one might ask what determines which cells will be initially activated to become part of the fear learning or fear memory process? Or, what determines which biochemical, electrical, and physiological changes will take place within cells that will permit an organism to differentiate learning/memory experiences over time.

After all, if the same cellular components (e.g., c-AMP, serotonin, PKA, CREB, etc.) are thought to be at the heart of memory formation, then how are those components put together in distinct packages that would enable an organism to differentiate among memories? Or, what determines the pattern of synaptic connectivity that will take place and which can be said to hold – allegedly – this or that form of memory/learning, and what is it about the structural or dynamical character of enhanced synaptic connectivity that gives expression to memory?

One might also critically reflect on the nature of the differences between the original existential circumstances that led to the – alleged – formation of a fear memory, and the quality of that memory relative to the actual event. People who suffer from PTSD have vivid, intense, flashbacks, and, consequently, there seems to be a dimension of intensity associated with such flashback memories that is comparable to the original circumstances out of which the memories arose.

However, memories are not always as vivid and intense as the original circumstances from which they were derived or on which they are based. So, the fact that a given memory in a mouse is activated doesn't necessarily explain – in and of itself – why such a memory should necessarily lead to the response of freezing, and, therefore, one is left with the possibility that something might be going on in the experiment other than what Ramirez and Liu are hypothesizing is the case.

Mice appear to have some degree of awareness or consciousness. How do cellular and synaptic changes generate phenomenology or how does phenomenal experience arise out of those changes?

When a mouse receives a shock to its feet, does the mouse experience fear or does it experience pain? Or, is the mouse experiencing stress?

There is a behavioral response in mice known as "freezing". This consists in a set of behavioral dispositions in which the mouse remains very still and, possibly, vigilant when immersed in a given existential situation that is considered threatening in some way.

Once a mouse has been shocked and, then, subsequently, exhibits, freezing, this doesn't necessarily mean that the mouse is experiencing fear or remembering fear while in the condition of freezing (although this might be the case). Instead, the mouse might be exhibiting a form of coping strategy (which could be instinctual rather than learned) that is intended to either help avoid subsequent shocks or deal with the pain of having been shocked, and if so, perhaps the primary phenomenological component under such circumstances is merely

| Explorations |

397

heightened vigilance with an inclination in the mouse toward escaping or avoidance when possible.

Alternatively, freezing in mice might represent a state of shock. Possibly, a mouse that is exhibiting freezing behavior might not either be in pain or in a state of fear, but, rather, is just stunned and directionless with respect to how to proceed or what to do next ... somewhat like a prize fighter who has been rocked by a punch and is merely trying to stay on his or her feet but with very little focused awareness concerning just what is going on around him or her.

A variation on the foregoing possibility is that 'freezing' in mice might be a response to stress rather than an expression of fear. Pulled in different direction by various internal and external forces, a mouse might freeze up, and, consequently, the associated phenomenological state is one of stress generated through conflict rather than fear.

The fact of the matter is that we don't know what is going on in the phenomenology of a mouse during the state of freezing. Is the mouse afraid, in pain, in shock, stressed, uncertain, vigilant, wanting to get away, remembering a previous, similar problematic experience, or is the mouse experiencing some combination of all of the foregoing possibilities? We don't know.

Freezing is a behavioral disposition that is exhibited by mice during certain circumstances. Freezing in mice is a coping strategy and/or an instinctual behavioral response.

Learning -- or memory formation -- might play some sort of modulating role with respect to how that behavioral response manifests itself within different circumstances. Nevertheless, we don't necessarily understand what is triggering the behavioral response of freezing or what the precise properties and dynamics of the triggering event are.

Is the freezing response being triggered by a memory? If so, how does the memory lead to the initiation of the behavior?

Moreover, mice have a more expansive repertoire of behavior than just freezing. Sometimes they fight and sometimes they take flight?

| Explorations |

What if the freezing is an indication that the mouse is uncertain about whether to pursue fighting or fleeing? What if the freezing indicates indecision rather than fear, stress, pain, or shock?

Perhaps, freezing means different things to a mouse in different circumstances. On some occasions, it might be an expression of fear, but on other occasions it might indicate stress, indecision, or a vigilant wait for the sort of information that might push the mouse toward fighting or fleeing.

We don't know what, if any, phenomenology is associated with that behavioral response. We don't know what, if anything, the cellular and synaptic changes that have been described by neuroscientists since the time of Kandel have to do with the generation of that phenomenology.

There is no neuroscientist on the face of the Earth who has yet been able to demonstrate how one goes from cellular changes in neurons to enhanced synaptic connectivity, and, then, is capable of proceeding on to demonstrate how the phenomenology of memories of a particular character and quality arise from those cellular and synaptic changes. All scientists have established so far is that there is a correlation between, on the one hand, certain kinds of biological events and, on the other hand, the appearance of behavior that seem to suggest that learning has taken place or that a memory has been formed, but, unfortunately, some scientists have jumped to unwarranted conclusions concerning the connection between biological activity and the phenomenology of experience.

Consider the following idea. One can probe the electronic intricacies of a television set all one likes – even down to the quantum level. However, such analysis will do nothing to tell one where the content and structure of the picture comes from that is made manifest through the television set.

As is the case with television sets, so too, biology, cell physiology, and synaptic connectivity might play a necessary supporting role with respect to the phenomenology of experience. Nonetheless, biology alone might not be sufficient to account for the character of the content that is given expression through the phenomenology of experience.

A television set plays a necessary supporting role with respect to being able to generate a picture on its screen but that same electronic device cannot account for why the picture has the content, structure, and informational quality it does. To account for the latter phenomenon, one needs to talk about television stations, writers, authors, directors, actors, producers, and viewers ... all of which exist beyond the horizons of the television set, just as a proper explanation for memory or learning might exist beyond the horizons of purely biological considerations – at least as those considerations are currently understood.

Let us return to the Ramirez/Liu experiment. Under normal circumstances, when a mouse is placed in an experimental box, the animal exhibits exploratory behavior ... sniffing and scurrying its way around the interior of the apparatus.

If the feet of the mouse are shocked during the exploratory process, the mouse, subsequently, might begin to display freezing behavior. According to Ramirez and Liu, the mouse has formed a memory of fear, and this state of fear leads to the behavioral response of freezing.

However, as indicated earlier, we really can't be certain of what is taking place within the phenomenology of the mouse. The mouse might be experiencing fear, but, as well, the mouse also might be experiencing a phenomenology of vigilance, avoidance, stress, shock, indecision, and/or pain along side of the fear or instead of such fear.

If shocked for a sufficiently long period of time with no possibility of escape, the mice also might come to exhibit the same sort of 'learned helplessness' that Martin Seligman discovered occurred with respect to dogs when the latter animals were exposed to inescapable shocks. Under such circumstances, the freezing might be a sign of learned helplessness rather than a state of fear per se.

Learned helplessness is a more complex phenomenological state than fear since it consists of the integration of a set of experiences rather than being a function of just one experience. Yet, the differences in phenomenological state between fear and learned helplessness both might end up being manifested through the same freezing behavior.

| Explorations |

Ramirez and Liu arrange for the genetically engineered channelrhodopsin switch to be activated through the application of a pulse of laser light. This sets in motion a series of cellular biochemical and physiological changes, and, then, freezing behavior is exhibited.

What actually has happened? Has a memory been activated and, then, that memory causes freezing behavior to appear?

Even if it is the case that a certain memory has, somehow, been activated through the laser 'flipping' of the channelrhodopsin switch, can one be sure that the biological situation isn't somewhat similar to a television set that has been switched on, and, yet, the picture which appears is not – strictly speaking – caused by the turning on of the television set? Rather, the turning on of the television set is little more than a necessary precursor for gaining access to a picture (memory) that is generated through an entirely different process occurring outside of the electronic circuits of the television set.

Does the laser-activation of those cells that were active during the process of memory formation (when the unfortunate mice were shocked) represent the recall of a specific kind of memory? Or, does the laser-activation of such cells merely set in motion a sort of 'learned reflex arc' or 'behavioral circuit' that results in freezing behavior without the middleman of memory mediating between laser pulse and the condition of freezing?

We see the pulse of laser light being applied. We see the freezing behavior.

Ramirez and Liu hypothesize that the two events are bridged by the experience of a memory of a specific kind that has been activated by a pulse of laser light. However, they are unable to provide a plausible explanation that can take a person step-by-step from the point of initiation (laser stimulation) to the terminal point of behavior and show that what was transpiring involves a memory of a certain kind and the existence of that specific memory caused the observed behavior.

The fact of the matter is that Ramirez and Liu can't even be certain what kind of memory was laid down during the process of shocking. They claim the memory is one of fear, but they can't prove this because they can't eliminate the possibilities that the memory that formed

| Explorations |

might have contained elements of stress, pain, shock, or indecision ... and not just fear.

Or, perhaps, fear was not part of the original memory phenomenology at all. For example, one might argue that the original memory was one of pain, not necessarily fear, and, therefore, fear is a secondary emotional response to the perception or anticipation of pain.

Did the laser-activation of cellular activity give expression to a memory of pain rather than fear? If so, then the title of their *Nature* article is, at best, misleading, and at worse, it is incorrect.

Moreover, if the original memory was of pain, then, how does the secondary event of fear come into the picture? How does laser-activation of a pain memory bring about an emotional response of fear that, in turn, brings about freezing behavior? Is the experience of fear a second memory different from the memory of pain, and isn't it possible that pain might be associated with other secondary phenomenological states (e.g., stress, flight, fight, vigilance, indecision, and shock) that could just as easily lead to a freezing response?

Ramirez and Liu can peer into the structure of their experimental situation only a little farther than their laser-activation of the channelrhodopsin. They know that such activation will set in motion a cascade of biochemical and physiological changes (the sort of changes explored by Eric Kandel and others), and they know that those changes will be followed by changes in synaptic connectivity.

However, they really don't understand what any of this cascade of molecular actually means other than the fact that, collectively speaking, such cascades are correlated with memory formation. The rest is all conjecture and speculation.

During the Boston presentation, Ramirez spoke of giving the mouse "a very mild foot shock". One wonders why a mouse would develop a fear memory if the shock were so "very mild"? Clearly, euphemistical language is being used to mask a process that is more painful than the phrase "very mild" might suggest.

Nothing was said during the Ramirez/Liu presentation (by either the researchers or the audience) with respect to the ethical issues entailed by treating animals in the way they were treated during the

| Explorations |

experiments that were the focus of the TED presentation. This was true both with respect to surgically altering the heads of the mice to accommodate a laser delivery system as well as in relation to shocking the mice, and, so, the ethical issues to which the researchers were vaguely alluding during their presentation apparently involved something other than the treatment of life forms within the lab.

When I was an undergraduate, I participated in an experiment involving the delivery of shocks, and the nature of the experiment was such that I was the one who delivered the shocks to myself. For me, there was a clear phenomenological difference between those shocks that were very mild and those shocks that were painful and might lead to a sense of fear, stress, shock, and/or anxiety if they were to continue.

In a rather startling expression of egocentricity, Ramirez/Liu appeared to be talking in terms of what they considered to be a very mild foot shock … with nary a spoken worry about what the mouse might have thought or felt about the whole affair. Nonetheless, the word that appears in the title of their Nature article is "fear" – the article title didn't say anything about 'a very mild shock memory recall, ' but, rather, used the phrase "fear memory recall".

Presumably, there is a difference in learning and memory formation with respect to different kinds of stimuli. The phenomenology of the experience involving "a very mild foot shock" is likely to be different than the phenomenology of an experience involving a shock deemed to be capable of generating a memory formation of fear.

So, even if one were to accept at face value everything that the two researchers said with respect to the nature of their experiment and the way in which it supposedly tapped into memory formation, there is a question that remains. Was the memory that was established in the mice one of fear, or of a very mild shock, or of something much more complex?

What exactly was in that memory? The researchers claim that the memory was one of fear, but even if this were true, that fear occurred in a context.

In other words, the shocks took place in an experimental apparatus within a laboratory. The air had a smell. The box had a smell. There were sounds. The box had a feel to it. There were visual qualities present within the box. The surgically implanted mechanism had a 'feel' to it.

The foregoing context served as horizon to the experience of the shock. The memory was not just a matter of the alleged fear but, as well, the memory involved certain aspects of the context surrounding the shock.

How are the foregoing sorts of contextual factors coded for with respect to either the cascade of cellular activities that occur in connection to memory formation or with respect to the subsequent alterations in synaptic connectivity? This is not an insignificant issue because, as we shall soon discover, it plays an important role within the Ramirez/Liu experiment.

More specifically, according to the two researchers, if one removes a mouse that has been shocked in one laboratory box and, in turn, places that mouse in another, different box, then the mouse will start out by behaving as any mouse tends to do when introduced into a new environment. In other words, the male or female mouse will begin to explore the box and will not exhibit freezing behavior. All of this changes when a laser is used to activate the channelrhodopsin membrane molecule in those cells that have been identified by the injected genetically engineered sensor-switch as having been active during the process of memory formation in the shock phase of the experiment.

When the laser is used to re-invoke the 'fear memory' by changing the three-dimensional conformation of the channelrhodopsin that leads to the flow of ions into the cell and sets in motion a cascade of biochemical and physiological events associated with memory, then mice that previously have been shocked will exhibit the freezing response. According to Ramirez and Liu, the mouse is being induced to remember the original experience of fear and responds accordingly – that is, the mouse freezes.

In their Boston presentation, Ramirez and Liu discuss how they have added a few wrinkles to their experimental design. For example, they talk about, first, taking surgically altered and genetically engineered mice and placing them in a blue box, and, then, identifying the cells that are active in the presence of such 'blueness'.

Before proceeding on with an account of the experiment, it seems to be appropriate to pause briefly and ask a question. How does one know that the cellular activity being identified by the researchers through their genetically engineered sensor-switch has to do specifically with blueness rather than some other feature of the experimental set-up, and, moreover, even if one were to accept the idea that the cellular activity has something to do with retaining a memory of blueness, once again, one can raise the question of what, precisely, such activity has to do with memory formation?

How – specifically -- is 'blueness' being encoded via the cascade of cellular events that are occurring during the learning of, or memory formation concerning, blueness, and how does this particular package or set of cellular events translate into unique changes in synaptic connectivity concerning the issue of blueness? Moreover, how is this aspect of learned or remembered blueness separated from, or integrated into, the context of other sensory experiences that form the context surrounding the experience of blueness?

In addition, one might ask why certain cells are selected for the memory of blueness, while other cells busy themselves with the memory of different sorts of sensory modalities. Or, one also might wonder how the work of an array of active cells concerning different facets of a experiential context become integrated to generate a unified phenomenological experience that can be understood in one way rather than another by a given life form. [By way of a personal aside, for reasons obvious and not so obvious, all of this talk about red and blue boxes led to my thinking about the contents of the so-called *Blue and Brown Books* of Ludwig Wittgenstein that I read as an undergraduate ... my memory seems to be somewhat colorblind].

Now, let's return to the Ramirez/Liu experiments. In the first stage of one of their experiments involving a blue box, nothing happens to the mice. They just get to explore the box.

In the next phase of the experiment, the mice are placed in a red box. While in the red box, a laser pulse activates the cells that were identified as being active during the blue-box experience, and, as well, the mice are given – I am quite certain – a very mild foot shock to

| Explorations |

generate a 'fear' memory that is now associated with a re-invoked or recalled memory of the blue box.

In the final state of this experiment, the mice are placed back in the blue box where they have never been shocked. Yet, as soon as the mice are placed in the blue box, they exhibit freezing behavior.

Ramirez and Liu maintain they have created a false memory in such mice. I have a little difficulty understanding how the two researchers arrived at their conclusion.

But, let's deal with first things first. Ramirez and Liu speak about an association being established between two things. On the one hand, there is the re-invoked memory of blueness, and, on the other hand, there is the shock that is given in the red box while the memory of blueness is re-invoked.

There is no false memory that is being created in the foregoing scenario. The association being established is not a false memory, but, rather, it constitutes the blending together of two facets of the red box context – namely, a shock and the experience of blueness.

This is an example of classical conditioning. One takes a stimulus – blueness – and pairs it with another stimulus – shock – to generate a behavioral response – freezing -- that can be initiated by the presence of blueness alone even without a shock being administered, and even though blueness had never before been experienced as being 'fear-stress-shock-pain-avoidance' related.

The mice are not misremembering the original experience of blueness. They have been taught something new during the time spent in the red box ... that is, they have been taught how the presence of blue can be threatening, and when the mice are placed back into the environment of the blue box, they are induced to enter into the condition of freezing because of what they learned in the red box.

Beyond the foregoing considerations, there is the problem of understanding the dynamics of association. How does the memory of association work?

Many individuals talk in terms of the capacity of various life forms to associate different aspects of experience whether through temporal and spatial juxtaposition. We all know that such a phenomenon is real, and we all note evidence of its presence through a wide variety of circumstances involving human beings and other life forms.

Nevertheless, no one really knows how it works. No one understands the dynamics of association, but, instead, we only acknowledge the result of those dynamics.

How does the memory of blueness and the memory of being shocked – very mildly -- enter into a new, modified understanding within the context of a the red experimental box that is capable of generating, say, the freezing response in mice? How does what happens in those cells that are active during the formation of a memory of blueness become intertwined with what happens in those cells that are active during the experience of being shocked?

One might suppose that there are many neuronal cells that are active during any given experience. Why is blueness singled out as the feature that is to be mixed with the sensory experience of being shocked?

Phenomena such as generalization do occur (as is evidenced by my previously noted aside concerning Wittgenstein's *Blue and Brown Books* in which some sort of 'colorblind' generalization took place in relation to the blue and *red* boxes of the Ramirez and Liu experiments). Various life forms do transfer certain aspects of learning or memory developed in one context to a broader array of contexts that are in some, as of yet, mysterious way acknowledged to be -- or arbitrarily designated as being -- similar to the original context of learning.

Unfortunately, we don't really know or understand much about how any of this actually works. We see all kinds of correlations, but we have little idea of how everything fits together and generates or causes this or that memory or this or that understanding or this or that belief or this or that instance of learning, and this remains true even with respect to the simplest of cases involving learning and memory formation such as in instances of: habituation, sensitization, association, conditioning, or generalization.

The experiments conducted by Ramirez and Liu really haven't gotten us any closer to understanding the specific dynamics of either memory, learning, or how the phenomenology surrounding such experience arises. More specifically, their work hasn't helped demonstrate how to bridge the gap between, on the one hand, changes in the internal biochemistry or physiology of neurons and synaptic connectivity, and, on the other hand, the actual, causal dynamics of learning and memory as a function of the former material changes.

Furthermore, Ramirez and Liu have not been able to explain in a plausible, consistent, rigorous, coherent fashion how changes in neurons and synaptic connectivity become manifested in phenomenological, conscious states that are characterized by differential qualities that are integrated into a unitary sense of experience concerning reality. In addition the foregoing considerations are quite independent of whether such unified phenomenology accurately reflects the nature of some aspect of that reality.

Ramirez and Liu only have provided us with some more correlations. These might be interesting correlations, but, in the end, that is all they are.

The methodological techniques that have been devised by and are used by Ramirez and Liu to demonstrate the existence of certain correlations are quite innovative. Nonetheless, the bottom line on all this ingenious innovativeness is that nothing which they have said in their TED talk or in the corresponding articles gets us any closer to understanding how the dynamics of memory and learning work, and, certainly nothing that they have said demonstrates the truth of the underlying philosophical premise that mind can be shown to be a function of purely material events ... events that can be tinkered with.

This leads to a further issue. Toward the end of the Boston TED talk, Xu Liu talked about how we are living in very exciting times in which science is not tied down by any arbitrary limits with respect to the prospect of progressing in our understanding and knowledge concerning such phenomena as memory and learning. In effect, science is bound only by our imaginations.

Unfortunately, the imaginations of some people are more problematic and disturbing than are the imaginations of other people. The Defense Department subsidizes a great deal of the scientific work that is taking place in academia and in the corporate sector (both are integral parts in the military-industrial complex), and, as luck would have it, the people who are in control of that Department imagine all kinds of things with respect to the arbitrary uses to which scientific research can be put -- uses that end up killing, maiming, hurting, and enslaving people ... both foreign and domestic.

Although, in my opinion, the research of Ramirez and Liu has not demonstrated the generation of false memory, that research has revealed some possible techniques for interfering with the minds of life forms. How long will it be before the research of people like Ramirez and Liu is weaponized and applied against whomever the people in power deem to be appropriate subjects.

We don't live just in the exciting times about which Liu enthuses. We also live in very perilous and authoritarian times ... times in which all too many governments are quite prepared to do whatever is necessary to stay in power, control resources, and induce citizens to serve that power. Ramirez and Liu are very naïve if they believe their research is only about scientific progress, and they also are in denial if they suppose that they do not have a moral responsibility with respect to the possible applications of their work.

Speaking vaguely about the ethical implications and ramifications of their research work after the fact has got things backward. They should have been concerned about those implications before they did their research, and, in fact, those ethical deliberations should have impacted their decision about whether, or not, such research should have been pursued at all.

The Ramirez/Liu research dredged up memories within me of Michael Crichton's book: *The Terminal Man*. Like the scientists in the book, all too many neuroscientists today are full of swagger and arrogance with respect to their technical proficiency and ingeniousness, and, unfortunately, like the scientists in Crichton's book, all too many of them appear to be ignorant of their own ignorance concerning the many lacunae between what they believe they know and the actual nature of reality.

The scientists in Crichton's book believed they knew what they were doing. They didn't, and their ignorance cost the lives of quite a few fictional people.

The neuroscientists of today seem to believe they know what they are doing. This is not necessarily the case, and the problematic

| Explorations |

ramifications of that ignorance might manifest itself in potentially tragic ways only after problems of one kind or another have arisen.

The many physicists who worked on the Manhattan project believed they knew what they were doing. Few of them grappled with the horrors of Hiroshima or Nagasaki before the fact except, perhaps, Oppenheimer who quoted from the Bhagavad-Gita after witnessing the Trinity test: "Now I am become Death, the destroyer of worlds".

There were many physicists and other scientists who worked to bring nuclear technology into the real world. Those scientists seem unconcerned – before the fact -- about the possibilities of Three Mile Island, Chernobyl, and Fukushima becoming future realities, or about the problems surrounding the disposal of nuclear wastes, or the use of depleted uranium as weapons of mass destruction.

T.S. Eliot said: "Where is the wisdom we have lost in knowledge? Where is the knowledge we have lost in information?" Ramirez and Liu, along with a great many other researchers have a lot of information but do not seem to possess much in the way of either knowledge or, more importantly, wisdom concerning the ethical implications of what they are doing.

More specifically, I worry about people – such as Ramirez and Liu – who believe they understand what is going on with their experiments when this just might not be the case. The ramifications of ignorance are possibilities to which the foregoing discussion have lent some degree of credibility.

In the first chapter of this book, evidence was put forth concerning the terrible consequences that have ensued, and are continuing to ensue, from the self-serving arrogance of the pharmaceutical industry with respect to its psychoactive concoctions that are based on a form of technical wizardry that is entirely devoid of any real understanding concerning the human mind, but, is, instead, rooted in a bevy of correlations that are not understood. Yet, quite recklessly, the pharmaceutical industry and the FDA are permitting -- if not rushing -- all manner of drugs into the market that are generated through spurious science in their attempt to create life-time dependencies (rather than cures) with respect to this or that psychoactive drug ... many of which entail potentially horrendous properties.

| Explorations |

As people such as Joanna Moncrieff (*The Myth of the Chemical Cure*) a psychiatrist from England, and Peter Breggin (*Medication Madness*), a psychiatrist from the United States, have pointed out, neuroscientists have very little understanding of how psychoactive drugs metabolize within human beings or how the actual dynamics of the 'effects' of those drugs take place. The existence of side effects lends support to the foregoing claim.

I know of no pharmacological study that begins with a set of predictions concerning the precise array of side effects that will arise in conjunction with the use of a given psychoactive agent. Scientists do not make such predictions because they don't actually know what happens in people when those drugs are taken.

For instance, there are many scientists and clinicians who speak in terms of the idea of "chemical imbalances' being the cause of various emotional and mental problems, and this mythology is present in the marketing campaigns for an array of pharmaceutical products being advertised on television. Let's consider the case of SSRI – that is, selective serotonin re-uptake inhibitors.

I don't know of any neuroscientist who has provided a convincing argument about how the absence of serotonin causes depression or how the absence of serotonin leads to the sorts of symptoms that are associated with clinical depression. Moreover, there is also the rather embarrassing fact that when independent, double blind studies are done concerning the efficacy of SSRIs, those drugs have been shown to be no more effective than placebos.

In his book *Embracing the Wide Sky*, Daniel Tammet (introduced earlier) claims that scientists now know (is this the same kind of 'knowing' that scientists previously had with respect to serotonin?) that antidepressants work not because those drugs help maintain high levels of serotonin in certain synaptic spaces of the brain but, instead, antidepressants work because they enhance the production of trophic factors (a class of proteins that includes molecules such as NGF or Nerve Growth Factor) that assists neurons to grow. Even if antidepressants do lead to the production of greater numbers of trophic factors, how does that production alleviate the symptoms of depression?

| Explorations |

Currently, there is no theory of which I am aware that credibly and viably accounts for why the problematic growth of neurons leads to depression (if this is what happens) or accounts for how such problematic nerve growth begins in the first place. Moreover, if depression is due to the problematic growth of certain groups of neurons, someone will have to come up with an explanation for why Electric Convulsive Therapy (ECT) -- which tends to destroy the growth of neurons -- appears to sometimes help relieve some of the symptoms of depression despite such destruction.

Moreover, just what is it that the enhanced growth of certain groups of neurons accomplishes? How does that growth alleviate the symptoms of depression, and, if enhancing the growth of neurons is all that antidepressants do, then, how does one explain the onset of 'medication madness' (see the work of Peter Breggin) in people who take antidepressants.

Finally, if scientists and doctors didn't initially know what was going on when people took antidepressants (after all, according to Tammet, it was only later that scientists discovered that antidepressants allegedly worked not because of the presence of serotonin but because of the stimulation of trophic factors like NGF), then why were doctors prescribing or administering so-called antidepressants at all? There seems to be a very unethical dimension to the practice of prescribing and administering drugs when the metabolic ramifications that ensue from the consumption of those drugs are not understood.

As Peter Breggin, Joanna Moncrieff, and others have documented in considerable detail, antidepressants seem to work by masking problems, not curing them. In the process, such psychoactive agents tend to dull, if not destroy, many facets of emotional life, consciousness, and human sensitivity.

Unfortunately, all too many so-called professionals seem to have mistaken the loss of one's humanity for the alleged effectiveness of a given drug with respect to a change in a user's symptom profile. Certain symptoms might disappear, but other problems surface, and people become so caught up in the former phenomenon that they fail to see the emergence of the latter kinds of problems.

Scientific methodologies are one thing. Conjecturing about the significance and meaning of the experimental results that are run through those methodologies is quite another issue altogether.

In line with the foregoing comments, I have a lot of concerns about the work of Ramirez and Liu because I am not convinced that they understand what they are doing ... anymore than I believe that all too many scientists know what they doing when it comes to psychoactive drugs like SSRIs. For example, I do not believe that Ramirez and Liu have developed a theory of memory or learning per se although Ramirez and Liu certainly believe that they are working at the cutting edge of such a theory.

Seemingly, what they have is a series of conjectures based on a problematic understanding about, and interpretation of, the correlational dimensions of their own experiments along with the experiments of other individuals working in the area of mind/brain research. The issue before us is the following one.

Are neuroscientists on the right track with respect to their attempt to reduce mental phenomena to some set of physical dynamics and, therefore, the work of researchers like Ramirez and Liu represent important steps along an inevitable path that will take us to the promised land of full understanding and a complete explanatory account of how mental phenomena are all functions of underlying biological events? Or, alternatively, are neuroscientists on an asymptote path that generates ever more tantalizing correlations that will never permit them to reach the promised land of complete explanations and, instead, will only enable them to provide flawed accounts of mental phenomena?

I believe the foregoing critical analysis of the Ramirez and Liu experiments leads to more than a few questions about just what it is that neuroscientists know with respect to the nature of mental phenomena such as memory formation. Maybe, eventually, they will reach the promised land of 'Full Explanations', but right now they are stuck in the entangled underbrush that populates the land of descriptions that are based on proliferating correlations, and they don't seem to have much, if any, real understanding, knowledge, or wisdom concerning the actual nature of the mind.

The Computational Mind

There are many individuals today who believe that the brain and the mind are synonymous entities. For such people, the term "mind" is just a more philosophical and archaic way of referring to the material and physical activities of the brain.

In other words, before the science of neurophysiology arose, the word "mind" was used as a catchall sort of notion that encompassed whatever theories (philosophical, theological, mythological, and/or psychological) that, supposedly, were associated with, or attempted to account for, mental phenomenology. However when the disciplines of information science, molecular biology, evolution, and neuroscience began to dominate the cognitive landscape, the brain was considered as the source and cause of all mental phenomenology, and, consequently, the word "mind" was relegated to being merely a linguistic reminder of how people in the past used to approach such phenomenology.

Since the advent of computers, many neurophysiologists (but not necessarily all of them) also often likened the activities of the brain/mind to an information-processing medium. Within such a context, reasoning, thinking, interpreting, and understanding are construed as computational processes without necessarily implying that the brain is just some kind of computer.

From the computational perspective, the brain constitutes a set of specialized modules that solve certain kinds of problems that are important for survival. Such modules are described as being the end product of natural selection, and, therefore, some proponents of the computational perspective claim that natural selection helps to design the computational modules inherent in the brain.

"Evolutionary psychology" is a phrase that certain individuals use (the term was coined by the psychologist Leda Cosmides and the anthropologist John Tooby) as a way of referring to the foregoing perspective. When engaged through those sorts of filters, psychology becomes a process of trying to reverse engineer the modules of the brain to understand how those processes serve evolutionary interests.

In general terms, evolutionary psychologists believe that the modules of the brain arose over long periods of time as a result of:

| Explorations |

Copying errors during the process of replication, and/or mutational events, and/or the combinatorial powers of sexual reproduction that individually, or collectively, resulted in a capacity that was selected because of its ability to fit in with existing, material conditions and, thereby, assist not just the organism possessing such capabilities to survive but, more importantly, if that capacity was transmitted to other members of the general species population to which that individual belonged, then such a capacity would render the gene pool of that population to be more evolutionarily viable.

To say that natural selection is responsible for the designing of the brain (or any of its modules) is misleading. The foregoing claim would still hold even if evolutionary theory were someday discovered to give expression to an accurate depiction concerning the origin of life together with the processes of speciation that has been alleged to ensue from that origin … which, as pointed out in Chapter Two, is a very contentious proposition.

A biological capacity can only be selected if, in a given environmental and ecological context, that capacity is functional (or, at least, not dysfunctional). Although the functionality of a given biological capacity is due to the interactional dynamics of both the nature of such a capacity as well as the nature of the environment in which that capacity emerges, nevertheless, the environment has had nothing to do with that capacity having the properties it does since those properties are, supposedly, largely due to the vagaries of: copying errors due to chance happenings, random mutations, and the luck of the draw with respect to reproductive combinatorics.

The "design" of the biological capacity that allegedly arises out of the foregoing array of random events exists <u>prior</u> to its being selected by the state of environmental conditions. Indeed, the prevailing environmental circumstances select that design precisely because it is compatible with existing environmental conditions.

On occasion, some evolutionary biologists misuse the term "evolutionary pressure" in an attempt to explain why a given biological capacity arises in a given set of environmental circumstances. However, not only is this sort of terminology rather somewhat Lamarckian in character, and, therefore, at odds with a Darwinian approach to evolutionary theory, but, even more importantly, the foregoing terminology (i.e., evolutionary pressure) is not supported by any plausible, evidentially based account concerning the specific nature of the dynamics that permits the environment to "pressure" an organism to come up with new capacities that are compatible with a given environment.

Of course, after a string of events involving natural selection takes place, there is a sense in which one might talk about the properties of the organism (or population) that constitute the focal point of that kind of series of selection events as having been shaped, to a degree, by the environmental circumstances that continue to support the existence of an organism or population with those kinds of properties. Nonetheless, the foregoing sense of shaping only involves the determination of which features are being selected and has nothing to do with designing those features ... the "designing" process has taken place before natural selection begins to act, and such existing designs are what natural selection acts on.

Notwithstanding the foregoing considerations, treating the mind as being a function of computational processes is intended to give emphasis to the idea that the brain processes information. The patterns, relationships, meanings, and logical currents inherent in that information can be studied – or so it is argued – independently of the media through which those properties arise.

According to advocates of the computational theory of mind, such an approach permits a long-standing puzzle in philosophy and psychology to be solved. More specifically, the computational theory of mind supposedly permits one to bring together two very different kinds of things into one, consistent, and coherent explanatory account – that is, non-material ideas such as intention, beliefs, and meaning can be translated into material processes within the brain (and vice versa).

In other words, beliefs, ideas, intentions, and meanings give expression to information. Moreover, from the perspective of the computational theory of mind, Information can be instantiated in the form of symbols that represent physical realities ... such as the firing of neurons and the process of configuration and re-configuration of synaptic circuits.

Thus, the activities and processes of the brain give expression to ideas, beliefs, values, intentions, and meanings. Seemingly ethereal entities like intention and meaning cause concrete, material, physical events in the form of brain processes ... and vice versa.

The structural character of ideas, meanings and intentions give expression to patterns of information. The structural character of neuronal action potentials, synaptic spaces, and glial cells give expression to patterns of information.

Information – which consists of a patterned sequence of symbols – becomes the common medium linking mental phenomenology and brain activity. Information flows through both the ethereal realms of mental phenomena and the physical/material realms of brain events.

According to the computational theory of mind, patterns of information can be encapsulated in programs that reflect the way in which those patterns of information might have been generated through an appropriately organized series of steps. That is, patterns of information can be translated into programs or algorithms that constitute a set of steps that are able to generate or recreate such patterns.

However, as Dick Martin, one of the main characters in the old television show '*Laugh In*', used to say: "Au contraire!" There are some problems roaming the interstitial spaces of the foregoing outline – brief though it might be -- concerning the computational theory of mind.

On the surface, the theory seems compelling and intriguing. Yet, when one probes beneath its surface a little, some of the initial impression of the theory's compelling and intriguing sense of shininess begins to fade and tarnish.

For instance, one can agree with the computational theory of mind that Ideas, thoughts, intentions, meanings, and beliefs can be described as a flow of information. Furthermore, the activities of neurons, synaptic spaces, and glial cells also can be described as a flow of information.

What is unclear is what one flow of information has to do with the other flow of information. For example, while the activity of a radio can be described as a flow of information, and, as well, while the signals being sent out by a radio tower or radio station can be described as a flow of information, the activities that are generating

| Explorations |

417

the signal are not the same as the activities which are receiving that signal and rendering it audible.

The two kinds of information do overlap with one another like Euler diagrams. Nonetheless, outside the spaces where the two kinds of information intermingle with one another to give expression to an audible radio program, the nature of the information that makes a radio receiver functional and the nature of the information that makes a radio program signal possible involve very different kinds of information.

The computational theory of mind is assuming that the activities of the brain contain the same kind of information as various ideas, meanings, and intentions do. However, this is not necessarily the case since the flow of information through the brain might be more like the activities underlying the functioning of a radio, whereas the flow of information running through ideas, beliefs, and intentions might be more like the activities that are underlying the generating and transmission of the original radio signal.

Now, admittedly, we don't know whether, or not, the foregoing similes are accurate. That is, we don't know if the brain is like a radio receiver, and we don't know if thoughts, beliefs, and intentions are like signals that are generated elsewhere but are being received by the brain.

However, that is precisely the point. Since we don't know how, on the one hand, thoughts and beliefs are possible, and, on the other hand, we don't actually know what is entailed by the activities of the brain (other than the generation of action potentials, the release of neurotransmitters, the dynamics of glial cells, and the configuration of synaptic spaces), we just can't assume our way to what the character of that relationship between mental phenomenology and brain activities will be, and, for the most part, the computational theory of mind appears to be doing just that ... namely, assuming that the same kind of information is flowing through both mental phenomenology and the activities of the brain.

Yes, there might be a flow of information running through thoughts/intentions and, as well, through brain activities. We just don't know whether the kinds of information running through the two sides of the issue being considered are equivalent to one another (as is

| Explorations |

418

assumed – not proven – to be the case by the computational theory of mind), or whether -- like the relationship between a radio receiver and the signals such a device is receiving from a radio station or tower (and despite the fact that the latter two kinds of activity are capable of interacting with one another) -- those two kinds of activity are complementary to one another and are not equivalent to each other.

The activities of a radio can be represented as a flow chart of information-containing steps to which a functioning radio gives expression. The information processing capacity of a radio can be represented as a program or patterned sequence of steps.

The activities of a radio station that lead to the generation of a signal can be represented as a flow chart of information containing steps to which a functioning radio station gives expression. The information processing capacity of a radio station can be represented as a program or patterned sequence of steps.

Nonetheless, the two foregoing programs are not the same. The flow of information that is contained in each of the two representational programs involves different steps and different dynamics and different patterns of organization.

Do thoughts cause brain events? Perhaps.

Do brain events cause thoughts? Possibly.

However, the causal character of the relationship between thoughts and brain events is not necessarily because -- as the computational theory of mind assumes – those two dimensions give expression to the same kinds of information. The computational theory of mind has not proven that, on the one hand, brain states and, on the other hand, thoughts, intentions, beliefs, meanings and the like are one and the same ... rather, that theory assumes this is the case.

Until the computational theory of mind can demonstrate that brain states give expression to, say, thoughts (and vice versa), then, the foregoing theory has not really solved the aforementioned puzzle concerning the causal relationship between mind and brain. Until the foregoing equivalency has been demonstrated, then the computational theory of mind has not shown that thoughts cause brain states or that brain states cause thoughts, but instead the computational theory of mind is using linguistic sleights of hand (i.e., the same term –

"information" -- is being used to refer to potentially different kinds of phenomena) in order to give the impression that the patterned information contained in thoughts, beliefs, intentions, and meanings is the same sort of informational currency that is flowing through the brain.

One should also keep in mind that the idea of 'information' is a medium of description and not necessarily a mode of ontology. Thoughts can be <u>described</u> in terms of informational content (as can brain events), but, <u>ontologically speaking</u>, thoughts are not necessarily a function of information, anymore than the activities of the brain can be reduced to being a function of information.

For example, words are linguistic symbols that give expression to information. In addition, words can be used to describe both mental phenomenology and brain activities, but neither mental phenomenology nor the activities of the brain are necessarily reducible to language, anymore than mental phenomenology and brain activities are necessarily reducible to flows of information despite the fact that both mind and brain can be described through the concept of information. Seemingly, the computational theory of mind has difficulty differentiating between such nuances of possible meaning.

From the perspective of the computational theory of mind, the modules of the brain -- that is, the specialized biological networks consisting of: Neuronal action potentials, glial cell activity, neurotransmitter dynamics, and synaptic configuration processes -- are constructed by means of an underlying algorithmic recipe inherent in the information of the genome. Such genetic information gives expression to a developmental system that is responsible for the unfolding of those specialized modules at the right time, and in the right place, and with the right set of components and capabilities.

During the brain's developmental process, an array of neuronal modalities must be fashioned and different kinds of glial cells must be constructed. For example, neurons and glial cells must be equipped with the right kind of membrane proteins as well as with a capacity to release neurotransmitters and gliotransmitters under the right circumstances and with the right kind of functional shapes to enable those transmitters to attach to the right kind of membrane proteins.

| Explorations |

In addition, neurons and glial cells must be induced (via the construction of paths made from the right kinds of chemical molecules) to migrate to their appropriate 'homes' within the architecture of the brain. Once settled, neurons must be induced to send out axon processes and dendritic branches to be able to communicate with appropriate neural networks in other parts of the brain as well as be able to lend assistance to the construction of various kinds of synaptic circuits, while glial cells must be induced to form networks of gap junctions that permit glial cells to communicate with one another as well as to be able to be sensitive – to some degree – to the dynamics of neurons.

How did the blueprint for the foregoing developmental process arise? No one knows.

Even if one assumes that such a blueprint came together through a process of evolutionary steps (and there is no compelling theory that explains what those steps were or when and how they occurred), nevertheless, no one knows why that blueprint has the properties it does or precisely what those properties accomplish, if anything, as far as the contents of mental phenomenology are concerned. Does the genomic blueprint for the brain enable ideas to be generated and intentions to be formed and judgments to be made, or does the genomic blueprint give expression to a very elaborate receiving device that, within limits, filters, frames, and modulates the signals it receives, but is not necessarily capable of producing the contents of mental phenomenology?

If the genomic blueprint for the brain is not capable of enabling the brain to generate either a screen of awareness and/or the phenomenological contents that play on such a screen, then, certainly, a huge problem is left behind – namely, how does one account for consciousness and the mental contents of consciousness. However, at the present time, that problem cannot be addressed adequately by merely assuming that the genomic blueprint underwrites something like a computational theory of mind.

If we don't know how the genomic blueprint for the brain arose, and if we don't know what, if anything, the blueprint for the brain has to do with the generation of consciousness and the contents of consciousness, and if we don't know how the modules of the brain acquire their specialized computational capabilities, then it becomes quite difficult to judge the value of any given edition of a computational theory of mind. Given the many things that we don't understand about how the genomic blueprint for the brain came to be or what, exactly such a blueprint is capable of accomplishing, can one really reverse engineer the contents of consciousness and in the process come to understand how the specialized modules of the brain made such contents possible or what functions they serve?

One can come up with an indefinitely large number of theories about how evolutionary forces might have generated the blueprint for the human brain. One can come up with an indefinitely large number of theories about why various modules of the brain have the capacities they do? One can come up with an indefinitely large number of theories about how the properties of the brain might be able to generate consciousness and/or the contents of consciousness. One can come up with an indefinitely large number of theories about how consciousness and the contents of consciousness arise through means other than the activities of the brain.

The problem is that we do not possess a sufficient understanding of the process of evolution (if that is what is directing things), or the nature of the brain, or the nature of mental phenomenology, or the nature of the universe to be able to identify which of the foregoing indefinitely large numbers of theories best reflects the available data. All manner of computational theories of mind are possible, but we have no reliable means of navigating our way through those possibilities to locate the 'right' one because too many fundamental issues concerning the nature of evolution, the brain, consciousness, mental phenomenology, and the universe are unknown.

Are beliefs, meanings, assumptions, ideas, values, judgments, inferences, insights, intentions, and interpretations various kinds of computations of the brain, and, if so, what kind of computations are they? Or, do the computations of the brain involve other kinds of activities that are related to, but different from, the dynamics that underlie the generation of beliefs and the other contents of mental phenomenology (much as a radio and the signals it receives are related to, but different from, one another)?

| Explorations |

The difference between information and noise is the presence or absence, respectively, of order. Any given computational theory of mind will have difficulty justifying its existence if that theory cannot account for the origins and nature of the order that renders its computations possible or cannot determine whether such computations are even possible as a function of what developmental genomics enable the brain to do.

Consider the following possibility. Intelligence, in general, could be considered to be a computational module, or one might divide that general capacity into an array of sub-specializations that collectively give expression to that general capacity.

Whether considered as one dynamic capacity or as a collection of specializations, from the perspective of the computational theory of mind, intelligence is a function of the way that neurons, glial cells, neurotransmitters, gliotransmitters, and synaptic circuits interact. Moreover, such interaction gives expression to the possibilities that the underlying genomic blueprint for the brain sets in motion through the processes of development as well as through the manner in which the millisecond-to-millisecond transactions of the brain unfold in accordance with the guidance of the genomic blueprint in terms of both general and specific forms of modulating influences.

One small, but important, dimension of intelligence involves the process of making assumptions in order to be able to engage various aspects of experience. Assumptions can play important catalytic, heuristic roles in the development of understanding by providing one with a conceptual place to stand as one works out the implications of such possibilities ... possibilities that might be difficult to conceptualize without the starting point provided by assumptions.

Mathematical systems, sciences, philosophies, and theologies all employ certain kinds of assumptions to which, for better or worse, individuals commit themselves. However, everyday life also is woven together by a variety of assumptions that help bridge the gap between what is known and what is not known.

Assumptions also help shape what we believe we know. If those assumptions are proven to be false or turn out to lead to problematic consequences, then, one will be required to rework the conceptual

| Explorations |

landscape that has been built, in part, through the presence of assumptions.

Assumptions provide vectored starting points from which to launch exploratory expeditions that seek to reach the promised land of understanding. Assumptions help to frame experiential data and invest that data with a sense of meaning. Assumptions purport to explain why a given phenomenon is the way that it is. Assumptions offer opportunities through which to test the nature of reality against the perspective to which an assumption gives expression. Assumptions can lead to fruitful, heuristically valuable results even if such assumptions turn out to be false or problematic.

The foregoing paragraph outlines what assumptions can do. However, what makes assumptions possible? How do assumptions arise?

The computational theory of mind maintains that assumptions emerge as a result of the interactional dynamics of neurons, glial cells, neurotransmitters, gliotransmitters, and synaptic circuitry that have been made possible by the potentials entailed by the genomic blueprint that helps govern the processes of life. The previous sentence outlines -- in a fairly clear manner -- a general outline concerning the emergence of assumptions from the perspective of the computational theory of mind.

The devil is in the details. This is because, so far, no one has been able to show how some set of specific brain dynamics, together with the potentials of the underlying genetic blueprint, are capable of giving expression to something as seemingly simple as the process of making an assumption.

Are assumptions insights of some kind? Are they intuitions?

Are assumptions inferences? Are they imaginative guesses concerning the possible nature of reality?

Are assumptions computations? If so, what kind of computations are they, and what makes such computations possible?

Do assumptions arise, somehow, as a function of the genomic blueprint for the brain? If so, how does this work, and how did the capacity to make assumptions become encoded in the DNA that gives expression to the blueprint for the brain?

| Explorations |

Or, do assumptions emerge through the dynamic potential of the neural networks that are put in play by the underlying genomic blueprint that governs the activities of the brain? If so, what are the specific details governing that process of emergence?

The computational theory of mind is rooted in many assumptions. That perspective employs assumptions concerning the nature of origins, evolution, mind, brain, computations, and theories.

If that theory cannot account for how assumptions are possible in terms of its own perspective, then, what, really, does such a theory have to offer? Is the computational theory of mind anything more than a set of empirical data framed, filtered, shaped, oriented, and ordered by a set of assumptions that is rooted in ignorance concerning the origins of such assumptions?

Are the assumptions we choose as heuristic tools through which to engage experience a matter of genetics and/or environment and/or something else? From the perspective of the computational theory of mind, how do human beings acquire the capacity to generate assumptions and, then, choose to use them in an attempt to explain, or frame, or theorize, or filter, or prove the nature of reality?

What combination of action potentials, glial cell dynamics, synaptic reconfigurations, and flow of neurotransmitters and gliotransmitters generates an assumption and the choice to implement that assumption? What determines that such an assumption will have one kind of structure and content rather than some other kind of structure and content?

Over the last 15-20 years, an array of interesting things have been discovered about what used to be referred to as junk DNA ... "junk" because no one could figure out what, if anything, it encoded for, and, consequently, most scientists dismissed the molecular material as genetic flotsam that merely constituted accumulated residue left over from generations of coding errors, jumping genes, and the like. In the light of recent research, however, an increasing proportion of so-called "junk DNA" is being shown to have functional value through the manner in which it provides instructions about how, when, and where the genetic blueprint expresses itself.

Perhaps, allegedly junk DNA is camouflaging the manner in which the computational character of the mind operates. Maybe such components of mental phenomenology as: consciousness, choice, imagination, creativity, language, reasoning, thinking, and understanding are functions of the instructional guidance contained in what previously had been considered to be nothing but junk.

When one is ignorant, anything seems to be possible. We are ignorant because proof has not, yet, surfaced with respect to how any of the foregoing computational possibilities correctly account for the phenomenology of mental spaces.

Furthermore, even if such a proof (or set of proofs) were forthcoming, there still would be a canyon-sized hole in the computational theory of mind's account of cognition. More specifically, ultimately, the computational theory of mind is rooted in evolution, and, consequently, advocates of that theory must be able to provide a plausible account of how such instructional and computational wherewithal became encoded in the human genome.

Currently – and as previously indicated -- the computational theory of mind does not have a plausible and viable account of how the genetic blueprint is able to generate the computational processes that constitute such phenomena as consciousness, reasoning, intelligence, imagination, creativity, understanding, and language. Furthermore, that theory does not possess a plausible and viable account of how such computational capabilities came to be encoded in the genetic blueprint for the brain.

Moreover, if the genetic blueprint does not provide strict instructions (via, say, what was formerly known as "junk DNA) for the running of cognitive, computational dynamics (such as choosing and making assumptions), then the computational theory of mind will have some computational work of its own to do. In other words, the computational theory of mind will have to provide an account of how the genetic blueprint for the brain creates the <u>potential</u> for generating mental phenomenology through the manner in which the genetic blueprint enables neurons, glial cells, gap junction networks, neurotransmitters, gliotransmitters, and synaptic circuitry to give expression to the dynamics through which the computations emerge that underwrite mental phenomenology.

| Explorations |

The lexicon of mental phenomenology includes terms such as: awareness, ideas, beliefs, values, judgments, intentions, emotions, reasoning, interpreting, and understanding. Presently, the computational theory of mind cannot account for the nature of the computations that generate the phenomena to which the foregoing terms allude, anymore than that theory can account for the nature of the computational process that makes assumptions possible.

| Explorations |

The Minnesota Study of Twins Reared Apart explores what happens when individuals who are from the same set of identical twins are raised in different environmental contexts and, then, that research is compared against what happens when individuals who are from the same set of fraternal twins grow up in different environments. Some interesting findings have been discovered.

For example Jim Lewis and Jim Springer are one of the sets of identical twins that were studied in the aforementioned research project. Their lives apart began at the age of four weeks, and they were not reunited until approximately 39 years later.

Both of the Jims shared some remarkable similarities despite having been raised in different circumstances. For instance, both of them married and divorced a woman named Betty ... presumably the Betty in question was different in each case.

Both Jims had a dog named "Toy". They both were fathers of boys named James with middle names that differed by only one letter, 'I' ... Alan versus Allan.

They both owned Chevrolets. Each of the two individuals was employed as a part-time sheriff, and they each spent their vacations in Florida.

The two Jims also exhibited pretty much the same pattern of behavior with respect to smoking and drinking. In addition, the two individuals both began to suffer headaches around the same time in their lives – age 18.

Not everything was the same between them. For instance, one of the Jims preferred to express himself orally while the other Jim was inclined toward writing things out in order to express himself.

Their hairstyle preferences were also different. One Jim likes to have sideburns and slick his hair back, while the other Jim lets his hair fall across his forehead and does not maintain sideburns.

There were other identical twins involved in the aforementioned study that exhibited their own sets of similarities. For example, there were two females who had been separated from one another at the age of six weeks and were not reunited for another fifty-plus years.

They both had been haunted by the same nightmarish dream for years. The dream consisted of having fishhooks and doorknobs stuffed in their mouths and, then eventually, dying of suffocation.

Although one might anticipate that identical twins would share some similar physical characteristics – for instance, being prone to headaches or being inclined toward similar behaviors with respect to, say, smoking -- nonetheless, issues involving overlapping behavioral tendencies with respect to nightmares, cars, vacation spots, and occupations, or the virtually identical character of the names for a spouse, child, and dog are a little more puzzling. Equally intriguing is the fact that there are some differences in how such twins comport themselves in certain areas of their lives since if everything is a matter of genetics, as one might assume, then how do such differences arise?

Are the choices that the two Jims made in conjunction with the name of the women they marred and divorced a function of genetics? Are the choices the two individuals made with respect to the kind of job, car, or place where they vacationed a matter of genetics?

Is choice a function of genetics? If so, how does the phenomenology of choice arise out of genomic dynamics?

Moreover, if choice is a matter of genetics, then, how does one account for the differences in choices that are made by identical twins? How do environment and genetics interact to give expression to such computational differences?

Are the only two options we have to decide the foregoing issues a matter of genetics or environment ... nature versus nurture? Does an individual bring anything of his or her own to the human condition that permits her or him to choose independently of nature and nurture?

Prior to the work of such experimental physicists as John Clauser, Stuart Freedman, Alain Aspect, Michael Horne, Anton Zeilinger, and a few others, the notion that two entities might be able to 'communicate' with one another in an apparently instantaneous-like manner seemed rather far-fetched. While I will have more to say on this topic later in the book, for present purposes, I will just draw your attention to the empirically proven fact that photons have been experimentally demonstrated to be 'in touch' with one another in ways that seem to

| Explorations |

be independent of the capacity of the speed of light to be able to transmit some sort of signal across the distance separating those quantum objects.

Since the time (1905) when Einstein's special theory of relativity first entered the consciousness of physicists, scientists have accepted the idea that nothing travels faster than the speed of light. Thus, if that understanding is correct, then what is one to make of an array of well-designed and well-executed experiments which have demonstrated that two quantum entities which previously had interacted with one another apparently can -- to some degree -- continue to communicate with each other despite the fact they have become separated by a distance that cannot be traversed by a signal traveling at the speed of light within the time frame being considered?

In English, the phenomenon is known as "entanglement". In general terms, the underlying principle appears to be that once, say, two photons interact with one another, then even when those quantum entities become separated from one another by distances that cannot be traversed by signals traveling at the speed of light within a given framework of measurement, nonetheless, those photons appear to still be causally connected such that if a change occurs to one of the entangled quantum entities, that change will be reflected, as well, in the behavior of the other entangled quantum object.

To be sure, the differences between human beings and a couple of quantum objects are indefinitely great. However, if quantum objects that once interacted with one another are capable of staying in touch with each other after being separated, then, perhaps it could also be the case that identical twins who interacted with each other for even a period as little as 4-6 weeks might continue to be entangled in certain ways with one another following separation, and, as a result, some of the choices of one twin might influence the choices of the other twin.

The foregoing idea is not being introduced as an explanation for why identical twins sometimes exhibit such extraordinary similarities in their choices. Instead, it is being mentioned to provide a concrete context through which to entertain the possibility that there might be more forces acting upon us than can be accounted for by genetics and the immediate environment.

| Explorations |

In 1980 John Searle introduced a thought experiment that attempted to point out what he considered to be a problem with the computational/information processing approach to the idea of what it means to have an understanding of something. More specifically, among other things, the computational or information processing theory maintains that understanding is just a matter of running an appropriate program (the algorithmic processing of information) under the right circumstances in order to, say, solve a problem, whereas opponents of the computational theory contend that understanding involves more than just being able to run the right program at the right time in order to obtain a certain kind of result.

Searle's thought experiment is often referred to as the Chinese Room Argument. The thought experiment begins when a human being who does not know, understand, or speak Chinese is placed in a room that has a variety of boxes containing Chinese characters (this serves as a data base).

The individual also is provided with a book of instructions that tells him what to do with the characters stored the boxes when pieces of paper -- with characters on them -- are slipped under the door to the Chinese room. Unknown to the person in the room, the squiggle-like markings on the paper are Chinese characters, and, in addition, the individual in the room does not know that the instruction book which she or he has been given is a program that gives expression to some form of artificial intelligence ... a form that is designed to assist the individual in the room to arrange the characters in the boxes so that they constitute appropriately crafted answers that are written in Chinese to questions that are being asked in Chinese in relation to a story (which, presumably, has been written or spoken in Chinese).

There is a general procedure that is followed by the person in the Chinese Room. First, a slip of paper with squiggles on it is slid into the room through the small space between the bottom of the door and the floor of the room.

The individual in the room picks up the piece of paper (the input), looks at the squiggles, and, then, consults the instruction book and the characters in the box to find out what to do when such squiggles appear on a slip of paper (this gives expression to a kind of information processing). Next, depending on what that individual finds in the instruction book, the person follows the instructions that are provided and writes down the indicated squiggles on a piece of paper, and, when necessary, slips those pieces of paper with squiggles on them beneath the door leading to another room (the output).

Over time, the individual in the Chinese Room gets quite proficient at finding out what to do when different pieces of paper with various squiggles on them are slipped into the room. Based on the answers that are received in relation to the questions that are slipped beneath the door, the person (or persons) on the other side of the door from the Chinese Room has (have) come to believe that the individual in the Chinese Room speaks Chinese.

The individual in the Chinese Room is doing nothing but: (1) taking pieces of paper with squiggles on them that have been written by someone else; (2) using the squiggle characteristics to locate the relevant sections of the instruction book and the characters in the boxes that deal with those kinds of squiggles; (3) following the instructions given in the book involving those squiggles to be able to provide an output that is relevant (according to the instruction book) to those squiggles, and (4) returning – to the other room -- a piece of paper with squiggles that have been manipulated in accordance with instructions provided by the book. Consequently, although the individual is providing apparently satisfactory answers as far as the question-askers are concerned, nonetheless, the person in the Chinese Room does not really understand what is going on as far as the meaning of the slips are concerned that are being received and sent.

He didn't understand Chinese at the beginning of the experiment. He doesn't understand Chinese at the end of the experiment.

On the surface, what is taking place in the Chinese Room appears to constitute evidence that the Turing Test has been passed. In other words, the person who is sliding pieces of paper containing questions written in Chinese under the door to the individual in the Chinese Room comes to believe that whoever is answering those questions is a conscious being who understands Chinese sufficiently well to be able to answer questions about a given story in a intelligible and satisfactory manner.

Searle argues that the Chinese Room Argument demonstrates that one can arrange a set of circumstances involving a computational

| Explorations |

432

system – that is: (1) A data base; (2) a program; (3) an input; and (4) an output -- which is capable of fooling people and inducing those individuals to believe they are dealing with a conscious, intentional, intelligent agent and, thereby, pass the Turing Test. Yet, despite the capacity of the previously outlined computational system to be able to pass the Turing Test, that computational system does not understand the nature of the Chinese characters that are being processed.

The foregoing argument involves some issues that are being conflated with one another when they should be kept separate. As a result, the computational/information processing aspect of things becomes somewhat muddled.

One can acknowledge that Information processing is taking place within the Chinese Room. However, only part of that processing involves some discernible computational properties – namely, the program in the instruction book.

Nevertheless, one cannot necessarily prove that the <u>creation</u> of such a program is the result of a computational process. Presumably, the program didn't write itself.

One or more human beings did the coding. Therefore, whether, or not, the cognitive processes that led to the writing of the program are computational in nature is a separate issue.

Moreover, the program contained in the instruction book and the collection of Chinese characters stored in the boxes that are in the Chinese Room are only capable of generating an answer because of the cognitive activity of the human being in the room. This cognitive activity includes: Rummaging around for the correct characters in the boxes (assuming no mistakes are made during this facet of information processing), and, then, the individual has to find the appropriate parts of the program in the instruction book (assuming no mistakes are made during this part of information processing), and, then, the individual has to interpret the instructions in the book to arrange the characters in a certain pattern (and, again, assuming that no mistakes are made during this facet of information processing).

Consequently, there are two modalities of information processing in the Chinese Room. The first modality – the instruction book -- is static, at least partially computational (i.e., the form of the program in

| Explorations |

and of itself), and it needs to be activated by a human being (or in some other way), while the second modality of information processing is active and is self-regulating – namely, the human being. Nevertheless, neither of the foregoing modalities is necessarily fully computational in character since we don't understand the nature of the dynamics through which those modalities of information processing have been created and/or operate.

Among the conclusions that John Searle draws with respect to the Chinese Room Argument is that the processing of information does not necessarily give expression to active understanding of the information that is being processed. In other words, the presence of activities of information processing that contain, at least to a degree, some computational elements (in the form of the instruction book) does not necessarily guarantee the presence of understanding concerning the information that is being processed.

To be sure, an artificial intelligence program that is sufficiently sophisticated might be able to fool human beings into believing that a given program has the capacity to understand and be aware of what is taking place during any series of blind exchanges between the individual and the program. Nonetheless, according to Searle, the capacity to process information through the manipulation of symbols (syntax) cannot necessarily be equated with the presence of understanding, consciousness, intention, or other expressions of intelligence concerning the meaning (semantics) of those manipulations.

The book of instructions in the Chinese Room does not understand the instructions that are written in it anymore than the pieces of paper on which squiggles are written understand the nature of the squiggles written upon them even though those squiggles constitute an algorithm of sorts (a question) written in Chinese. It also is quite clear that the person or person who wrote the instruction book does, in fact, understand Chinese or else the instructions in that book -- when properly followed -- would not have provided intelligible answers to the questions being asked via the slips of paper being slid beneath the door into the Chinese Room.

On the other hand, the individual in the Chinese Room who is reading the book of instructions is able to understand the nature of the instructions being written (assuming that the instructions are written in a language that the person can understand) ... otherwise that individual could not produce results that satisfied people in the next room who are asking various questions. What makes things work in the Chinese Room is the ability of the person in the Chinese Room: (1) To be aware of the contents of the instruction book; (2) to be able to read/understand those instructions; to be able to manipulate the indicated squiggles in the required way, and (4) to be able to slip such results under the door at the indicated times.

What the individual in the Chinese Room is doing is processing information using the pieces of paper in conjunction with the contents of an instruction book. The issue is not whether, or not, that individual is processing information but, rather, the issue is how is that person able to do what that he or she is doing in the Chinese Room.

Is that individual using computational techniques to process such information? If the person in the Chinese Room is using computational processes to be aware of, focus on, read, understand, interpret, and write in accordance with the directives of the instruction book, then, irrespective of whether that individual can understand Chinese, the person is operating in a manner that is consistent with the computational theory of mind.

At the present time the problem is that we don't know if the cognitive processes being used by the individual in the Chinese Room are, or are not, computational in character. That is: We do not know whether, or not, consciousness is a computational process? We do not know whether, or not, intelligence is a computational process? We do not know whether, or not, reasoning is a computational process? We do not know whether, or not, language is a computational process? We do not know whether, or not, the process of understanding is a computational process?

To contend that, currently, we do not know whether, or not, any of the foregoing capacities are computational in nature means that if such computational programs exist in human beings, then, at the present time, we don't know what they are. In other words, we don't know what sequential -- or in parallel -- combinations of neurons, glial cells, synaptic circuitry, neurotransmitters, and gliotransmitters will generate consciousness, or intelligence, or reasoning, or reading, or understanding, or writing. Moreover, we don't know what the nature of the DNA computational processes are (assuming they do exist) that would enable appropriate algorithms to arise through such genomic coding that were, in turn, capable of giving expression to mental phenomenology of one kind or another.

Searle's Chinese Room Argument demonstrates that not all instances of information processing necessarily entail an understanding of everything that is being processed – for example, knowledge of Chinese. Theoretically, one could process information involving Chinese symbols without knowing any Chinese, but whether, or not, the capacity to process information -- that underlies and makes possible what is taking place in the Chinese Room – is computational in nature is a separate issue.

Searle has not shown that what the person in the Chinese Room is doing demonstrates that the computational theory of mind is wrong. In fact, what the person in that Room is doing might actually be the computational theory of mind in action, but, currently, we lack the evidence needed to prove or disprove that possibility.

Awareness, intentionality, and understanding do not necessarily have to be <u>directly</u> present in the modalities of information processing that run in accordance with a set of computations. Nonetheless, awareness, intentionality and understanding tend to be <u>implicitly</u> present in contexts involving information processing by virtue of the fact that the program exists at all ... in other words, presumably such a program did not come into existence through its own efforts). Thus, computers can carry out a program and still not necessarily be aware of 'themselves' or the programs being run through it.

However, as indicated earlier, the jury is still out on whether, or not, the manner in which human beings process information is computational in nature. Furthermore, the jury is still out on whether, or not, the genome consists of a set of computations that generate mental phenomenology and its contents.

There is a further issue related to the foregoing considerations. Let us imagine that somewhere down the temporal line an individual discovers that understanding is, indeed, a function of computational processes involving the way, for example, that the generic blueprint for the brain gives expression to itself through the dynamics of

| Explorations |

436

physical-chemical processes but, nonetheless, the individual within whom those computations are occurring is not aware that they are being carried out but, instead, is only aware of the results of those computations.

Is the <u>awareness</u> of those results necessarily computational in character? In other words, even if one were to acknowledge that the generation of a given kind of understanding were computational in character, does such an acknowledgement necessarily force one to conclude that awareness of those results must also be computational in character?

Conceivably, a distinction might be able to be drawn between consciousness and the contents of consciousness. In other words, even if the contents of consciousness were computational in nature, this would not necessarily automatically mean that the phenomenology in which those computational results appeared was also computational in character.

The foregoing scenario is like the Chinese Room. The brain (a possible modality of computational information processing) represents the instruction book or program, and consciousness represents the individual in the Chinese Room who works with that program to provide answers for the person in the next room who is asking questions.

Given the foregoing possibility, consciousness is said to be aware of a state of understanding that it did not produce (just as the individual in the Chinese Room is aware of an instruction book and a set of boxes with Chinese characters that the individual did not produce). One of the questions arising in conjunction with the scenario being outlined above is the following one: Is the computational processes of the brain aware of what it is doing at the time it is doing it? Or, considered from a slightly different perspective, could the brain pass the Turing Test even though there is an absence of awareness or understanding present in the brain with respect to the nature of the computational processes that are taking place?

Searle wanted the Chinese Room Argument to distinguish between, on the one hand, the kinds of information processing that went on in a computer and, on the other hand, the sorts of information processing that take place in a human being. He wanted to show that computer programs are not, in and of themselves, necessarily capable of consciousness and intentionality, whereas human beings, in and of themselves, do exhibit consciousness and intentionality.

The Chinese Room Argument addresses the former issue but not the latter one ... or, at least, not completely. In other words, while Searle has shown that the kind of information processing that involves at least some computational features (such as in a program or a computer) does not necessarily entail understanding of the information that is being processed, nonetheless he has not shown that the information processing that takes place in human beings is necessarily aware of itself ... only that awareness of some kind is present.

Searle does not know what makes such consciousness possible. Furthermore, he does not know what makes the understandings that appear in consciousness possible.

Human beings can pass the Turing Test. Nevertheless, they do not necessarily have any more understanding of how such understanding and concomitant awareness are possible than the person in the Chinese Room understands the information involving Chinese that she or he is processing.

Searle assumes that biology -- unlike computers and algorithms/programs -- produces consciousness and understanding. However, he has not shown that this is the case.

He only demonstrates that there are circumstances in which information processing takes place in a way that could pass the Turing Test despite the fact there is no understanding present with respect to the nature of the information that is being processed. Consequently, unwittingly (and indirectly as far as the purpose of his Chinese Room Argument is concerned), Searle's argument has led to a problem.

The thrust of his argument is not capable of resolving the problem that ensues from his thought-experiment. Indeed, Searle has created for himself the very problem with which he wished to saddle the computational theory of mind – namely, just because human beings can pass the Turing Test, this does not necessarily mean that human beings understand, or are aware of, the nature of the information processing (which might or might not be computational in character) that is taking place within the brain and that might, or might not, be responsible for consciousness, intentionality, intelligence and so on.

| Explorations |

The Nature of the Unconscious

In February 1997, *Science* published an article by a group of researchers at the University of Iowa. The title of the article was: "Deciding Advantageously Before Knowing the Advantageous Strategy."

The contents of the foregoing article discussed an experiment involving the development of strategies for maximizing winnings in a given set of circumstances. Those circumstances involved four decks of cards, two of which were blue in color while the other two decks were red in color, and, in addition, each card – from each of the four decks – carried a value that represented a gain or a loss of money.

Furthermore, the researchers knew ahead of time that while an experimental subject occasionally might be able to earn a lot of money by choosing cards from the red decks, more often than not, the red cards would lead, over time, to the loss of money. The blue cards, on the other hand, entailed only relatively small gains, but those gains were fairly consistent.

The individuals conducting the experiment wanted to know how long it would take before a given subject would realize that choosing the blue cards was more likely to lead to monetary gains whereas choosing cards from the red decks was likely to undermine a subject's attempt to maximize winnings. There were several stages to the experiment.

During the first phase of the experiment, a general group of people was tested. Such individuals began to suspect there is something problematic about the cards in the red deck when approximately 50 cards have been selected, and by the time 80 cards have been selected, most of the individuals participating in the first stage of the experiment, are able to accurately describe the nature of the problem.

Although people in the general group suspect – around the 50 card juncture – that there might be a problem with the cards in the red deck as far as maximizing winnings is concerned, they usually are not able to articulate what the nature of that problem is at that time. They just know they are becoming more inclined toward choosing cards from the blue deck, and another 30 cards, or so, will have to be selected before the penny drops, so to speak, and the subjects are able to indentify the precise nature of the problem involving cards from the red decks and, as well, are able to specify the nature of that problem.

The second stage of the foregoing experiment focused on the responses of individuals who liked to gamble. Aside from the distinguishing feature of liking to gamble, the other primary difference between the two groups is that the hands of the individuals in the gambler group were hooked up to an apparatus that measured the dynamics of the sweat glands in the palms of their hands, both with respect to heat and stress.

The glands in the palms of the hands of the gamblers began to sweat after about 10 cards. Moreover, the behavior of the gamblers began to change around the same time ... that is they began to favor cards from the blue deck over cards from the red deck.

Therefore, some 40 cards prior to the time when individuals from the gambler group of subjects or from the general group of subjects would consciously begin to suspect there might be some kind of problem entailed by selecting cards from the red deck, and 70 cards prior to the point when those individuals would be able to articulate what the nature of the problem was, 'something' in those individuals knew there was a problem with cards from the red deck and, as a result, such awareness led to changes in behavior that were not being instigated by the conscious minds of those individuals ... in other words, individuals from the gambler group were favoring cards from the blue decks, but those people were not aware this was taking place.

The 'something' that seemed to be aware of what was going on prior to the time when "normal consciousness" was aware of the problem involving cards from the red deck is sometimes referred to as the "adaptive unconscious." This terminology seems rather curious.

While normal consciousness appears to be unaware of what is going on, the so-called adaptive unconscious seems to have a keen insight into what is transpiring. The foregoing awareness is sufficiently keen to bring about an alteration in a person's behavior in order to reflect, and be able to profit from, such an understanding.

What seems to be acting in an unconscious manner is the normal, surface, waking consciousness. What seems to be conscious are the dynamics that are taking place out of sight from allegedly normal, surface, waking consciousness.

The Iowa experiment gives expression to the presence of an inverted perspective. What is normally considered to be conscious is, instead, unconscious, while what is usually considered to be unconscious is, actually, quite aware of what is transpiring.

In the second stage of the foregoing Iowa experiment, 'normal' consciousness seems to be in something of a stupor and lacking the requisite intelligence to be able to figure out what is going on. Yet, 10 cards into the experiment, another part of human understanding – something that is, allegedly, unconscious -- grasps the situation.

Why is the adaptive unconscious being referred to as the unconscious when the capabilities it is manifesting in the experiment seem to indicate otherwise? Why is surface awareness being referred to as conscious behavior when that awareness is so obviously oblivious to what is taking place before its very eyes?

Antonio Damasio, a neurologist, led the Iowa research group that devised the foregoing experiment. Among other things, Dr. Damasio has a scientific interest in a segment of the brain known as the ventromedial prefrontal cortex.

A variety of data implicates the ventromedial prefrontal cortex of the brain as having some degree of responsibility for helping to render judgments that shape behavior. For example, that area of the brain seems to be involved in processes of differential diagnosis with respect to prioritizing incoming information concerning how to proceed amidst various possibilities in a given set of circumstances.

Patients with damage to their ventromedial prefrontal cortex were run through the aforementioned experiment involving four decks and two kinds of colored cards. Those patients performed differently than did either the general ('normal') group or the gambler group.

Like the people in the gambler group, the individuals in the group with damaged ventromedial prefrontal cortices had the palms of their hands hooked up to a monitor so that the activity of their sweat glands could be measured. However, unlike the individuals in the gambler group, the people in the ventromedial prefrontal cortex patient group displayed no hint of glandular activity during the experiment.

Can one assume that the absence of any sign of glandular activity in the patients with damage to their ventromedial prefrontal cortex was because those patients were not aware of some sort of problem involving the red colored cards? Not necessarily, since one, or another, dimension of cognition in those patients still might have been aware of the problem with the red cards but, for whatever reason, the signal that induced sweating in the palms of the gamblers was blocked in the case of the patients with damage to their ventromedial prefrontal cortex.

In addition, unlike the other two experimental groups, individuals with damage to their ventromedial prefrontal cortex also did not seem to exhibit any intuitional sense -- at around the 50-card mark -- that something might be amiss with the red cards. Nonetheless, how or when the foregoing fact was determined is somewhat unclear.

Conceivably, the individuals in the patient group might not have considered the presence of that information to be very high priority and, as a result, it was not reported because it was loss amidst lots of other information and not because there had been no experience of such an intuition. Or, perhaps, at some point the patients did have such a 'hunch', but because that experiential information was not flagged as being important to them, it was not converted into a long-term memory and, therefore, if the individuals in the patient group were asked about whether, or not, they had any intuition concerning the situation, they might not have remembered what they actually had experienced.

Finally, even after the members of the patient group arrived at a 'conscious' understanding of the problem entailed by the red cards, their behavior did not change. In other words, they did not take advantage of that understanding to maximize their winnings.

To be sure, something is being disrupted in patients with damage to their ventromedial prefrontal cortex, but what – precisely -- that 'something' is isn't necessarily clear. Whatever it is, unlike Damasio, I'm not convinced that the problem is one involving decision making per se ... although decision-making might be affected by whatever the foregoing problem entails.

Participating in an experiment involves making a decision, and, yet apparently, decisions were made to begin to participate and decisions were made to continue to participate. Choosing cards from decks of cards involves making decisions, and, yet, cards were selected. Responding to the questions of the researchers involves making decisions, and, yet, answers appear to have been given.

If an individual didn't care about maximizing winnings, then it might make sense that despite coming to grasp the significance of the red and blue cards, such an individual would not necessarily use that understanding to help him or her to maximize winnings about which the person didn't care. If a person were indifferent to a hunch that something was amiss with the red cards, then, why bother to remember a fleeting instance of phenomenology that appeared to be unimportant? If a person were indifferent to maximizing winnings, then why bother to induce the glands in the palm to sweat ... sweating is a sign of tension, or concern, or stress, so, why would an individual who doesn't care about winning bother to sweat?

Considered from a different perspective, one also might suppose that decisions are, in fact, being made with respect to the filtering of information concerning the experiment. However, if an individual is uninterested, or unmotivated, or indifferent to the idea of maximizing winnings, then, such an individual might appear to be having difficulty with decision making when she or he fails to use new understanding to benefit himself or herself.

Nonetheless, deciding to rate certain kinds of information as being unimportant with respect to the issue of devising strategies to maximize winnings is not necessarily the same as being unable to make decisions at all. The Iowa researchers might have pre-conceived ideas about what constitutes evidence of a decision having been made and, as a result, they might not recognize the presence of certain kinds of decisions that run contrary to their expectations about what a decision looks like.

Notwithstanding the foregoing considerations, even if one were to agree with Dr. Damasio that the ventromedial prefrontal cortex was connected, somehow, to the process of making judgments and decisions with respect to the relative importance of incoming information in relation to an ongoing set of circumstances as well as with respect to the sort of behavior that would best address those circumstances, there are some questions that need to be asked. Those

| Explorations |

questions all concern the role of the ventromedial prefrontal cortex in the process of decision-making.

How does a network of neurons, glial cells, synaptic circuits, neurotransmitters, gliotransmitters, and gap junctions in the ventromedial prefrontal cortex make decisions concerning the relative importance of incoming information? How does such a network prioritize that sort of information? Where do the values come from that establish what the priorities are? How is incoming experiential information interpreted to determine its relative importance? What is sufficiently aware of incoming experiential information to be able to make the foregoing sorts of determinations?

What if the ventromedial prefrontal cortex is not responsible for making such decisions but, rather, is merely a medium for transmitting certain kinds of signals involving those decisions? If the ventromedial prefrontal cortex is responsible for decision-making, we, currently, have no idea how that cortex does what it does.

Conceivably, the reason why no one has, yet, come up with a plausible account about how networks of neurons, glial cells, and the like are capable of making such decisions is because those networks don't actually possess the capacities that are being attributed to them. Decision-making might be done in some way that occurs outside the dynamics of the brain, and the reason why the ventromedial prefrontal complex is associated with such processes is because that segment of the brain has some kind of a role to play with respect to translating into biological terms information from the non-brain-based dynamics being alluded to ... a biological dynamic that supports/receives such information processing signals without being responsible for generating the kinds of information processing signals that give expression to decision-making.

Assuming that the brain is responsible for intelligence, decision-making, evaluation, interpretation, judging, prioritizing, and so on might appear to be a far simpler proposition than supposing that there could be some undiscovered realm (possibly of a physical nature) that lies beyond the brain that is responsible for phenomenology and its contents even as the brain plays some sort of complementary and/or supportive role with respect to that phenomenological dynamic. Nevertheless, the foregoing assumption is simpler only if it is actually

| Explorations |

the case that the brain is responsible for: Phenomenology, its contents, and the capabilities that make those phenomenological contents possible ... something that, at the present time, seems to be a long way away from being demonstrated.

Many of the fundamental features of the quantum world were discovered gradually over a period of 75 years, or so, because, among other things, the assumptions that were made along the way about the nature of atomic phenomena didn't make sense in the light of empirical data. While it might still be the case that researchers will discover a conceptual Rosetta-like Stone to decode how neurotransmitters, gliotransmitters, synaptic circuits, neurons, glial cells, and gap junctions interact to produce the phenomenology of consciousness and its contents, nonetheless, it might also be the case that the assumption that the brain underwrites all mental phenomena could be wrong in part, or entirely, even as the brain does have its role to play with respect to those phenomena ... and, today, that role is only partially understood.

Modern imaging technology – which is rapidly evolving with the passage of time – is giving better and better resolution concerning the precise nature of the dynamics of the brain that are implicated in one, or another, cognitive process (and the aforementioned ventromedial prefrontal cortex is just one of many networks that could be mentioned in this respect). However, as such resolution continues to improve and as the focus of imaging technology narrows the scope of the field being examined, the brain networks being considered are shrinking in size and, yet, those shrinking networks are being burdened with the responsibility of having to explain considerable complexity and specialization as a function of smaller and smaller networks of brain circuitry.

Up until relatively recently, researchers have been pointing to the existence of billions of neurons and glial cells in the brain, along with the on-going dynamics of trillions of synaptic connections, to account for consciousness and other mental phenomena. However, as imaging technology zeros in on smaller and smaller networks of the brain (such as the ventromedial prefrontal cortex) in order to account for specialized mental phenomena, a possible problem begins to rear its head.

| Explorations |

More specifically, if various kinds of mental phenomena are not caused by the complexity of billions of cells and trillions of synaptic circuits interacting with one another but, rather, are the result of the properties of particular, dynamic circuits of limited size (relatively speaking), then, researchers might have to re-think how such, relatively small circuits are responsible for behavior of considerable complexity.

For example, on the basis of various statistical methods, some people (e.g., Stephen Waydo) have estimated that a given concept might involve the firing of just 1/1000th (a million neurons) of the available neurons (approximately a billion neurons) in the medial temporal lobe. Other individuals (e.g., the recently deceased Jerome Lettvin) have suggested that specific concepts might involve the firing of no more than 18,000 neurons.

While there is certainly a difference in size between a network involving a million neurons and a network involving 18,000 neurons, in either case, one is no longer talking about billions of cells and trillions of synaptic connections. How did a million neurons (and associated synaptic connections) or 18,000 neurons (and associated synaptic connections) come to represent or give expression to a particular concept?

Within such relatively restricted fields of consideration, what differentially regulates the flow of neurotransmitters and gliotransmitters amidst an array of neurons, synaptic circuits, and gap junctions to generate one concept rather than another? What induces synaptic circuits to reconfigure themselves to help give expression to one kind of concept rather than another kind of concept?

Within such relatively restricted fields of consideration, what is responsible for integrating those concepts into a decision circuit (for example, in the ventromedial prefrontal cortex) that leads in one direction rather than another? How do neurons, glial cells, synaptic circuits, gap junctions, neurotransmitters, and gliotransmitters interact to produce an evaluation, interpretation, or prioritizing of incoming information so that decisions emerge from such restricted fields of consideration.

The aforementioned Iowa research concerning the experiment involving four decks and two colors of cards bearing different values supposedly indicates that subjects are making complex evaluations in an unconscious manner. Furthermore, the foregoing research also indicates that individuals who have some sort of damage in their ventromedial prefrontal cortex are unable to make the same sort of evaluations, and, therefore, the ventromedial prefrontal cortex is identified as the location where such unconscious evaluations/prioritizations are made for the purpose of making decisions concerning the problem with the red cards relative to the blue cards.

Aside from the previously outlined reservations about what, exactly, the nature of the deficit might be in people with damage to their ventromedial prefrontal cortex, one might also question the description of whatever it is that is capable of discerning a difference between the values of the blue cards and the red cards in the Iowa experiments as being an <u>unconscious</u> process.

'Something' is aware of the differences between the red cards and the blue cards. 'Something' is keeping tract of what happens over time with respect to both kinds of cards. 'Something' is evaluating such differences in an intelligent, reasoned manner. 'Something' is actively influencing behavior so that individual subjects (other than ventromedial prefrontal cortex patients) will be able to take advantage of such understanding so that winnings will be maximized.

None of the foregoing activity qualifies as being unconscious. To be sure, such activity does take place outside the awareness of so-called normal, waking consciousness, but this only means there are several kinds of consciousness that are capable of operating simultaneously in human beings.

If we identify with so-called normal, waking consciousness, then every other form of consciousness that is occurring within us will seem alien and other ... as unconscious in nature. However, such an interpretation of what is transpiring is merely a biased take on what the evidence is telling us.

The unconscious realm is not what is figuring out what is going on with the red cards in the experiment. The unconscious in not what generates a correct 'hunch' concerning what has been discovered that bubbles into view within so-called normal, waking consciousness.

| Explorations |

The unconscious realm in gamblers is not what permits them to figure out what is going on after selecting just ten cards. Instead, a conscious, intelligent, reasoned understanding of the experimental situation is taking place, and one of the ways in which that assessment is disclosed to so-called normal, waking consciousness is through the activity of sweat glands in the palms of the hands of the gamblers.

The sweating palms are trying to tell normal, waking consciousness something. However, normal, waking consciousness is too busy engaging incoming information from its own, limited perspective, and, therefore, the form of consciousness that actually knows something has to assume responsibility for modifying behavior in a way that will maximize winnings even though normal, waking consciousness doesn't understand what is taking place.

There is no unconscious dynamic taking place because the activity that is being described as giving expression to the unconscious could not do what it does if it actually were unconscious. Indeed, how can that which is supposedly unaware of the incoming information (e.g., the four decks of cards experiment) evaluate the significance and value of that information in such an intelligent manner?

The principles underlying the value of the blue and red cards were understood before waking consciousness understood what those principles entailed. Consciousness is present in a manner that is being manifested through different modalities.

Normal waking consciousness might believe that it is the chief operating officer as a function of the sense of 'self' that has been constructed through an array of biases, assumptions, expectations, beliefs, interests, needs, hopes, and past choices that regulate and govern what takes place in (and what is granted access to) normal, waking consciousness. However, evidence – such as that produced through the Iowa experiments – indicates that so-called normal, waking consciousness is not the only form of consciousness that is operating. (These issues will be discussed further in the final chapter of *Final Jeopardy: The Reality Problem, Volume II.*)

Because normal, waking consciousness has developed the false belief that it should be in control of things, other conscious modalities have to struggle to find ways of influencing what transpires in the form of awareness that is known as 'normal, waking consciousness'. This struggle comes in the form of such things as: Sweating palms, hunches, intuitions, insights, or, finally, by inducing surface awareness to acknowledge the correctness of a conscious understanding (e.g., concerning the difference between red cards and blue cards) that has been present for quite some time but -- due to the inclination of normal, waking consciousness to try to control the flow of both focal awareness as well as the contents of consciousness -- so-called normal, waking consciousness has resisted the attempts of the other modalities of consciousness to inform and modulate the understanding of normal, waking consciousness.

Once the waking form of consciousness becomes inclined toward certain biases, beliefs, and assumptions, then, other modalities of consciousness encompassing data (ideas, values, and feelings) that run contrary to the framework of so-called waking consciousness tend to be relegated to compartmentalized mental spaces that form along the horizons of normal, waking consciousness. Such relegated forms of consciousness are referred to as being unconscious.

However, there is nothing of an unconscious nature that is taking place in such modalities of awareness. The evidence from experiments such as those performed by the aforementioned Iowa researchers indicates as much ... and due to its own agenda in such matters, the only source of resistance to the foregoing reality is normal, waking consciousness.

There are many, many experiments that could be cited in place of the aforementioned Iowa research (and the Bibliography for this book references some of that material) which all point in the same direction as the Iowa research. In other words, there are numerous experiments that – like the Iowa four decks of cards experiment -- supposedly demonstrate the existence of the unconscious when the data from those experiments actually provide evidence concerning the existence of modalities of intelligent awareness or consciousness that run parallel to so-called normal, waking consciousness but, under certain circumstances are also able to engage, inform, and modulate normal, waking consciousness.

Normal, waking consciousness gives expression to working memory. Such consciousness constitutes the bench of awareness on which recent and on-going experiences are processed and through which beliefs, values, expectation, ideas, emotions, motivations, and interests, are constructed (i.e., turned into learning or long-term memory) and that, in turn, serve as filters that frame the way working memory is inclined to engage future experiences.

Various modalities of awareness – besides working memory – simultaneously seek to modulate the perspective of working memory by processing incoming data and forwarding that information to working memory. A dialectical dynamic takes place between working memory and those other modalities of awareness to determine which kinds of information will get to shape – at least for the moment – the hermeneutical perspective that will filter and frame the current understanding or interpretive orientation of working memory through which experience is engaged.

For example, emotions give expression to modalities of awareness that seek to modulate working memory or normal, waking consciousness according to the perspective of a given emotion. Moreover, there are, generally speaking, three broad categories of emotions that seek to induce working memory to filter and frame experience in certain ways.

On the one hand, there are problematic emotions such as: jealousy, envy, anger, greed, anxiety, apathy, despair, depression, lust, rage, and hatred. On the other hand, there are constructive emotions such as: love, compassion, empathy, patience, charitableness, gratitude, and remorse.

Finally, there are emotions that might be constructive or problematic depending on circumstances. Among this third category of emotions are the following possibilities: hope, grief, joy, shame, trust, desire, contentment, fear, confidence, curiosity, passion, and courage.

According to modern neuroscience, the amygdala is the heart of emotional life. If the amygdala (there are two of them) are: Removed, disconnected from the rest of the brain, or if there is some sort of damage to those structures of the brain, then, the individuals so affected tend to suffer from various forms of affective blindness or dysfunctional emotionality.

While clinical and experimental evidence might indicate that when the amygdala in human beings or animals are, in some way, defective,

| Explorations |

451

and, as a result, those organisms are observed to exhibit emotional deficits of one kind or another, nonetheless, such facts do not necessarily mean that the amygdala are responsible for generating emotions. The amygdala could act as receivers for emotional signals from elsewhere, and, if this were the case, then, when the amygdala are defective, such dysfunctional organs would disrupt the reception of such signals and, in the process, yield a condition of affective blindness even though those organs are not responsible for the generation of emotions.

One reason for thinking in the foregoing manner revolves around the fact that no one has, yet, come up with a plausible explanation for how the dynamics of neurons, action potentials, glial cells, gap junctions, neurotransmitters, gliotransmitters, hormones, and synaptic circuits generate the phenomenological feeling and flavor of different emotions. We might all agree there is a neurochemistry that is associated with the presence of emotions, but there is almost no agreement about how: Neurochemistry generates emotion; or, how various networks of neurochemistry arose in order to give expression to different kinds of emotional experience; or, how neurochemistry 'knows' what emotions to generate in a given set of circumstances; or, how – or if – neurotransmitters such as serotonin, dopamine, cortisol, GABA, oxytocin, and so on are capable of producing feeling in human beings (or animals); or, how the nuances of emotion are differentially constructed through various circuits in the amygdala.

From the perspective of normal, waking consciousness (i.e., working memory), emotions seem to impinge from the outside. Working memory is unaware of how or why such emotions arise or where they come from, and, therefore, working memory considers such interlopers as products of the great unknown ... that is, the unconscious.

Nonetheless, there is an active awareness flowing through any particular emotion that gives expression to an understanding concerning the potential significance that on-going experience might have in relation to the interests of something (e.g., a parallel system of intelligent awareness) that is not necessarily a function of working memory. Of course, certain emotions can, and do, serve the interests of working memory, but even then, emotions often seem to be aware of the significance of what is transpiring in on-going experience (from the perspective of the hermeneutical orientation of such emotions) and, as a result, enter into the awareness of working memory without necessarily being called for by working memory.

When emotions disturb normal, waking consciousness, they frequently (but not always) come as uninvited and unwelcome outsiders. Such emotions seem to operate independently of the dynamics of working memory/waking consciousness, and, yet, there is a dimension of intelligence (not always of a constructive nature) to such emotions that gives expression to different kinds of evaluations or judgments (according to the nature of the emotion) concerning what is taking place in working memory.

The phenomenon of "thin slicing" is rooted, to some extent, in our emotions. 'Thin slicing' refers to the process of rendering judgments about situations based on a limited amount of information, and such judgments are a function of being able to perceive the presence of certain kinds of patterns of behavior or properties in a given situation that capture – when done correctly – something important about a person or a set of circumstances.

For instance, Wendy Levinson conducted research that was geared toward trying to discover what the differences are, if any, between doctors that got sued on multiple occasions and doctors that have never been sued. She listened to hundreds of conversations between doctors and their patients, and she noticed a pattern that might account for why some doctors got sued, while other doctors did not get sued.

More specifically, she noticed that doctors who did not get sued tended to display certain characteristics ... characteristics that were not in evidence – or to the same degree -- among the physicians who got sued on multiple occasions. For example, doctors who did not get sued spent an average of three minutes, or longer, with their patients than did doctors who were likely to be sued.

Moreover, the doctors who had not been sued spent their minutes with their clients emphasizing active listening in which individuals were encouraged to talk about their condition. In addition, those doctors tended to joke and laugh a lot more with their patients than did doctors who had been sued on multiple occasions.

| Explorations |

453

The 'thin slicing' that patients/clients did in relation to their doctors had to do with how the doctor made them feel. Doctors that were willing to spend a little more time with their clients and who were willing to use that time to show interest in the lives and conditions of their clients and who were willing to laugh and joke with their patients were not likely to be sued, whereas doctors who tended to de-emphasize or lacked the foregoing qualities were the ones who got sued.

For the most part, individuals spend only a limited amount of time with their doctors over the course of many years. So, visits lasting 15 to 20 minutes constitute only a very small sampling of the millions of minutes that are entailed by the life of a doctor.

Doctors who do not get sued do not necessarily give better medical information or treatment to their clients than doctors who do get sued, and individuals from the former group are not necessarily better doctors than individuals from the latter group are. There are doctors who make medical mistakes who never get sued, while there are very competent doctors who get sued irrespective of whether they have made a mistake.

Nalini Ambady, a psychologist followed-up on the research of Wendy Levinson. Dr. Ambady listened to the Levinson recordings and selected two conversations from each doctor/client relationship.

Dr. Ambady reduced those conversations to ten second segments. She, then, filtered the smaller, audio segments in such a way that the content of the words were removed from the audio recordings while the rhythm, intonation, and pitch of those ten second conversations were retained.

The next step of her research involved having judges evaluate those clips and rate them for the presence of qualities such as: Hostility, warmth, and dominance. Once those ratings were made, Dr. Ambady discovered that she was able to use those judgments to differentially distinguish between doctors who were, and were not, likely to have been sued.

Doctors -- based on just the pitch, rhythm, and intonation of what they said – who were judged to exhibit qualities such as warmth were in the group of doctors who had not been sued. Doctors who were judged to display qualities such as dominance – again based on just the intonation, rhythm, and pitch of what was said – were in the group of doctors that had been sued multiple times.

The 'thin slicing' of the judges in the experiment conducted by Dr. Ambady was fairly extreme. Nonetheless, it served as an accurate predictor of who had, and who had not, been sued.

Similar 'thin slicing' experiments have been done in conjunction with being able to predict whether marriages will, or will not, be successful and whether someone is, or is not, a good teacher. Gavin De Becker wrote a book entitled: *The Gift of Fear* that explored how learning to attend to certain kinds of 'thin slicing' emotional assessments that take place outside of the activities of waking consciousness could protect a person against being killed, raped, or physically assaulted in some way.

Human beings engage in such 'thin slicing' all the time. On the basis of very little information, we make judgments or evaluations – especially emotional ones -- concerning people and situations.

The judgments and evaluations that are being made through the process of 'thin slicing' are not unconscious. There is an intelligent awareness present in those 'thin slicing' judgments/evaluations – to which normal, waking consciousness/working memory is not necessarily privy (except indirectly through physical responses such as sweating palms, or through hunches, intuitions, and feelings) – that often are capable of accurately assessing the nature or character of what is transpiring in the on-going experiential activity being processed (to a degree) by working memory.

Now, not all instances of thin slicing are necessarily accurate reflections of what is taking place. There are all kinds of ways that thin slicing can be influenced, corrupted, and thwarted by the biases, fears, anxieties, beliefs, values, interests, and so on that frame waking consciousness or working memory.

However, irrespective of whether the process of thin slicing manages to accurately capture some facet of on-going experience or whether that process fails to grasp what is going on in on-going experience, the phenomenon itself gives expression to a form of awareness (outside the awareness of working memory) in which various kinds of assessments, evaluations, and/or judgments are being made according to certain kinds of logic and reasoning and that is taking place in conjunction with what is transpiring in normal waking consciousness/working memory. In other words, there are parallel modalities of intelligent awareness that are operating side-by-side in the same individual, and while the dynamics underlying thin slicing are aware of what is taking place in normal, waking consciousness, the latter is unaware of what is transpiring in conjunction with such thin slicing dynamics (or only vaguely so through the presence of physical indicators – such as sweating palms – or through the presence of intuitions, hunches and other kinds of feelings).

The so-called unconscious is not unconscious. Instead, waking consciousness/working memory has engaged in an inaccurate form of thin slicing and, as a result, has come to the conclusion that what is taking place outside of its sphere of awareness must be of an unconscious nature, but, in reality, the only thing that is unconscious is normal waking consciousness (or working memory) relative to all the other modalities of conscious activity that are taking place within the individual but beyond the narrow, compartmentalized horizons of working memory.

Emotions give expression to a hermeneutical assessment of some aspect of on-going experience. Some of those assessments are largely problematic (e.g., hatred, jealousy, despair, rage), while other emotional assessments are largely constructive (e.g., love, compassion, patience, and empathy), and still other emotional assessments, depending on circumstances, are either problematic or constructive (e.g., hope, courage, trust, and contentment).

Emotions are centers of active awareness that communicate hermeneutical perspectives capable of informing us about ourselves and about the world in a way that cannot necessarily be grasped through rational analysis. Moreover, emotions – whether of a problematic or constructive nature -- engage experience in a manner that often tends to be far more intense than most forms of reasoned-based engagement.

Indeed, feeling the truth of something is often a quite different kind of experience than is the experience of understanding that same thing intellectually. However, there are experiences involving

| Explorations |

456

intellectual insights or epiphanies (Eureka moments) that give expression to experiences that encompass intensity on both the emotional and rational level, but the emotional component of that experience is a function of a separate emotional evaluation or assessment of the significance of the intellectual breakthrough.

Even when certain emotions generate a problematic assessment of an on-going experiential context, there is still a form of logic – problematic though it might be – that flows through such emotional evaluations. Emotions are not blind, but, instead, they always operate out of a certain hermeneutical orientation.

Unfortunately and all too frequently, some emotions are very narrow and rigid in the perspective to which they give expression. As a result, emotions are often blind or indifferent to other points of view -- emotional or intellectual – and such emotions might be referred to as being egocentric.

The kind of understanding to which emotions give expression is done through feeling rather than through thinking. Nonetheless, there is an awareness and modality of intelligence that is present in such feelings, and, therefore, emotions constitute centers of awareness that are capable of evaluating experiential situations according to the rules and principles governing such centers ... rules and principles that vary from emotion to emotion.

Emotions are centers of rule or principle governed awareness that run in parallel with the activities of normal waking consciousness (i.e., working memory). Emotions are aware (although filtered and framed by their own hermeneutical perspective) of what is transpiring in ongoing experience, but normal, waking consciousness tends to be unaware of what is transpiring in different emotional centers until waking consciousness begins to be besieged by emotions expressing their point of view and insisting that normal, waking consciousness become cognizant of that perspective.

When Eleanor Longden began university in 1999, there were at least two dimensions to her personality. On the one hand, she was intelligent, competent, and full of energy, but, at the same time, she also was frightened of almost everything, perpetually anxious, haunted by a sense of emptiness, and very unhappy.

| Explorations |

At a certain point she began to hear a Voice. The Voice would make comments and observations about what was going on in Eleanor's life and the Voice seemed to be coming from a source that was separate from what Eleanor, at that time, considered to be her 'self' ... her person.

The Voice would come and go. Sometimes it stayed for a few days commenting on pretty much everything Eleanor did, and, then it would go away, only to come back at a later time.

The visits of the Voice became more frequent. The stays became longer.

For the most part, the Voice was just a relatively neutral town crier concerning the events in Eleanor's life. At times, however, the Voice would express things with an emotion that had been present in Eleanor but that had gone unexpressed in some given set of circumstances.

In time, Eleanor had an emotional and mental breakdown. She was diagnosed as being schizophrenic.

Largely because of the negative way (fear, distrust, suspicion) through which other people began responding to the label of schizophrenic that had been attached to her, Eleanor began to respond to the Voice in the same negative fashion and became hostile toward the presence of the Voice and its running commentary. Even the so-called 'professional' assistance she began to receive -- after hospitalization and being diagnosed as a schizophrenic -- encouraged Eleanor to view the Voice as a symptom of madness rather than as being a part of herself that might have something to teach her concerning the problematic ways in which she was engaging life and thinking about herself.

As Eleanor became more antagonistic and resistant toward the Voice, the Voice reflected those feelings back to her. Eventually, the Voice was replaced by many voices, all of which were demanding in an incessant and manipulative manner ... including attempting to induce Eleanor to hurt herself.

She began to have terrifying, macabre visions. Delusions arose in her that became more extreme over time.

| Explorations |

Fortunately, at a certain point during her mental distress, Eleanor came in contact with some individuals (e.g., members of the Hearing Voices Movement that is shaped and inspired by the work of Sandra Escher and Marius Romme) who were able to induce her to take a more constructive approach to her condition. Among other things, they helped her to entertain the possibility that the voices she was hearing were merely a means through which the awareness of past traumas to her being had been trying to communicate meaningful – if not important -- content to her waking consciousness or working memory.

However, the form of communication through which various centers of traumatized awareness within her engaged her working memory was largely metaphorical and emotional in nature. She had to learn how to interpret or decode what was being communicated to her, and she had to learn how to become receptive, within certain limits, to what was being communicated.

Eleanor gradually discovered how to work co-operatively and constructively with her voices. Boundaries and conditions had to be set, but within such a framework, constant progress was made.

Over time, she learned that each of the voices she heard gave expression to different traumas from her past. Furthermore, she came to understand that the more menacing, hostile, and aggressive a given voice was, the more traumatic and painful were the experiences to which such a voice gave expression.

Although the voices never went away, Eleanor's manner of engaging the voices changed in a radical fashion. The more she became able to be a compassionate witness to the traumatic experiences that were being communicated through her voices and the more she became an active listener to their grievances, then the more the voices began to calm down and express themselves in benign ways.

Eleanor's ideas about schizophrenia also changed. She did not consider schizophrenia to be the result of genetics or some sort of chemical imbalance but, instead, she felt that schizophrenia encompassed the mind's deeply felt reaction to a set of past – and, perhaps, even on-going -- traumas, abuses, and existential losses of one kind or another.

| Explorations |

459

Eleanor Longden went on to successfully complete her undergraduate work and, as well, to earn a master's degree in psychology. She is active in doing research and participates in the process of helping other people who hear voices to discover how to heal themselves by learning how to listen to and engage their voices.

Her story is unique, but it does not constitute an isolated incident of recovery. Marius Romme, a Dutch psychiatrist, has edited a book entitled: *Living with Voices: Fifty Stories of Recovery* (PCCS Books, 2013). In addition, Eleanor Longden and Dirk Corstens have written an article with the title: '*The Origins of Voices: Links Between Voice Hearing and Life History in a Survey of 100 Cases*' that will appear in a forthcoming book: *Psychosis: Psychological, Social, and Integrative Approaches*.

The voices that were communicating with Eleanor Longden were not forces of the unconscious. They were centers of awareness concerning issues of trust, betrayal, fear, abuse, neglect, trauma, and loss.

Those centers were aware of what was, and had been, transpiring in her life. However, Eleanor's waking consciousness was not aware of what was taking place in those centers of consciousness until first, the Voice, and, then, other voices began to give waking consciousness or working memory an earful.

When Eleanor's working memory learned how to engage those centers of awareness, the seeds of recovery began to be sown. Recovery involved a process of getting centers of awareness that simultaneously were running parallel to one another to become engaged in co-operative and constructive forms of communication.

Irrespective of what other mental and physical components might be present, a person's manner of responding to abuse, trauma, loss, fear, and so on is often deeply emotional. Those emotions give expression to existential, hermeneutical understandings or perspectives that are keenly aware of what is transpiring and/or what has transpired in a person's life.

Although identity diffusion disorder is considered to involve different kinds of mental issues than schizophrenia does, nonetheless, as far as the perspective that is being outlined in this section is concerned, there are, potentially, some important overlapping themes. More specifically, in those individuals who suffer from identity diffusion disorder, there are different personalities – somewhat akin to the role that voices play in schizophrenia – that tend to operate in parallel with one another and, with the exception of so-called normal, waking consciousness or working memory, those personalities (or voices in the case of schizophrenia) do seem to have varying degrees of awareness involving one another and, especially, they seem to have an awareness of what is taking place in waking consciousness or working memory despite the fact that the latter kind of awareness does not reciprocate with respect to being aware of what is transpiring in relation to the other personalities (or voices in the case of schizophrenia).

In schizophrenia, the voices are the ones who are trying to initiate a conversation of some kind with working memory. They do so by intruding into the mental space of normal, waking consciousness.

During identity diffusion disorder, various personalities that have arisen attract the attention of working memory in other ways. Rather than merely intrude into the mental space of waking consciousness through the use of voices, the other personalities hijack working memory and compartmentalize normal, waking consciousness to such a degree that the latter is not able to form memories concerning on-going experiences and, therefore, is unaware of what has taken place during the temporal framework within which the hijacking occurred.

Sooner, or later, however, what takes place during those instances of hijacking -- together with the lack of memory of normal, waking consciousness concerning such episodes -- tends to lead to life complications of one kind or another. Those complications become the doorway through which the contributions of different personalities -- like the contribution of different voices in schizophrenia -- serve as metaphorical clues that are to be decoded (with the assistance of another human being ... such as a therapist) in order to uncover existential problems of abuse, betrayal, trauma, loss, and emotional damage.

There is a certain amount of controversy surrounding the diagnosis of identity dissociative disorder. The disorder – to whatever extent it exists – appears to occur much less frequently outside of the United States than it does in America.

For example, in Japan and India, the disorder is considered to be non-existent. Moreover, in England, the incidence of identity dissociative disorder seems to be fairly rare.

To be sure, the processes through which symptoms and mental conditions are interpreted or diagnosed in different parts of the world tend to vary. Consequently, at least some cases of identity diffusion disorder might occur in Japan or India but those conditions are engaged and understood in a different manner than is the case in the United States, and as a result, the same condition in two different, geographically and culturally separated localities might be labeled in alternative ways in countries and cultures that are separate and distinct from one another.

Notwithstanding the foregoing considerations, in the United States, diagnosed cases of identity diffusion disorder have mushroomed over time. For instance, between 1930 and 1960, there were, on average, only two cases per decade that came to the attention of mental health workers, but in the 1980s, tens of thousands of cases were being reported.

Furthermore, whereas the cases of identity diffusion disorder (previously referred to as multiple personality disorder) between 1930 and 1960 tended to involve only 2-3 personalities, the number of personalities being reported in the 1980s exploded right along with the rapidly increased numbers of the disorder that, supposedly, were being diagnosed. In the 1980s clients were reportedly exhibiting between 3 and 12 distinct personalities rather than the 2-3 personalities that had been reported in cases between 1930 and 1960.

Were there thousands of cases involving identity dissociative disorder that were occurring between 1930 and 1960 and, for whatever set of reasons, simply, went undiagnosed? Possibly!

However, some psychologists believe that identity dissociative disorder is a cultural phenomenon that has been induced into existence by the way in which many therapists and psychologists have talked clients into believing that the latter individuals suffer from identity diffusion disorder. As was discovered in conjunction with false memory syndrome, research has demonstrated that the way in which questions are asked by a therapist or psychologist can shape the beliefs and understanding of the individual who is being asked the questions, and this might also be the case with respect to the issue of identity diffusion disorder.

While the explosion of diagnosed cases involving identity diffusion disorder that began in the 1980s could be, to a considerable extent, an iatrogenic-like phenomenon (that is, a problem generated through the process of psychological/medical diagnosis and/or treatment), this does not necessarily mean that all diagnosed cases of identity diffusion disorder are spurious. The cases that were reported between 1930 and 1960 might be few in number (6-7), but this all took place long before the diagnostic frenzy of the 1980s, and, therefore, those earlier cases were not necessarily induced by the physicians and therapists who were treating such individuals. Moreover, although many of the alleged cases of identity diffusion disorder that were diagnosed in the 1980s might have been therapist-induced, this does not necessarily mean all diagnosed cases were therapist induced.

Actual cases of identity diffusion disorder might be rare. However, there is no evidence to show that such a condition does not exist. Rather, the available evidence only indicates that the disorder might be far less prevalent than is often believed to be the case.

Finally, while according to the perspective of DSM-V (Diagnostic and Statistical Manual of Mental Disorders, 5th edition) identity diffusion disorder is considered to give expression to a different kind of malady than schizophrenia, nonetheless, the underlying parallels in the roles that appear to be played by voices and personalities (outlined earlier) is suggestive. Possibly, voices and personalities are variations on an underlying mental mechanism and, as a result, there might not be as much of a difference as DSM-V's diagnostic categories tend to indicate between certain aspects of schizophrenia (e.g., conditions involving hallucinations and delusions to give metaphorical expression to underlying trauma) and identity diffusion disorder (which uses personalities to give metaphorical expression to underlying trauma).

Let's engage the issue of the unconscious from one last perspective. More specifically, let's consider some of the results from split-brain research.

| Explorations |

The term "split-brain" alludes to a surgical procedure in which the corpus callosum (the extensive band of intermingled nerve fibers and glial cells that connect the two cerebral hemispheres of the brain) is severed, isolating the two hemispheres from one another. Such a procedure is sometimes carried out in relation to patients who suffer from seizures that cannot be treated in any other way.

A number of decades ago, clinicians discovered that disrupting the flow of information across the corpus callosum from one hemisphere to the other often resulted in the significant reduction in seizure activity. No one seemed to understand why the procedure worked, but because it led to the lessening of seizure activity, it was considered to be a pragmatic solution for a difficult and serious problem that previously had resisted other kinds of medical treatment.

However, given the radical nature of the procedure and despite the fact that the procedure had beneficial medical results, researchers were interested in trying to map out what, if any, collateral damage might have occurred as a result of the surgical procedure. This is where split-brain research enters the picture.

For many (but not all) individuals, the left hemisphere of the brain tends to play a dominant role in, among other functions, the understanding and production of language. On the other hand, the right hemisphere, among other functions, tends to control and sense what takes place in relation to the left side of the body.

The corpus callosum connects the two hemispheres. Scientists believe that information concerning what is happening in a given hemisphere is transmitted to the other hemisphere via the corpus callosum.

So, what happens to cognitive functioning when the information bridge between the two hemispheres is removed through the severing of the circuitry that previously linked the two hemispheres with one another? Dr. Michael Gazzaniga, among others, wanted to find out what, if anything, happened to cognitive functioning in such surgically treated patients.

The foregoing research revolved around the way human eyes are hooked up to our brains. Our visual system sends information to both hemispheres, but the nature of that information depends on which side of a person's visual system processes that information.

Information – such as an image or word – that is presented to the left of a given fixed point in the visual field will be sent to the right hemisphere. Information that is presented to the right of that fixed point in the visual field will be transmitted to the left hemisphere.

Generally speaking, individuals who have not been subjected to the split-brain surgical procedure will be able to use information from both sides of the visual field, relay that information to the appropriate hemisphere (based on the way the visual system is wired) and, then, via the corpus callosum, such information is exchanged between hemispheres and a holistic, visual picture is assembled. The foregoing situation is different for those people who have undergone split-brain surgery.

In the latter individuals, when an image is presented to the right of the aforementioned fixed point of the visual field, that information travels to the left hemisphere (where, in most people, language operations tend to reside), and, consequently, the individual will be able to give the word that corresponds to the object or word that is seen. However, if an object or word is presented to the left of the aforementioned fixed point of the visual field, the information will travel to the right hemisphere and the person will be unable to name the object.

In individuals who have not undergone split-brain surgery, whatever part of the visual system is projected to one hemisphere will be shared with the other hemisphere via the corpus callosum. In individuals who have gone through split-brain surgery, such information cannot be shared via the corpus callosum, and, therefore, the right brain doesn't have access to the linguistic facilities of the left-brain, and, as a result, the seen object goes unnamed even though it is visible.

In split-brain patients, the right hemisphere does have access to visual information concerning what has been presented to the left of the visual field. However, in order to be able to give expression to the presence of such information, some non-verbal means will have to be used in order to be able to elicit such information.

For example, suppose a banana or the picture of a banana had been presented to the left portion of the visual field. If the individual were subsequently shown pictures of fruit, including one involving a banana, the banana could be picked out to reflect what had been seen.

Even more interesting things happen in relation to split-brain patients if two different images are presented simultaneously to each half of the visual field. In one of the experiments, the image of a chicken claw was presented to the left part of the visual field, while a snowy scene was shown to the right half of the visual field.

The pictures that subsequently were presented to the subject included the picture of a chicken and the picture of a snow shovel. If a subject was asked to use his or her right hand (controlled by the left hemisphere) to select the picture that best reflected the nature of the image that had been flashed earlier to the right side of the visual field (a chicken claw that was relayed to the left hemisphere), then, the person would point to or select the picture of the chicken, but if the individual were asked to use her or his left hand (controlled by the right hemisphere) to select the picture that best represented what had been shown, previously, to the left side of the visual field (a snowy scene that was transmitted to the right hemisphere), then, the subject would choose the shovel.

In the latter case, if the subject was asked to explain why the shovel was selected, the individual would engage in confabulation – that is, the individual would invent a story to give a 'rational' account of why the given choice of picture had been made. For instance, the person might say something to the effect of needing to be able to shovel out the waste material that had been left by the chickens.

The subject's explanation for why the picture of the shovel was selected was intended to permit that individual to give an answer that seemed to make sense to the language-dominant hemisphere. Nevertheless, there was knowledge or understanding associated with right hemisphere activity that influenced what was selected with the left hand.

The latter kind of knowledge or understanding was not unconscious. It just couldn't be verbalized.

| Explorations |

There was an intelligent awareness associated with the understanding present in the right hemisphere (concerning a snowy scene) that could induce a subject's left hand to pick the appropriate image (the shovel) from among the pictures being presented that best reflected or was most appropriate in relation to the information that earlier had been flashed to the left side of the visual field and that was, then, transmitted to the right hemisphere. Such understanding could not be put into words and, therefore, working memory had no linguistic way to give expression to that understanding, and, yet, the actions of the subject demonstrated that such understanding was present in working memory.

Language plays such a significant, dominant role in filtering and framing experience that when we have no words to express an understanding – such as in the foregoing split-brain experiment – it might seem as if such understanding is of an unconscious nature. However, this is not the case since that understanding is present, aware, and intelligent yet is operating through a different -- but parallel and simultaneous -- modality of consciousness than the left hemisphere does.

In another split-brain experiment, the researchers wanted to probe emotional responses to images that were presented to subjects. For example, in one of these experiments, the left sides of the visual fields of subjects were exposed to a film that showed one individual throwing another person into a fire, and, this means, that such information will show up in the right, largely non-linguistic hemisphere of the subject.

When asked what they saw, subjects might say something to the effect of: "I'm not sure", or "there was some kind of flash" or, "there were some trees with red leaves ... like in the fall." In addition, the subjects would indicate that they found the experience disturbing, upsetting, scary, unsettling, and the like.

There are several interesting dimensions to the foregoing responses. Even though the linguistic descriptions were sketchy and somewhat off the mark, nonetheless, those descriptions reflected, in a limited and somewhat distorted way, what the subjects had seen even though the right visual field of those subjects had not been presented

| Explorations |

with any imagery concerning the situation in which one person had thrown another individual into a fire.

If the corpus callosum of the subjects had been severed, how did the left hemisphere have enough understanding of the situation to be able to give descriptions that – although limited and distorted – were appropriate to the imagery in the film that had been presented to the left side of the visual field and, therefore, supposedly only was transmitted to the right, non-language dominant hemisphere? How did the understanding associated with right hemisphere information get transmitted to the language dominant left hemisphere if the corpus callosum had been surgically severed?

Moreover, putting aside issues concerning the linguistic descriptions of what had been seen, the language-dominant left hemisphere is giving entirely relevant linguistic responses to the emotional content of the images in the film that were presented to the left portion of the visual field and which were transmitted to the right hemisphere. Again, how did the language-dominant left hemisphere gain access to the emotional understanding associated with the visual information that had been transmitted to the right hemisphere if the corpus callosum had been severed?

Conceivably, one possible explanation is that not all of the bands of fiber in the corpus callosum were necessarily severed. If so, then, although limited in number, those fibers might have been sufficient to transmit at least some information from one hemisphere to the other.

However, there is no evidence to indicate that the foregoing correctly accounts for how the left hemisphere appeared to have access to, and an understanding of, information that, supposedly, only was available to the right hemisphere. Thus, while it is possible that some sort of leakage was taking place between cerebral hemispheres via still intact fibers of the corpus callosum, this is only a conjecture.

Another possibility is that working memory has access to information from both the right and left hemispheres, but not all of that information is necessarily capable of being translated into a linguistic format. If this were the case, then, linguistic responses might be shaped, to varying degrees, by information and understanding that is present but that is difficult to translate properly into linguistic terms.

| Explorations |

Seemingly, the left hemisphere is aware of some aspect of phenomenology that is being shaped by information coming from the right hemisphere. Moreover, there is sufficient awareness in the left hemisphere concerning that information to permit the language centers in the left hemisphere to be able to provide a limited, distorted, but not entirely irrelevant description of the visual information that was sent to the right hemisphere. Furthermore, there is sufficient awareness of that information to enable the left hemisphere to provide an entirely relevant description of the emotional content of the experience arising in conjunction with the imagery presented through the left side of the visual field that would end up in the right hemisphere.

Since the early experiments of Michael Gazzaniga, a lot of research has indicated that the brain is not necessarily as lateralized (which occurs when cerebral hemispheres have specialized functions distinct from one another) as once was believed to be the case. While there might be dominant aspects to certain dimensions of hemisphere activity, the non-dominant hemisphere might have a lot more going for it – including in relation to linguistic activity -- than previously had been thought.

Irrespective of what, ultimately, might be going on cognitively in split-brain patients, the main thrust of the foregoing discussion is to indicate that there can be parallel systems of awareness that simultaneously impact working memory. These parallel systems involve forms of understanding that cannot always be translated into linguistic terms and, yet, they are intelligent, aware assessments of on-going experience.

| Explorations |

A Few Notes on Consciousness

Within consciousness, there are different elements that simultaneously reflect both aspects of reality as well as give expression to dimensions of unreality. Our task is to try to differentially sort out those two sources of information as best we can, and the degree to which a given individual is successful with respect to the foregoing task tends to have a considerable impact on how that person proceeds through life.

For example, consider the relationship between the biological activity of our eyes and what we see. The two are not necessarily the same.

Our eyes contain photoreceptors that transduce different wavelengths of light into various kinds of electrochemical signals. In addition, the biological dynamics of the eyes are capable of identifying differences of contrast in a visual scene that allows boundaries to be detected and through which a great deal of information concerning the nature of the world can be deduced and/or inferred.

The band of fibers leading from the eye to various areas of the brain is known as the optic nerve. The foregoing bundle of fibers transmits electrochemical signals that carry visual information concerning the world.

The visual signals carried by the optic nerve are in the form of various kinds of patterns. Subsequently, different portions of the brain assemble those patterns in a way that generates a holistic, integrated representation of the visual information that entered the human brain through the eyes.

According to modern neuroscience, the visual information flowing through the optic nerve is delivered to the thalamus ... a region of the brain that, among other things, plays a role in processing sensory information. After the thalamus has done its thing in relation to such visual information, that information is forwarded to the primary visual cortex that is the gateway to approximately 30 other cortical areas that, in succession, continue to process the visual information that has been routed through, first, the optic nerve, and, then, the thalamus.

Some of the cortical areas being alluded to earlier are specialists in detecting edges. Other cortical areas specialize in the detection of:

| Explorations |

470

Corners, lines, movement, contours, curves, direction of movement, color and many other dimensions that might, or might not, be connected to the visual information that originally entered the eyes.

Eventually, all of the foregoing cortical processing activity is integrated into a visual representation that contains information such as shape, contours, size, contrasts, distance, and color concerning the aspect of the world that had been engaged by the eyes. During the foregoing set of processing activities, many kinds of interpolation and extrapolation are involved.

The representation produced through the processing of visual information is rooted in all manner of interpretation and distortion. For example, the world is (at least) three-dimensional, and, yet, the retina begins with a two-dimension rendition of – at a minimum -- a three-dimensional world.

As the two-dimensional nature of the retinal information is further processed by the visual system, many guesses, interpretations, approximations, and inferences are made. Perception is more akin to an artistic representation of reality than it is a photographic-like process.

In fact, in many ways the human visual system consists of a very low-resolution arrangement. More specifically, each optic nerve gives expression to the collective efforts of approximately one million axon processes that are bundled together and collectively referred to as the optic nerve.

The foregoing facts mean that each optic nerve carries, roughly, a megapixel of information. Given that, today, many relatively cheap smart phones are able to take photographs that contain 8 megapixels, or more, of information, then, relatively speaking, the optic nerve is a low-resolution phenomenon.

Yet, the quality of human phenomenology seems to give expression to very rich kinds of visual experiences. How does such a relatively low-resolution process yield results that appear to be so richly textured?

Of course, part of the issue is that it is hard to understand just what the quality of our visual ability is when this is all that we experience. We feel that our visual experience is very rich, but this might only be because we don't know what we are missing when it comes to those sorts of experiences.

For example, human beings are trichromats. In other words, there are three kinds of cones (color-oriented photoreceptors) in the retina of the eye that are capable of perceiving combinations of three colors -- red, blue, and green -- that range between 390 and 700 nanometers in wavelength.

There also are organisms (including certain, reptiles, amphibians, arachnids, and fish) that are believed to be tetrachromats. Thus, in addition to having photoreceptors that perceive colors such as green, blue, and red, the foregoing sorts of organisms also are able to see light in the range of 10 to 400 nanometers, and as a result, they can see ultraviolet colors.

There are also are organisms (such as butterflies and certain birds) that appear to possess five kinds of photoreceptors, several of which appear to be capable of receiving colors in wavelengths that fall outside of human visual abilities. They are referred to as pentachromats.

The visual experience of tetrachromats and pentachromats appears to be richer than that of human beings. Thus, although human visual experience seems to be quite rich when considered only in its own terms, this sense of richness might only be because we tend to be biased by the limits of our capacity to engage the world visually.

There are other kinds of biases affecting human visual experience. For example, human beings cannot actually see the color that has been labeled "magenta" (a sort of soft, purplish red), and, instead, the human visual system tends to fill in such a gap in color vision with a blend of its own that is similar to magenta without actually being magenta (i.e., the human visual system engages in a certain amount of confabulation or visual fabrication).

The inclination of the visual system to engage in its own version of confabulation (memory, at times, also exhibits this sort of behavior) is not limited to inventing a color to fill in for, say, magenta. There also is a great deal of evidence to indicate that the sensory system fills in, or invents, details for quite a few facets of experience that are not actually captured by our sensory capabilities.

| Explorations |

For example, consider the McGurk effect that was stumbled upon accidentally in 1976 by Harry McGurk and his research assistant, John MacDonald. They were engaged in research that sought to determine how the language behavior of infants was affected by different developmental stages.

At one point during their research, they arranged for a technician to dub a video with a set of phonemes (basic units of sound) that were different from the ones actually uttered by the individual who was speaking in the video. When the dubbed video was run, the two researchers perceived the presence of a third phoneme that was different from either the phonemes that were actually spoken or the phonemes that was dubbed into the video.

For instance, let us suppose that the person in the video said: "Da, da, da". If one closes one's eyes (and, as a result loses the visual information involving the movements of the videoed individual's mouth) one might hear: "Ba, ba, ba".

On the other hand, if one turns off the sound for the video and just watches the movement of that individual's lips, one might perceive something different. For example, one might believe one is seeing the person in the video say: "Ga, ga, ga".

In effect, a perceptual illusion of sorts takes place. This illusion occurs when an auditory element in one sound is associated with visual information involving another sound, and, in the process, gives rise to the perception of a third sound.

The McGurk effect is quite strong. In other words, even when a person knows what is going on, nonetheless, that person still might remain under its sway.

Nonetheless, not everyone is subject to the McGurk effect to the same degree. Individuals who are good at integrating sensory information tend to be more prone to the effect (the visual data such individuals receive alters the manner in which they perceive sound), whereas individuals with, say, brain damage (and, therefore, might have trouble with integrating sensory information), might be less susceptible to that effect.

The foregoing considerations tend to raise a few questions. For instance, one wonders how the human species acquired the capacity to

| Explorations |

473

fill in or generate details that were not actually sensed such as occurs in conjunction with the magenta phenomenon, and, to some extent, is also present in the McGurk effect. One also wonders how such acquired capabilities often are able to confabulate in a seamless-like fashion that does not appreciably interfere with being able to understand what is taking place in the world.

Of course, there are times -- such as in the McGurk effect when one is trying to understand what someone is saying – when our capacity to confabulate sensory data might interfere with our ability to determine the nature of the aspect of reality that is being engaged. And, yet, that kind of interference is often of a limited and minor nature, and, consequently, our capacity to confabulate doesn't necessarily get in the way of being able to make accurate contact, to varying degrees, with different facets of reality.

The foregoing wonderment also leads to further questions. For example, earlier in this section, mention was made of the 30, or so, cortical regions involved in the processing of visual information coming from the retina and its photoreceptors (cones and rods) via the optic nerve, and, consequently, one also would like to know how those cortical regions of specialized visual processing came into being and, as well, one would like to know how the cognitive capacities came into being that are able to integrate all that visual information into a representation that actually corresponds, within limits, to elements of reality that are on-going in the world along – and, presumably, beyond -- the horizons of visual engagement.

In addition to the specialized capabilities within cortical regions of the visual system that are processing subsets of patterned visual data (such as contours, edges, lines, movement, and so on), there also are an array of interpretations that assign meaning, value, significance, beliefs, and judgments concerning what is being visually processed into a representation, of some kind, that alludes to a world or realm of reality beyond such a representation ... a hermeneutical representation that might, or might not, faithfully reflect – to varying degrees – that which is being represented. Consequently, one also wonders how the capacity (capacities) arose to hermeneutically engage the raw data of visual experience ... or, the raw data of sensory experience in general.

| Explorations |

The origin(s) of the capacity (capacities) to process raw visual data into a workable representation of that which helped give rise to such raw data is steeped in mystery. The origin(s) of the capacity (capacities) to confabulate missing details into a seamless-seeming phenomenology is also shrouded in mystery ... as is the origin(s) of the capacity (capacities) to generate hermeneutical and epistemological renderings that are intended to account for why experience has the qualitative characteristics to which it appears to give expression.

Consciousness consists of a phenomenological medium populated by contents of one kind or another ... a surface that has the capacity to reflexively engage itself to varying degrees. Consciousness also seems to consist of a deeper set of processes that appear to be generating – seemingly with some degree of awareness and intelligence -- the structural features of 'surface' phenomenology for if that process of generation were not rooted in an intelligent awareness of some kind, one has difficulty understanding how completely blind, random, automated and computational sets of processes (whose origins are unknown) could generate experience that has an intelligible relation with that (i.e., reality) to which such experience alludes.

Flowing through all of the foregoing considerations is the need to be able to distinguish between truth and falsehood – between, on the one hand, reality or truth and, on the other hand, illusion, delusion misperception, or misinterpretation. Human sensory capabilities have limits, and human processing of what is sensed involves a certain amount of confabulation, interpolation, extrapolation, inference, expectation, and assumption, and, finally, the means through which raw data becomes transformed into a representation of reality is surrounded by clouds of unknowing, and, yet, somehow -- within one, or another, level of intelligent, reflexive awareness -- human beings come to have demonstrable epistemological relationships with that which makes experience possible.

The foregoing relationship can be corrupted because it is subject to the distorting influences of illusion, delusion, bias, error, and confabulation. And, yet, if the issue of corruption were the whole story, then, we could not possibly know there are such things as illusions, delusions, biases, confabulations, or errors.

| Explorations |

475

Up until a few years ago, many neuroscientists believed that nothing much went on in the brain when, say, an individual was not engaged in any sort of overt, mental activity but was just idling or resting. Or, said in a slightly different fashion, neuroscientists were of the opinion that whatever might be taking place in the brain during such "down" periods was little more than random noise.

Modern neuroimaging techniques have indicated that there seems to be more going on in a so-called idling or resting brain than previously was believed. Apparently, when people aren't doing anything in particular or when they are anesthetized and waiting for an operation of some kind, different regions of the brain are engaged in various forms of patterned chatter in which signals of different kinds are being transmitted from one region to another.

The aforementioned resting state represents a form of baseline activity within the brain, and it is now referred to as the 'default mode network' (DMN). Conscious activity appears to constitute a move away from the activity of the default mode network.

To understand what the last sentence of the previous paragraph means, let us begin with an interesting fact. The resting state consumes approximately 20 times the amount of energy than is used when some sort of specific, conscious response is made in relation to a given stimulus.

One might suppose that such a differential in energy consumption between the resting state and conscious activity is somewhat counterintuitive. However, there are, at least, several ways to interpret such differences in energy usage involving conscious activity and the DMN.

For example, prior to directed conscious activity, various parts of the brain might be operating like military operatives who are scouting different regions of the experiential landscape and, periodically, reporting to one another about whether, or not, anything is going on in their sector that might be worthy of attention. Such on-going, cyclic reporting activity is likely to consume a fair amount of energy.

Alternatively, the DMN activity of the brain might serve as something akin to an electrified grid. Such a grid automatically identifies when there is some manner of physical or mental stimulus breach in any particular sector, and, once again, this sort of constant electronic monitoring would consume a fair amount of energy.

In either case, once a 'sentry' has reported that there is some sort of sensory or conscious activity in a given sector or if a 'breach" of the electrical grid arises in some given region of the brain, the chatter tends to die down and lends support to the newly emergent activity in accordance with whatever the nature of the report or breach might be. Consequently, prior to the report of a 'sentry' or a breach of the grid, a lot more energy is likely to be used than when the field of possibilities is narrowed down to focus on a specific instance of mental activity.

The idea that the brain's electrical activity is always busy doing 'something' is not a new one. What is new is that such activity might have some role to play with respect to prepping, priming, and/or organizing mental activity in some fashion.

Nearly a hundred years ago – back in 1920s – Hans Berger, inventor of the electroencephalograph, argued in a number of articles that the brain never really rests but is continuously engaged in activities of various kinds ... some of those activities are electrical in nature. His perspective – although not his invention – was largely ignored.

The limits of what neuroscience could discover by means of the electroencephalograph were exceeded during the latter portion of the 1970s with the advent of PET scans. Positron-emission tomography uses oxygen uptake, glucose metabolism, and blood flow as indices to measure neural activity.

In 1992, fMRIs were introduced. Functional magnetic resonance imaging uses the differential magnetic properties of blood-rich and blood-poor activities in the brain to measure neural activity.

Use of PET scans and fMRIs led some neuroscientists to believe that the brain didn't seem to do much except when it was engaged in specific sorts of mental tasks. Such an impression might have been an artifact of the kinds of experiments that were being conducted in which two kinds of activity might have been tested against one another in order to try to pin down which area of the brain was more involved in, say, reading aloud rather than reading to oneself.

| Explorations |

Early PET and fMRI cognitive research was not concerned with what the brain did in the absence of an assigned task. Such research focused on contrasting different kinds of task-oriented activity in order to be able to map the brain according to what metabolic activities took place in which regions of the brain during various kinds of focused tasks.

Eventually, however, cognitive researchers began to take a look at what was occurring in the brain apart from the relatively localized nature of the activity that was switched on while performing some particular form of mental or behavioral activity. Among other things, such research discovered that the focalized neural activity associated with the performance of specific tasks tended to increase the amount of energy being consumed by the brain by less than 5 % relative to the baseline of energy consumption that was taking place independently of such mini-spikes in energy consumption.

Some researchers (e.g., Marcus Raichle) referred to baseline energy consumption as the 'dark energy' of the brain. This term was used because despite being elusive and relatively intangible -- except in terms of gross energy consumption measurements – the dark energy of the brain appeared to dominate the activity of the brain ... as its astrophysical counterpart seems to be doing with respect to the universe.

In the middle of the 1990s, a research group led by Dr. Marcus Raichle discovered that a certain region of the brain (medial parietal cortex) -- which seems to have something to do with memories involving personal events in an individual's life -- underwent a decrease in activity level relative to the resting state when some other region of the brain was occupied with performing a given task. The portion of the medial parietal cortex that exhibited the greatest drop in neural activity under the foregoing circumstances was dubbed the MMPA ... the letters stood for the 'medial mystery parietal area'.

Other investigators have replicated the foregoing research. Moreover, the foregoing findings were extended to several other regions of the brain (e.g., the medial prefrontal cortex that appears to play a role with respect to the so-called mirror neuron phenomena).

The principle underlying such discoveries seems to be that the brain is engaged in on-going activity even when an individual is resting. Yet, when the need for more focused activity arises, then, the baseline energy consumption in areas that are not involved in such focal activity appears to decrease.

The acronym BOLD is often used in conjunction with fMRIs. The former letters stand for: Blood oxygen level dependent.

BOLD signals tend to fluctuate or cycle approximately every ten seconds in areas of the brain that – relatively speaking – are at rest. Initially, the BOLD signals were considered to constitute random electrical noise in the brain and were subtracted from the imaging process in order to better enhance the resolution of the brain activity being focused on in conjunction with the performance of some given task.

However, beginning in 1995 discoveries were made that changed the way that cognitive scientists interpreted what was taking place in the brain with respect to the possible significance of so-called baseline resting activity. More specifically, first, a group of researchers led by Dr. Bharat Biswal, found that when a person is not engaged in any specific mental or behavioral task, the aforementioned 10 cycle, slow waves fluctuated in unison in the areas of the right and left hemispheres that controlled left and right-handed movement respectively. Next, a few years later, another research group found the same sort of ten cycle, slow waves in the DMN – i.e., the aforementioned default mode network – of individuals who were at rest.

The foregoing slow wave cycles showed up not only when individuals were at rest, but they also showed up under other conditions. For example if a person were in a light sleep or was under a general anesthetic, the same slow wave cycles occurred.

Another set of researchers, using a different detection methodology, had been studying a form of electrical activity in the brain that is known as SCPs or slow cortical potential. The research team investigating the groups of neurons that exhibited SCP, cyclic, electrical activity found that SCPs were identical with BOLD signals.

There are many frequencies of electrical cycling in the brain. Those frequencies range from the relatively slow cycles of SCPs and

| Explorations |

479

BOLD signals (10 cycles per second) up to frequencies involving more than 100 cycles per second.

Researchers, such as Matias Palva, have shown that a rise in SCPs tends to be followed by an increase of activity among electrical signals involving other kinds of frequencies. Pinning down what any of this ultimately means, however, continues to be elusive.

Apparently, each neural network/circuit appears to give expression to its own, unique electrical SCP (slow cortical potential) signature. As a result, different neural networks are ready to spring into action when called upon to do so.

According to some researchers, the DMN (Default Mode Network) which is responsible for consuming so much energy during the resting state, plays a role like that of a musical conductor with respect to all of the foregoing neural networks or circuits (which are like individual instruments or musicians) that consist of signature frequencies which can be called on to perform, or be silenced, as required by the DMN. How the DMN knows how to organize all of the foregoing activity or how the DMN knows how to call on – or silence – a given signature frequency at the right time and for the appropriate amount of time is not known.

An international team of researches did discover in 2008 that by observing electrical activity in the DMN, they could predict – as much as 30 seconds ahead of time -- when subjects in a scanner apparatus were going to make mistakes in some assigned task. The sign that an error would be forthcoming was indicated when (a) the DMN's activity increased, and (b) the activity in the neural network/circuit associated with directed awareness decreased.

What caused DMN activity to increase or what caused a given kind of focal activity to decrease is not known. Whether the increase in DMN activity caused focal activity to decrease, or whether the decrease in focal activity caused DMN activity, is not known.

One might also question whether, or not, the brain and/or mind is ever really at rest. Based on my own observations of what takes place in my mind – at least on the surface – there don't seem to be many instances of resting or inactivity.

Quite apart from whatever tasks of life might require my attention, daydreaming, thinking, remembering, planning, considering possibilities, critically reflecting on the events of life, worrying, and so on, all seem to follow upon one another in an almost seamless stream of sequential, conscious events that emerge one after another, stay for awhile, and, then, disappear ... even as I go about fulfilling the requirements of life.

Conceivably, DSM might give expression to the brain activity that is associated with the constant chatter that is taking place mentally as a sort of default mode of activity. However, when we focus on something specific, this marks a departure from the regularly scheduled programming of one's mental life (such as daydreaming, remembering, worrying, and so on), and, as a result, energy consumption goes up slightly due to this increased focal activity, but there also will be a decrease in the activity of background mental activity that is unrelated to on-gong focal engagement of some task.

Filtered through the foregoing prism, the aforementioned 2008 international study can be re-interpreted. More specifically, the reason why researchers can predict that an error is going to be made by subjects up to 30 seconds prior to the mistake being made might be because the decrease in focal activity and the increase in DMN activity indicates that some sort of default activity (e.g., daydreaming, remembering, worrying, and the like) is competing with focal activity and, as a result, undermining the efficacy of the latter ... thereby increasing the likelihood that a mistake will ensue.

Moreover, one doesn't necessarily have to conclude that the changes in the electrical cycles of the DMN are disrupting focalized electrical cycles. Instead, the transitions in electrical activity with respect to both the DMN, as well as the circuits involving focalized activity, might merely be neural correlates that reflect the manner in which the phenomenology of mental life is undergoing various kinds of conflicting or competing fluctuations. Since we don't know what the relationship is between the dynamics of brain activity and the phenomenology of mental life, one cannot automatically assume that one understands the significance of the transitions in electrical activity in the DMN or in certain neural circuits that are involved in focused forms of activity.

Transitions in the electrical activity of different regions of the brain serve as markers or indicators concerning the presence of certain kinds of behavioral phenomena. However, we are not, yet, in any position to state scientifically that the presence of such markers or indicators is causal in nature.

Finally, there is a certain amount of evidence indicating that such mental disorders as depression, schizophrenia, and Alzheimer's might be functionally related to the sort of activity that is taking place in the DMN. For example, individuals who have been diagnosed as being clinically depressed seem to show a decrease in connectivity between a certain facet of DMN activity and regions in the brain associated with emotions, whereas individuals who have been diagnosed as schizophrenic exhibit an enhanced level of signaling activity within the DMN.

Do changes in the signaling activity of the DMN constitute a cause of mental disorders such as depression and schizophrenia? Or, do changes in the signaling activity of the DMN reflect the presence of forces that are disrupting DMN activity ... forces that are a function of something other than changes in DMN activity?

Changes in the electrical activity within the DMN might well serve as a diagnostic tool for detecting the presence of such disorders as schizophrenia, depression, and Alzheimer's. Nonetheless, being able to diagnose the presence of some sort of disorder is not necessarily coextensive with understanding the etiology of the disorder being diagnosed.

Some neuroscientists believe that the DMN is at the heart of a system that is capable of organizing how, when, where, and why the so-called dark energy of the brain is used. Even if foregoing belief turns out to be true, one still won't necessarily be in a position to be able to account for: (1) how the DMN knows how to allocate its energy, or, (2) what, precisely, such organizational activity accomplishes with respect to the phenomenology of everyday experience, or, (3) how the DMN came to acquire such capabilities.

| Explorations |

In 1985 Benjamin Libet, an American neuroscientist, released a paper entitled: "*Unconscious cerebral initiative and the role of conscious will in voluntary action*". The paper consisted of an overview and analysis of experiments that had been conducted by Libet ... experiments that revolved around the apparent differences between, on the one hand, the point in time when a subject's brain indicated that a choice had been made and, on the other hand, the time when a subject indicated that his or her subjective state of mind was conscious of having made a choice.

Neuroscientists had known since the 1960s that voluntary motor action follows the emergence of a 'readiness potential' or RP. An RP consists of a slow, negative transition in electrical potential that takes place, on average, about 800 milliseconds before a subsequent motor behavior occurs.

Did the subjective awareness of choosing to move, say, a finger take place: Before, simultaneously with, or after a related finger-movement RP signaled its presence? An inquiring mind (i.e., Libet) wanted to know.

Libet's experiment needed to make three kinds of temporal measurement. He needed to know: (1) When a person subjectively was aware of choosing to do something (designated as 'W' – for "will" -- in the experiment); (2) when the readiness potential occurred that preceded the action chosen (labeled 'RP' in the experiment), and (3) when the actual action took place (designated as 'M' – for movement – in the experiment).

Determining the values of 'M' and 'RP' in any given experimental trial was relatively easy to measure. Electrodes attached to muscles revealed the value of 'M', and 'RP' was determined by averaging the shift in negative electrical potential that was exhibited by a subject over a number of trials (40) involving movement of a certain kind.

The method that Libet used to measure the point in time when a subject became aware of having made a choice to flex her or his wrist was a little bit more complicated. A clock face was displayed on a screen, and the face of the clock was swept once every 2.56 seconds by a spot of light.

| Explorations |

483

The experiment required the subjects to indicate where the spot of light was on the face of the clock when they were aware of having chosen to flex their wrist. Several independent means were used prior to running the experimental trials to ensure the reliability of the subjects' estimates concerning when their choices had been made, and, on average, the subjects indicated that the choice to move their wrists was made approximately 120 milliseconds before M -- that is, the movement – occurred.

Surprisingly, Libet discovered that the RP (readiness potential) showed up prior a subject's awareness of having made the choice to move his or her wrist. The average value of that differential was 350 milliseconds.

In other words, 350 milliseconds before a subject was aware of choosing to flex her or his wrist, an RP (indicating that movement was imminent) was present. If choice is what causes movement, then, why did the awareness of having made a choice follow the appearance of electrical potential in the brain ... an electrical potential which indicated that the wrist movement was about to take place?

Libet – as the aforementioned title to his article suggests – believed that the cause of the wrist movement resided in the unconscious. Conscious awareness of choice came after the brain's change in electrical potential indicated that a movement of the wrist was imminent, and, therefore, conscious activity (W) could not be considered to cause that (i.e., RP) which clearly came before such activity.

As a result, Libet raised a question in conjunction with his experiment. Does consciousness have anything to do with the choices that are made?

Libet did seem to believe that subjective consciousness might have the capacity to assent to, or veto, the 'unconscious' choice that was made prior to the emergence of subjective awareness of such a choice. However, if this is the case, Libet did not explain how the assenting or vetoing process took place in subjective consciousness.

More importantly perhaps, whatever questions (and interpretive responses) Libet might have had with respect to his experiment there

| Explorations |

are some questions, apparently, that he did not ask himself. For example, what transpired before the RP emerged?

Libet assumed that what took place prior to the emergence of the RP was of an unconscious nature. However, he had no idea what actually was occurring during the period that occurred prior to the appearance of the RP.

How is an 'unconscious' process capable of being aware of the nature of an experiment, and how does such an 'unconscious' understanding know when or how to respond? Can we assume that working memory – i.e., normal, waking consciousness – is the only form of awareness that is present?

The earlier discussion involving split-brain research (along with the 'hearing voices' issue in schizophrenia, the idea of personalities in identity dissociative disorder, as well as the four decks of two-colored cards experiment performed by Damasio) indicated there might be parallel, active modalities of awareness taking place within us simultaneously. Isn't it possible that some other locus of awareness makes the choice to, say, flex a wrist and that information concerning such a choice is transmitted to working memory within a time frame that only shows up in a subject's working memory dominated awareness after the appearance of the RP?

We think we know who we are. Supposedly, we are the entity that is trying to construct an understanding of experience through the activities of working memory.

Attention is dominated by the activities of working memory. In fact, attention is dominated by the activities of working memory to such an extent that we become inclined to identify with such activities and, in the process, we often shy away from looking too closely at what is transpiring beyond the horizons of working memory because this sort of scrutiny tends to lead to: Problems, questions, doubt, uncertainty, instability, anxiety, confusion, and a sense of losing touch with that which we have deluded ourselves into believing we are ... i.e., working memory.

Libet's experiment suggests there is something deeper in us that has the capacity to be aware of circumstances and make relevant choices concerning those circumstances ... a 'something deeper' that

| Explorations |

appears to be somewhat different from – and, perhaps, to some degree independent of -- that which transpires in working memory. This 'deeper something' is not unconscious but, rather, the nature of working memory is such that it tends to give expression to a form of awareness that has blinders on and, therefore, is not aware of lots of other things that are going on within the mind ... things that are going on in a quite intelligent, understanding, willful, and conscious manner.

It is working memory that is relatively unconscious. Every so often, however, working memory notices experiential data – such as in the Libet experiment -- which alludes to the possibility of dimensions of reality that might exist beyond the limited horizons of working memory, and, what working memory does with such disturbing/exciting information will go a long way toward determining whether – and how -- the great unknown will be engaged or largely ignored ... if not actively denied by working memory.

| Explorations |

Some Closing Remarks

As indicated in the Introduction to this book, if a person were so inclined (which, for reasons noted over the last four hundred-plus pages, I am not) such an individual could embrace science -- as is -- and, as well, that individual could adopt the general perspective of neuroscience and the theory of evolution -- as is -- without necessarily having to make all that many conceptual adjustments concerning the possible nature of the relationship between God and the universe.

For instance, one might maintain that the processes of evolution are merely the way in which God brought about the origin of life and, as well, the way through which God permitted life to unfold and radiate across different eras, epochs, periods, and conditions. Or, one might maintain that science is an important means of seeking the truth and, therefore, is completely consonant with a Supreme Being Who gave emphasis to the importance of pursuing truth in whatever way it might be most likely to be discovered with the least amount of distortion ... something that seems to be at the heart of most, if not all, authentic spiritual traditions but is not something that is necessarily at the heart of many kinds of theological systems that often tend to be more dedicated to their own ideological orientations than they are to uncovering the truth.

However, I believe that sufficient considerations have been put forth in the previous four hundred and fifty-five pages to induce a critically reflective individual to question whether, or not, either the practice of science, in general, or the pursuit of evolutionary theory and neuroscience, in particular, give expression to disciplines that are necessarily dedicated to uncovering the truth concerning the nature of one's relationship with the universe or reality ... or whatever makes such a universe or reality possible.

Upon exploring matters (as has been done in the first part of this book) by means of the Burzynski affair, the SSRI issue, and the 'HIV causes AIDS' topic, one seems to arrive at the conclusion – after a little bit of critical reflection -- that a deeply troubling number of scientists do not appear to care about truth. Instead, under all too many circumstances, an embarrassing number of them appear to care more about profits, prestige, power, control, ego, delusional thinking, and career than they do about discovering the truth of things.

| Explorations |

Similarly, I am not quite sure to what extent one can maintain that evolutionary biologists and neuroscientists are more interested in discovering the truth than they are in pursuing their own ideological interests and agendas ... any more than one can claim that many theologians are committed to discovering the truth about the nature of reality rather than pursuing their own theological creations and agendas. As Chapter Two and Chapter Three of the current book have demonstrated, the theory of evolution, along with theories claiming that the mind is a function of the activities of the brain are not, yet, scientific theories, but, nonetheless, currently, both evolutionary theory and neuroscience are often portrayed as constituting scientific proof that all life has originated and developed as a function of evolutionary processes and that mind is nothing more than the activities of a brain that is governed by the dynamics of genomic operations that have been established through evolutionary processes.

What are the implications of the foregoing four hundred and fifty-five pages of discussion for the Final Jeopardy issue concerning the reality problem that was outlined in the Introduction to this book? The implications are quite straightforward: If an individual is going to permit his or her engagement of reality to be ruled by considerations of: Power, career, ego, greed, dishonesty, ideology, bias, control, ideology, ignorance, hatred, money, selfishness, injustice, arrogance, as well as delusional and magical thinking, then that individual is likely to place herself or himself – along with others -- in considerable jeopardy when it comes to trying to discover the truth about the nature of reality.

Without the truth, all decisions or judgments concerning the structural and dynamic character of reality, as well as the issue of Final Jeopardy, begin at no beginning and work toward no end. Any activity that refers to itself as being scientific and, yet, is lacking in objectivity, critical reflection, sincere curiosity, rigor, and demonstrable explanatory power does not give expression to science but, instead, gives expression to some form of hermeneutics sprinkled with technical considerations.

There might be legitimate differences of scientific opinion among various individuals concerning the issues that science explores. Nonetheless, there shouldn't be many, if any, degrees of difference

| Explorations |

489

among individuals who claim to be pursuing the truth through science with respect to their commitment to the basic moral principles of science.

The issues entailed by: the Burzynski affair, SSRIs, HIV, evolution, and neuroscience are not about agreeing to disagree scientifically with respect to this or that topic. Discussion of the foregoing themes throughout the previous pages of this book indicates that there appear to have been a variety of moral and/or epistemological departures, of one kind or another, that have plagued the process of science in a number of disciplines that carry important implications for understanding the nature of reality and for understanding how human beings might fit into such a framework.

Many people have died as a result of, and considerable pain has been inflicted in conjunction with, the first three topics noted above. In addition, many minds and hearts are being suffocated as a result of an array of ideas that trumpet evolution, along with many of the theories of neuroscience, as scientific fact (which is not necessarily the case ... nor are they necessarily worthy of being called scientific theories when it comes to issues of origins) but that, nonetheless, are being force-fed to the aforementioned suffocating minds and hearts with the assistance of schools, colleges, universities, the media, government, and the courts.

Science is not just an epistemological discipline. It is a moral one, as well.

In fact, one might go so far as to say that without a deep moral commitment in relation to a scientific pursuit of the reality problem, then even if the epistemological side of science should make some headway with respect to coming to understand – at least on a descriptive level --certain aspects of the nature of reality, nevertheless, whatever epistemological progress might be made in a context that is devoid of -- or deemphasizes -- morality will come back to haunt us all in one way or another.

Indeed, a sixth extinction event could be stalking life on Earth at the present time, and, in many respects (but not entirely since each of us has his or her role to play in this unfolding tragedy) the aforementioned extinction event has been set in motion by people who call themselves scientists but who fail to understand the

| Explorations |

epistemological and moral dimensions that are inherent in the process of science. In all too many cases, chemistry, biology, physics, medicine, and psychology have been set free from the moral underpinnings of real science and, in the process, the world and most, if not, all of its life forms have been placed in great jeopardy.

I like science. Anyone who reads this book and comes away with the impression that the author of this work is anti-science hasn't understood much of what has been said here.

Quite frankly, any person who might make the foregoing sort of judgment concerning my thoughts about science does not seem to understand very much about the nature of science. Moreover, this would be true irrespective of what that individual's academic credentials suggest is the case with respect to the issue of expertise.

There are individuals who were mentioned in this book's discussion of the Burzynski affair, the SSRI issue, and the HIV causes AIDS matter that, in my opinion, are real scientists. Unfortunately, most of those individuals do not belong to the mainstream of the so-called scientific community, and, moreover, those individuals often have been ignored, ridiculed, or punished in a variety of ways ... apparently a common and traditional form of reward for many real scientists.

While some of the individuals associated with the theory of evolution have, from time to time, done some good science, they also have often permitted some very unscientific tendencies – both epistemologically and morally -- to creep into their work as well. For example, to try to claim, at the present time, that evolution -- in any sense other than as a function of the principles of population biology -- is a matter of scientific fact or constitutes a scientific theory is about as unscientific as one can be because the proof required to back up such a claim is currently unavailable.

Among other things, this book has explored, in concrete terms, some of the methodological problems that permeate certain kinds of research involving cancer, SSRIs, and HIV. Such problematic research entails both epistemological, as well as moral, issues.

Maybe someday an individual will come along who will scientifically prove that Antineoplastons do not, and cannot, help cure various kinds of cancer. That day has not, yet, arrived.

Perhaps, at some point in the future, a person will be able to scientifically demonstrate that an absence of serotonin causes depression and that the presence of serotonin (and/or nerve growth factor – NGF) caused by the presence of SSRIs cures depression rather than just acting to mask the latter condition while simultaneously inducing some people to commit suicide or violent acts. However, the foregoing sort of future has not, yet, arrived.

While various forms of AIDS do exist in the world, those forms have not been proven – scientifically -- to be caused by HIV. Conceivably, this or that individual might, one day, show clear-cut, undeniable, scientific evidence that HIV not only exists, but, as well, that it causes AIDS. So far, this has not been accomplished.

Finally, let us be clear about something. At no point in this book have I said that evolutionary theory -- or the idea that brain and mind are identical with one another – could not be true in some sense. What I have said is that at the present time: (1) Any theory of evolution (considered as something other than a reflection of the principles of population biology) and, as well, (2) any theory of mind that treats mental phenomena as a strict function of brain dynamics do not – at this point in time -- constitute scientific facts, nor do they currently qualify as scientific theories.

The theory of evolution – in any sense other than that of giving expression to the principles of population biology -- is a philosophical, ideological, or hermeneutical theory. It is not a scientific theory.

The same sorts of things can be said with respect to any theory of mind that seeks to claim that mental phenomena are a function of brain activities. Irrespective of how many technical facts might be added to the conceptual stew, nonetheless, at the present time, any mind/brain identity theory gives expression to a philosophical, ideological, or hermeneutical framework and not to a scientific theory.

Possibly, a person will appear on the scene at some given point of time in the future who will be able to provide the evidence and proof needed to demonstrate that evolution (in a sense that extends beyond

| Explorations |

population biology) is true. That temporal juncture has not, yet, been reached.

The fact that the theory of evolution has not, yet, been proven to be true -- and, in fact, might never be proven to be true in any sense other than in the fairly limited way provided by the principles of population biology -- tends to open up the reality problem that is to be addressed through the Final Jeopardy challenge. However, this dimension of opening things up conceptually doesn't mean that anything or everything will constitute good responses with respect to the Final Jeopardy challenge.

For example, Chapter Three has explored a variety of issues involving glial cells, mirror neurons, memory, learning, the computational theory of mind, the nature of the unconscious, as well as some perspectives on consciousness. Although more and more of the modern discussion concerning cognitive functioning is dominated by neurobiology, molecular biology, and the belief that mind can be reduced to the activities of the brain, nonetheless, there seems to be less and less reason to accept such a perspective as an accurate reflection of the nature of reality, while at the same time there also appears to be a number of the reasons for rejecting – or, at a minimum, being cautious toward – such a theoretical perspective ... reasons and arguments that have been developed throughout the previous chapter.

Currently, there is absolutely no proof that the brain is responsible for generating consciousness, reason, values, creativity, understanding, meaning, or judgment. Demonstrating that the latter sort of capabilities exhibit deficits of one kind or another when particular sections or circuits of the brain are disrupted through injury, surgery, disease, or trauma is no more an indication that those sections and circuits are responsible for the generation of phenomenology and its contents than disrupting the electronics of a radio is an indication that the radio is responsible for the programming signals being received by that radio.

How – of if -- molecules (such as neurotransmitters, gliotransmitters, and hormones) generate: Meanings, values, beliefs, ideas, interpretations, feelings, and memories are not known. How action potentials, gap junctions, and synaptic circuitry – individually or collectively – are capable of generating phenomenology and its contents is not known.

There are many correlations that have been demonstrated involving brain activity and phenomenology. What is missing is proof that there is a causal connection between the two, and what is missing is proof concerning what the precise character of that causal relationship is.

At the present time, most, if not all, neuroscientists believe they are very, very close to being able to prove that the mind is a function of brain activity. Nonetheless, there might be something of the asymptote inherent in those sorts of beliefs, since despite a great many intriguing and impressive discoveries in the aforementioned field of research, nonetheless, the nature of the causal 'mechanisms' underlying phenomenology and the contents of phenomenology continue to elude the grasp of neuroscientists.

Moreover, even if someone came along and provided a means of showing that the mind and the brain were one and the same, there still would be an even more fundamental question to ask with respect to the dynamics of the brain. More specifically, how did such complex, intricate, ordered, networks of functioning come into existence in the first place, and, this, of course, brings us back to a variety of issues that pose some very difficult problems concerning origins that remain unsolved by the theory of evolution.

Research in neuroscience and psychology is important because, among other things, that work helps demonstrate all the ways in which understanding is colored, shaped, modulated, and oriented by emotional, perceptual, motivational, physical, and hermeneutical forces. However, the fact that such forces can be mapped and explored in ways that give expression, within limits, to certain kinds of truth indicates that despite the extent to which human beings are susceptible to bias, manipulation, illusions, undue influence, perceptual errors, and the like, nonetheless, human beings also have the capacity to rise above their epistemological vulnerabilities and latch on to portions of the truth.

Maybe someone, someday, will show how physical, material systems generate phenomenology and its contents. Perhaps someday, someone will prove how physical, material systems were able to evolve in order to be capable of underwriting the dynamics of a brain that made phenomenology and its contents possible.

I don't fear such a tomorrow. Indeed, I am ready to try to embrace the truth whatever it might turn out to be.

Today, however, I am confronted by a great deal of uncertainty and ambiguity with respect to the nature of the ultimate significance, value, meaning, and implications of research in neuroscience and psychology. Yet, today is when I have to jot down my Final Jeopardy response to the reality problem question (and, yes, I do realize that 480 pages, or so, is not exactly a matter of jotting).

Presently, as far as the human mind is concerned, the epistemological situation is a lot more fluid and amorphous than proponents of the mind/brain identity theory would have us believe. My Final Jeopardy response must seek to maintain a balance between what is known as well as what is not known.

As I indicated in the Introduction, even if I were required to accept as true the materialistic and physical assumptions that underlie modern neuroscience and that treat the mind as a function of brain activity, all that such concessions might require me to do is to rework some of my beliefs and understandings concerning the way things work in the universe. Currently, however, the foregoing sorts of 'truths' have not been established.

The findings of neuroscience and psychology have not forced humanity down an epistemological cul-de-sac concerning the nature of human potential. If anything, the discoveries that have taken place within neuroscience and psychology – when critically reflected upon (which, to some extent, has taken place in this book) – tend to indicate that there just might be much more to phenomenology and its contents than currently can be accounted for by neuroscience and psychology.

Reasoning, evidence, critical reflection, and science have all been utilized in this book to point out, and elaborate upon, an array of shortcomings in relation to a number of topics ... including the theory of evolution as well as a variety of issues in neuroscience. The way forward also will require the use of reasoning, evidence, critical reflection, and science (in both its epistemological and moral senses).

| Explorations |

495

The theory of evolution cannot -- in a step-by step fashion – currently account for the origin of: Life, or the DNA code, or anaerobic respiration, or aerobic respiration, or photosynthesis, or cyanobacteria, or archaea, or eukaryotic life forms, or endocytosis, or endosymbiosis, or any number of other possibilities ... including consciousness, intelligence, reason, language, creativity, curiosity, and talent. Notwithstanding the best efforts of evolutionary biologists and neuroscientists, issues involving origins concerning life and mind envelop us in mystery.

On the other hand, while we might be immersed in mystery, we also are surrounded by evidence. What often eludes us is the meaning or significance of that evidence.

We must learn to listen to the evidence. What is reality conveying to us by its very presence ... by its being one set of processes, rather than some other set of processes?

Attentive, focused listening requires a person to utilize all of his or her faculties in relation to: Exploring, reasoning about, questioning, rigorously probing, interpreting, critically analyzing, and feeling – yes feeling -- experiential data. I have tried to pursue such a process of listening through the pages of this book.

Listening in the foregoing way might not have given me all the answers ... or even any of them. Nonetheless, I believe a method of active listening has helped me to understand what not to do when engaging the problem of reality, and I also believe that active listening has helped me to appreciate that coming to understand what reality might not be is almost as important as coming to understand what reality is.

As a result, active listening has helped me to formulate part of my response to the Final Jeopardy challenge ... and that part is contained in the pages of this book. Those results have encouraged me to try to undertake more of that kind of listening in conjunction with a variety of other issues entailed by the reality problem that might find their way into printed expression at some point in the future ... if life co-operaes).

| Explorations |

| Explorations |

Bibliography

Articles

Jerry Adler, 'Erasing Painful Memories', pp. 56-61, *Scientific American*, May 2012.

Zeeya Mer Ali, 'Gravity Off The Grid', pp. 44-51, *Discover*, March 2012.

Ross D. Andersen, 'An Ear To The Big Bang', pp. 40-47, *Scientific American*, October 2013.

Zvi Bern, Lance J. Dixon and David Kosower, 'Loops, Trees and the Search for New Physics', pp. 34-41, *Scientific American*, May 2012.

Jan Bernauer and Randolf Pohl, 'The Proton Radius Problem', pp. 32-39, *Scientific American*, February 2014.

Yudhijit Bhattacharjee, 'Paranormal Psychologist', pp. 52-58, *Discover*, March 2012.

Leo Blitz, 'The Dark Side of the Milky Way', pp. 36-45, *Scientific American*, October 2011.

Deborah Blum, 'The Scent of Your Thoughts', pp. 54-57, *Scientific American*, October 2011.

Alan Burdick, 'The Sixth Sense: Time', pp. 8-11, *Discover Magazine – The Brain*, Spring 2011.

Kevin L. Campbell and Michael Hofreiter, 'New Life For Ancient DNA', pp. pp. 46-51, *Scientific American*, August 2012.

David Castlevechhi, 'Is Supersymmetry Dead?' pp. 16-18, *Scientific American*, May 2012.

Heather Chapin and Sean Mackey, 'A Transparent Trainable Brain', pp. 50-57, *Scientific American Mind*, March/April 2013.

Timothy Clifton and Pedro G. Ferreira, 'Does Dark Energy Really Exist?', pp. 48-55, *Scientific American*, April 2009.

Jennifer Crocker and Jessica J. Carnevale, 'Letting Go of Self-esteem', pp.26-33, *Scientific American Mind*, September/October 2013.

Tamara Davis, 'Is the Universe Leaking Energy', pp. 38-47, *Scientific American*, July 2010.

Felipe De Brigard, 'The Anatomy of Amnesia', pp. 39-41, *Scientific American Mind*, May/June 2014.

| Explorations |

Karl Deisseroth, 'Conrolling the Brain With Light', pp. 48-55, *Scientific American*, November 2010.

Peter B. deMenocal, 'Climate Shocks,' pp. 48-53, September 2014.

Theodosius Dobzhansky, 'Nothing in Biology Makes Sense Except in the Light of Evolution', pp. 125-129; March 1973.

Cara Feinberg, 'The Placebo Phenomenon', pp. 36-39, *Harvard Magazine*, January-February 2013.

Jonathan Feng and Mark Trodden, 'Dark Worlds', pp. 38-45, *Scientific American*, November 2010.

Douglas Finkbeiner, Meng Su, and Dmitry Malyshev, 'Giant Bubbles of the Milky Way', pp. 42-47, *Scientific American*, July 2014.

Tim Folger, 'Second Genesis', pp. 18-24, *Discover Magazine – Extreme Universe*, Winter 2010.

Tim Folger, 'How Can You Be In Two Places At Once?', pp. 56-61, *Discover Magazine – Extreme Universe*, Winter 2010.

Fred H. Gage and Alysson R. Muotri, 'What Makes Each Brain Unique', pp. 26-31, *Scientific American*, March 2012.

Avishay Gal-Yam, 'Super Supernova', pp. 44-49, *Scientific American*, June 2012.

Donald Goldsmith, 'The Far, Far Future of Stars', pp. 32-39, *Scientific American*, March 2012.

Alison Gopnik, 'How Babies Think', pp. 76-81, *Scientific American*, July 2010.

Andrew Grant, 'Night Ranger', pp. 32-35, *Discover Magazine – Extreme Universe*, Winter 2010.

Andrew Grant, 'Enter String Man', pp. 70-73, *Discover Magazine – Extreme Universe*, Winter 2010.

Ann Graybiel and Kyle S. Smith, 'Good Habits, Bad Habits', pp. 38-43, *Scientific American,* June 2014.

Trisha Gura, 'When Pretending Is The Remedy', pp. 34-39, *Scientific American Mind,* March/April 2013.

Katherine Harmon, 'Shattered Ancestry', pp. 42-49, *Scientific American*, February 2013.

Claus C. Hilgetag and Helen Barbas, 'Sculpting the Brain', pp. 66-71, *Scientific American*, February 2009.

Martin Hirsch, Heinrich Pas, and Werner Porod, 'Ghostly Beacons of New Physics', pp. 40-47, *Scientific American*, April 2013.

Courtney Humphries, 'Life's Beginnings', pp. 29-33; p. 74, *Harvard Magazine*, September-October 2013.

Ray Jayawardhana, ' Coming Soon: A Supernova Near You', pp. 68-73, *Scientific American*, December 2013.

Allan R. Jones and Caroline C. Overly, 'Mapping the Mind', pp. 56-63, *Scientific American Mind*, September/October 2010.

Mazen A. Kheirbek and Rene Hen, 'Add Neurons, Subtract Anxiety', pp. 62-67, *Scientific American*, July 2014.

Kent A. Kiehl and Joshua W. Buckholtz, 'Inside the Mind of a Psychopath', pp. 22-29, *Scientific American Mind*, September/Octrober 2010.

Christof Koch, 'Keep It In Mind', pp. 26-29, *Scientific American Mind*, May/June 2014.

Christof Koch, 'The Conscious Infant', pp. 24-25, *Scientific American Mind*, September/October 2013.

Christof Koch and Giulio Tononi, 'A Test For Consciousness', pp. 44-47, *Scientific American*, June 2011.

Morten L. Kringelbach and Kent C. Berridge, 'The Joyful Mind', pp. 40-45, *Scientific American*, August 2012.

Meinard Kuhlmann, 'What Is Real?', pp. 40-47, *Scientific American*, August 2013.

Robert Kunzig, 'Sticky Stuff', pp. 50-55, *Discover Magazine – Extreme Universe*, Winter 2010.

Robert Kunzig, 'The Unbearable Lightness of Neutrinos', pp. 62-69, *Discover Magazine – Extreme Universe*, Winter 2010.

Matthew Kurtz, 'A Social Salve For Schizophrenia', pp. 62-67, *Scientific American Mind*, March/April 2013.

Michael D. Lemonick, 'The Dawn of Distant Skies', pp. 40-47, *Scientific American*, July 2013.

Michael D. Lemonick, 'Big Bang', pp. 12-17, *Discover Magazine – Extreme Universe*, Winter 2010.

Noam I. Libeskind, 'Dwarf Galaxies and the Dark Web', pp. 46-51, *Scientific American*, March 2014.

Don Lincoln, 'The Inner Life of Quarks', pp. 36-43, *Scientific American*, November 2012.

Eleanor Longden, 'Listening to Voices', pp. 34-37, *Scientific American Mind*, September/October 2013.

Joseph Lykken and Maria Spiropulu, 'Supersymmetry and the Crisis in Physics', pp. 34-39, *Scientific American* 2014.

Bruno Maddox, 'Hypnotize Me', pp. 59-61, *Discover Magazine – The Brain*, Spring 2011.

Donald G. MacKay, 'The Engine of Memory', pp. 30-38, *Scientific American Mind*, May/June 2014.

Ronald Martin and Antonietta Quigg, 'Tiny Plants That Once Ruled The Seas', pp. 40-45, *Scientific American*, June 2013.

James L. McGaugh and Aurora LePort, 'Remembrance of All Things Past', pp. 40-45, *Scientific American*, February 2014.

Kat McGowan, 'The Second Coming of Sigmund Freud', pp. 54-61, *Discover*, April 2014.

Christopher P. McKay and Victor Parro Garcia, 'How To Search For Life On Mars', pp. 44-49, *Scientific American*, June 2014.

Michael Moyer, 'Is Space Digital', pp. 30-36, *Scientific American*, February 2012.

Steve Nadis, 'First Light', pp. 38-45, *Discover*, April 2014.

Perth Group, 'Perth Group's Comments on Emperor's New Virus, 2011.

Corey Powell, 'When a Slumbering Monster Awakes', pp. 62-63, *Discover*, April 2014.

Heather Pringle, 'The Origins of Creativity', pp. 36-43, *Scientific American*, March 2013.

Rodrigo Quian Quiroga, 'Brain Cells For Grandmother', pp. 30-35, *Scientific American*, February 2013.

Marcus E. Raichle, 'The Brain's Dark Energy', pp. 44-49, *Scientific American*, March 2010.

V.S. Ramachandran, 'True Vision', pp. 32-40, *Discover Magazine – The Brain*, Spring 2011.

Christopher J. Reed, Hunter Lewis, Eric Trejo, Vern Winston and Caryn Evila, 'Protein Adaptations in Archaeal Extremophiles' Hindawai Publishing Corporation, 2013.

Michael Riordan, Guido Tonelli and Sau Lan Wu, 'The Higgs At Last', pp. 66-73, Scientific American, October 2012.

Lawrence D. Rosenblum, 'A Confederacy of Senses', pp. 72-75, *Scientific American*, January 2013.

Lawrence D. Rosenblum, 'The Eighth Sense: Echo-Location', pp. 18-21, *Discover Magazine – The Brain*, Spring 2011.

Subir Sachdev, 'Strange and Stringy', pp. 44-51, *Scientific American*, January 2013.

Eric Scerri, 'Cracks in the Periodic Table', pp. 68-73, *Scientific American*, June 2013.

Caleb Scharf, 'The Benevolence of Black Holes', pp. 34-39, *Scientific American,* August 2012.

Terry Sejnowski and Tobi Delbruch, 'The Language of the Brain', pp. 54-59, *Scientific American*, October 2012.

Azim F. Shariff and Kathleen D. Vohs, 'The World Without Free Will', pp. 76-79, *Scientific American*, June 2014.

Michael Shermer, 'Darwin Misunderstood', page 34, *Scientific American*, February 2009.

Pawan Sinha, 'Once Blind and Now They See', pp. 48-55, *Scientific American*, July 2013.

Steven Stahler, 'The Inner Life of Star Clusters', pp. 44-51, *Scientific American*, March 2013.

Paul J. Steinhardt, 'The Inflation Debate', pp. 36-43, *Scientific American*, April 2011.

Ian Tattersall, 'If I Had A Hammer', 54-59, September 2014

Gary Taubes, 'RNA Revolution', pp. 46-52, *Discover*, October 2009.

Elizabeth A. Tibbetts and Adrian G. Dyer, 'Good With Faces', pp. 62-67, *Scientific American*, December 2013.

Giulio Tononi and Chiara Cirelli, 'Perchance to Prune', pp. 34-39, *Scientific American*, August 2013.

Vlatko Vedral, 'Living in a Quantum World', pp. 38-43, *Scientific American*, June 2011.

Hans Christian von Baeyer, 'Quantum Weirdness?' pp. 46-51, *Scientific American*, June 2013.

Bernard Wood, 'Welcome to the Family', pp. 42-47, Scientific American, September 2014.

Kate Wong, 'The Human Saga', pp. 37-39, *Scientific American*, September 2014.

Karen Wright, 'They Came From Outer Space', pp. 46-49, *Discover Magazine – Extreme Universe*, Winter 2010.

Rafael Yuste and George M. Church, ' The New Century of the Brain', pp. 38-45, *Scientific American*, March 2014.

Carl Zimmer, 'The Surprising Origins of Life's Complexity', pp. 84-89, *Scientific American*, August 2013.

Carl Zimmer, 'Calculating Minds', pp. 56-58, *Discover Magazine – The Brain*, Spring 2011.

Carl Zimmer, '100 Trillion Connections', pp. 58-63, *Scientific American*, January 2011.

Books

Stanley Aronowitz, *The Knowledge Factory: Dismantling the Corporate University and Creating True Higher Learning*, Beacon Press, 2000.

Lyndon Ashmore, *Big Bang Blasted!:The Story of the Expanding Universe and How It Was Shown to be Wrong*, Book Surge, 2006.

Halton Arp, *Seeing Red: Redshifts, Cosmology and Academic Science*, Apeiron, 1998.

Peter Atkins, *Four Laws: What Drives the Universe*, Oxford University Press, 2007.

Ian G. Barbour, *Myths, Models and Paradigms: A Comparative Study In Science and Religion*, Harper & Row Publishers, 1974.

John D. Barrow, *New Theories of Everything*, Oxford University Press, 2007.

John D. Barrow, *The Constants: From Alpha to Omega – The Numbers That Encode the Deepest Secrets of the Universe*, Random House, 2002.

Alison Bass, *Side Effects: A Prosecutor, A Whistleblower, and a Bestselling Antidepressant on Trial*, Algonquin Books, 2008.

Wayne Becker, Lewis J. Kleinsmith, and Jeff Hardin – with contributions from Gregory Paul Bertoni, *The World of the Cell*, Sixth Edition, Pearson Education, Inc., 2006.

Michael J. Behe, *Darwin's Black Box*, Touchstone, 1996.

Michael J. Benton, *When Life Nearly Died: The Greatest Mass Extinction of All Time*, Thames & Hudson, 2003.

Susan Blackmore, *Consciousness: An Introduction*, Oxford University Press, 2004.

Allan Bloom, *The Closing of the American Mind*, Simon & Schuster, 1987.

David Bohm, *Wholeness and the Implicate Order*, Ark Paperbacks, 1983.

C.J. Brainerd and V.F Reyna, *The Science of False Memory*, Oxford University Press, 2005.

| Explorations |

Peter R. Breggin, *Medication Madness: A Psychiatrist Exposes the Dangers of Mood-Altering Medications*, St. Martin's Press, 2008.

Harold I. Brown, *Perception, Theory and Commitment: The New Philosophy of Science*, The University of Chicago, 1977.

Truddi Chase et. al., *When Rabbit Howls*, Jove Books, 1987.

Brian Clegg, *Before the Big Bang: The Prehistory of Our Universe*, St. Martin's Press, 2009.

Brian Clegg, *The God Effect: Quantum Entanglement, Science's Strangest Phenomenon*, St. Martin's Press, 2006.

Frank Close, *The Infinity Puzzle: Quantum Field Theory and the Hunt for an Orderly Universe*, Basic Books, 2011.

Frank Close, *Antimatter*, Oxford University Press, 2009.

Francis S. Collins, *The Language of God: A Scientist Presents Evidence for Belief*, Free Press, 2006.

Brian Cox & Jeff Forshaw, *Why Does $E=mc^2$?*, Da Capo Press, 2009.

Robert P. Crease and Charles Mann, *The Second Creation: Makers of the Revolution in 20th-Century Physics*, Collier Books, 1986.

Antonio Damasio, *Self Comes to Mind: Constructing the Conscious Brain*, Pantheon Books, 2010.

Paul Davies, *Cosmic Jackpot: Why our Universe Is Just Right For Life*, Houghton Mifflin, 2007.

Richard Dawkins, *The God Delusion*, Houghton Mifflin, 2006.

Richard Dawkins, *The Selfish Gene*, Paladin, 1978.

Richard Dawkins, *The Blind Watchmaker: Why The Evidence of Evolution Reveals a Universe Without Design*, W.W. Norton & Company, 1987.

Daniel C. Dennett, *Darwin's Dangerous Idea: Evolution and the Meaning of Life*, Simon & Schuster, 1995.

Guy Deutscher, *Through the Language Glass: Why the World Looks Different in Other Languages*, Metropolitan Books, 2010.

Norman Doidge, *The Brain That Changes Itself*, Viking 2007.

Bart D. Ehrman, *God's Problem: How the Bible Fails to Answer Our Most Important Question – Why We Suffer*, Harper Collins, 2008.

A.C. Ewing, *A Short Commentary on Kant's Critique of Pure Reason*, The University of Chicago Press, 1938.

R. Douglas Fields, *The Other Brain*, Simon and Schuster, 2009.

Chester E. Finn, Jr., Bruno V. Manno, and Gregg Vanourek, *Charter Schools in Action: Renewing Public Education*, Princeton University Press, 2000.

Viktor E. Frankl, *Man's Search For Meaning – Third Edition*, Touchstone, 1984.

Elio Frattaroli, *Healing the Soul in the Age of the Brain: Why Medication Isn't Enough*, Penguin Books, 2001.

Tim Friend, *The Third Domain: The Untold Story of Archaea and the Future of Biotechnology*, Joseph Henry Press, 2007.

Harald Fritzsch (translated by Gregory Stodolsky), *The Fundamental Constants: A Mystery of Physics*, World Scientific Publishing Company, 2009.

Douglas Futuyma, *Evolution*, Sinauer Associates Inc, 2005.

John Taylor Gatto, *The Underground History of American Education*, The Oxford Village Press, 2003.

Michael S. Gazzaniga, *Mind Matters: How Mind and Brain Interact to Create Our Conscious Lives*, Houghton Mifflin Company, 1988.

Louisa Gilder, *The Age of Entanglement: When Quantum Physics was Reborn*, Alfred A. Knopf, 2008.

Malcolm Gladwell, *Blink: The Power of Thinking Without Thinking*, Little, Brown and Company, 2005.

Peter Godfrey-Smith, *Theory and Reality: An Introduction to the Philosophy of Science*, University of Chicago Press, 2003.

Rebecca Goldstein, *Incompleteness*, W.W. Norton & Company, 2005.

Nelson Goodman, *Ways of Worldmaking*, Hackett Publishing Company, 1978.

Martin L. Gross, *The Conspiracy of Ignorance: The Failure of Public Schools*, Harper Collins Publishers, 1999.

Stephen Hawking, *A Brief History of Time: From the Big Bang to Black Holes*, Bantam Books, 1990.

Robert M. Hazen, *Genesis: The Scientific Quest For Life's Origins*, Joseph Henry Press, 2005.

Nick Herbert, *Elemental Mind: Human Consciousness and the New Physics*, Dutton, 1993.

Nick Herbert, *Quantum Reality: Beyond the New Physics*, Anchor Press/Doubleday, 1985.

John Holland, *Emergence: From Chaos to Order*, Helix Books, 1999.

Dan Hooper, Dark Cosmos: *In Search of Our Universe's Missing Mass and Energy*, Smithsonian Books, 2006.

John Horgan, *Rational Mysticism: Spirituality Meets Science in the Search for Enlightenment*, Mariner Books, 2004.

John Horgan, *The Undiscovered Mind: How the Human Brain Defies Replication, Medication, and Explanation*, Touchstone Books, 1999.

James Davison Hunter, *The Death of Character: Moral Education in an Age Without Good and Evil*, Basic Books, 2000.

Marco Iacoboni, *Mirroring People: The New Science of How We Connect With Others*, Farrar, Straus and Giroux, 2008.

Robert Kane, *A Contemporary Introduction to Free Will*, Oxford University Press, 2005.

Stuart Kauffman, *Reinventing the Sacred*, Basic Books, 2008.

Robert Kegan, *The Evolving Self: Problem and Process in Human Development*, Harvard University Press, 1982.

George A. Kelley, *A Theory of Personality: The Psychology of Personal Constructs*, W.W. Norton & Company, 1963.

Alfie Kohn, *The Schools Our Children Deserve: Moving Beyond Traditional Classrooms and "Tougher Standards"*, Houghton Mifflin, 1999.

Manjit Kumar, *Quantum: Einstein, Bohr, and the Great Debate About the Nature of Reality*, W.W. Norton & Company, 2008.

Nick Lane, *Life Ascending*, W.W. Norton & Company, 2009.

Leon M. Lederman and Christopher Hill, *Symmetry and the Beautiful Universe*, Prometheus books, 2004.

Thomas Lickona, *Educating For Character: How Our Schools Can Teach Respect and Responsibility*, Bantam Book, 1991.

Lillian R. Lieber, *Infinity: Beyond the Beyond the Beyond*, Paul Dry Books, 2007.

Myron Lieberman, *Public Education: An Autopsy*, Harvard University Press, 1993.

David Lindley, *Uncertainty: Einstein, Heisenberg, Bohr and the Struggle for the Soul of Science*, Doubleday, 2007.

Mario Livio, *Is God a Mathematician?*, Simon & Schuster, 2009.

Stephen L. Macknik and Susana Martinez-Conde with Sandra Blakeslee, *Sleights of Mind: What the Neuroscience of Magic Reveals About Our Everyday Deceptions*, Henry Holt and Company, 2010.

Lynn Margulis and Dorion Sagan, *Microcosmos: Four Billion Years of Evolution From Our Microbial Ancestors*, Simon & Schuster, 1986.

Thomas O. McGarity and Wendy Wagner, *Bending Science: How Special Interests Corrupt Public Health Research*, Harvard University Press, 2008.

Thomas Metzinger, *The Ego Tunnel: The Science of the Mind and the Myth of the Self*, Basic Books, 2009.

Kenneth R. Miller, *Only a Theory: Evolution and the Battle for America's Soul*, Viking, 2008.

Melanie Mitchell, *Complexity: A Guided Tour*, Oxford University Press, 2009.

Leonard Mlodinow, *Subliminal: How Your Unconscious Mind Rules Your Behavior*, Pantheon Books, 2012.

Shannon Moffett, *The Three-Pound Enigma: The Human Brain and the Quest to Unlock Its Mysteries*, Algonquin Books, 2006.

Joanna Moncrieff, *The Myth of the Chemical Cure: A Critique of Psychiatric Drug Treatment – Revised Edition*, Palgrave Macmillan, 2009

Read Montague, *Why Choose This Book?*, Penguin Group, 2006.

Chris Mooney and Sheril Kirshenbaum, *Unscientific America: How Scientific Illiteracy Threatens Our Future*, Basic Books, 2009.

David G. Myers, Pyschology, 8th Edition, Worth Publishers, 2007.

Paul J. Nahin, *The Story of the Square Root of -1: An Imaginary Tale*, Princeton University Press, 1998.

| Explorations |

John G. Nichols, A. Robert Martin, Bruce G. Wallace, and Paul A. Fuchs, *From Neuron to Brain*, Sinauer Associates, Inc., 2001.

Debra Niehoff, *The Language of Life: How Cells Communicate in Health and Disease*, Joseph Henry Press, 2005.

Naomi Oreskes & Erik M. Conway, *Merchants of Doubt: How a Handful of Scientists Obscured the Truth on Issues from Tobacco to Global Warming*, Bloomsbury Press, 2010.

F. David Peat, *Einstein's Moon: Bell's Theorem and the Curious Quest for Quantum Reality*, Contemporary Books, 1990.

Richard Panek, *The 4% Universe: Dark Matter, Dark Energy, and the Race to Discover the Rest of Reality*, Houghton Mifflin Harcourt, 2011.

John Allen Paulos, *Irreligion*, Hill and Wang, 2008.

Lewis J. Perelman, *School's Out*, Avon Books, 1992.

Melody Petersen, *Our Daily Meds*, Sarah Crichton Books, 2008.

Steven Pinker, *How the Mind Works*, W.W. Norton & Company, 1997.

J.C. Polkinghorne, *The Quantum World*, Penguin Books, 1986.

Alfred S. Posamentier and Ingmar Lehmann, *The (Fabulous) Fibonacci Numbers*, Prometheus Books, 2007.

Helen R. Quinn and Yossi Nir, *The Mystery of the Missing Antimatter*, Princeton University Press, 2008.

Lisa Randall, *Warped Passages: Unraveling The Mysteries of the Universe's Hidden Dimensions*, Harper Perennial, 2005.

Hilton Ratcliffe, *The Static Universe: Exploding the Myth of Cosmic Expansion*, Apeiron 2010.

Hilton Ratcliffe, *The Virtue of Heresy: Confessions of a Dissident Astronomer*, Author House, 2008.

Darrel W. Ray, *The God Virus: How Religion Infects Our Lives and Culture*, IPC Press, 2009.

Richard Restak, *The Naked Brain: How the Emerging Neurosociety is Changing How We Live, Work and Love*, Harmony Books, 2006.

Mark Ronan, *Symmetry Monster: One of the Greatest Quests of Mathematics*, Oxford University Press, 2006.

Ian Sample, *Massive: The Missing Particle that Sparked the Greatest Hunt in Science*, Basic Books, 2010.

John W. Santock, *Life-Span Development*, 11th Edition, McGraw-Hill, 2008.

Joseph Schild - Editor, *The Big Bang: A Critical Analysis*, Cosmology Science Publishers, 2011.

Donald E. Scott, *The Electric Sky: A Challenge to the Myths of Modern Astronomy*, Mikamar Publishing, 2006.

Robert Shapiro, *Origins: A Skeptic's Guide to the Creation of Life on Earth*, Bantam Books, 1986.

Rupert Sheldrake, *The Presence of the Past: Morphic Resonance and the Habits of Nature*, Vintage Books, 1989.

Lee Smolin, *Three Roads to Quantum Gravity*, Basic Books, 2001.

Lee Smolin, *The Trouble With Physics: The Rise of String Theory, The Fall of a Science, and What Comes Next*, Houghton Mifflin, 2006.

James D. Stein, *Cosmic Numbers: The Numbers That Define Our Universe*, Basic Books, 2011.

Kathleen Stein, *The Genius Engine*, John Wiley & Sons, 2007.

Paul J. Steinhardt and Neil Turok, *Endless Universe: Beyond the Big Bang*, Doubleday, 2007.

Ian Stewart, *In Pursuit of the Unknown: 17 Equations That Changed the World*, Profile Books, 2012.

Ian Stewart, *Why Beauty is Truth: A History of Symmetry*, Basic Books, 2007.

Ian Stewart, *Flatterland: Like Flatland, Only More So*, Basic Books, 2001.

Martha Stout, *The Sociopath Next Door*, Broadway Books, 2005.

Martha Stout, *The Myth of Sanity*, Penguin Books, 2001.

Leonard Susskind, *The Black Hole War: My Battle With Stephen Hawking to Make the World Safe for Quantum Mechanics*, Little, Brown and Company, 2008.

Leonard Susskind, *The Cosmic Landscape: String Theory and the Illusion of Intelligent Design*, Back Bay Books, 2006.

Nassim Nicholas Taleb, *The Black Swan: The Impact of the Highly Improbable*, Random House, 2010.

Nassim Nicholas Taleb, *Fooled by Randomness: The Hidden Role of Chance in Life and in the Markets*, Random House, 2004.

Daniel Tammet, *Embracing the Wide Sky: A Tour Across the Horizons of Mind*, Free Press, 2009.

Nicholas Wade, *The Faith Instinct: How Religion Evolved & Why It Endures*, The Penguin Press, 2009.

Daniel M. Wegner, *The Illusion of Conscious Will*, Bradford Books, 2002.

David L. Weiner, *Reality Check: What Your Mind Knows, But Isn't Telling You*, Prometheus Books, 2005.

Peter Woit, *Not Even Wrong: The Failure of String Theory and the Search For Unity in Physical Law*, Basic Books, 2006.

Videos

Brent W. Leung (Director), *House of Numbers*, Knowledge Matters Ltd., 2009.

Brent W. Leung (Director), *The Emperor's New Virus*, Knowledge Matters, 2011.

Mark A. Levinson (Producer and Director) and David E. Kaplan (Producer), *Particle Fever*, Anthos Media in participation with PF Productions, 2014.

Erik Merola (Director), *Burzynski: Cancer Is Serious Business*, 2011.

Erik Merola, (Director) *Burzynski: Cancer Is A Serious Business – Part II*, 2013.

Erik Merola (Director) *Second Opinion: Laetrile At Sloan-Kettering*, 2014.

Gary Null (Writer/Director) *Seeds of Death: Unveiling the Lies of GMOs*, Gary Null and Associates, 2012.

Marie-Monique Robin, *The World According to Monsanto*, Institute for Responsible Technology, 2008.

Jeffrey M. Smith, *Genetic Roulette: The Gamble of Our Lives*, Institute For Responsible Technology, 2012.

Jeffrey M. Smith, *Your Milk On Drugs – Just Say No!*, Institute for Responsible Technology, 2008

Cevin Soling (Director), *The War On Kids*, Spectacle Films, 2009.

Bertram Verhaag (Writer and Director), *Scientists Under Attack: Genetic Engineering in the Magnetic Field of Money*, DENKmal-Films, Ltd., 2010.

www.ingramcontent.com/pod-product-compliance
Lightning Source LLC
Chambersburg PA
CBHW020623220526
45464CB00001B/5